LIPPINCOTT'S MANUAL OF
Psychiatric Nursing Care Plans

Judith M. Schultz, MS, RN
Senior Account Manager
Healthways, Inc.
San Francisco, California

Sheila L. Videbeck, PhD, RN
Professor, Nursing
Des Moines Area Community College
Ankeny, Iowa

NINTH EDITION

Wolters Kluwer | Lippincott Williams & Wilkins

Health

elphia • Baltimore • New York • London
os Aires • Hong Kong • Sydney • Tokyo

Vice President, Publishing: Julie K. Stegman
Supervising Product Manager: Betsy Gentzler
Editorial Assistant: Jacalyn Clay
Design Coordinator: Joan Wendt
Art Coordinator: Brett MacNaughton
Manufacturing Coordinator: Karin Duffield
Prepress Vendor: S4Carlisle Publishing Services

9th edition

9 8 7 6 5 4 3

Printed in China.

Library of Congress Cataloging-in-Publication Data

Schultz, Judith M.
Lippincott's manual of psychiatric nursing care plans / Judith M. Schultz, Sheila L. Videbeck.—9th ed.
    p. ; cm.
  Manual of psychiatric nursing care plans
  Includes bibliographical references and index.
  ISBN 978-1-60913-694-9 (alk. paper)
  I. Videbeck, Sheila L. II. Title. III. Title: Manual of psychiatric nursing care plans.
  [DNLM: 1. Mental Disorders—nursing—Handbooks. 2. Patient Care Planning—Handbooks. 3. Psychiatric Nursing—methods—Handbooks. WY 49]
  616.89'0231—dc23

2011051681

RRS1703

REVIEWERS

Dolores Bradley, MSN, BSN, RN, CNE
Nursing Faculty, Associate Professor
Farmingdale State College
State University of New York
Farmingdale, New York

Kay Foland, PhD, RN, CNP, CNS-BC, PMHNP-BC
Professor
College of Nursing
South Dakota State University
Rapid City, South Dakota

Jennifer Graber, EdD(c), APRN, BC, CS
Nursing Instructor
Stanton Campus
Delaware Technical Community College
Newark, Delaware

Mary Lou Hamilton, MS, RN
Nursing Faculty in Psychiatric Mental
Health Nursing
Delaware Technical Community College
Newark, Delaware

Elaine Kusick, MSN, BSN, RN
Instructor, Nursing
Butler County Community College
Butler, Pennsylvania

Ann Michalski
Associate Professor
Bakersfield College
Bakersfield, California

Alita Sellers, PhD, RN, CNE
Professor, Coordinator RN to BSN Program
West Virginia University, Parkersburg
Parkersburg, West Virginia

Karen Gahan Tarnow, PhD, RN
Clinical Associate Professor
University of Kansas School of Nursing
Kansas City, Kansas

PREFACE

The ninth edition of *Lippincott's Manual of Psychiatric Nursing Care Plans* continues to be an outstanding resource for nursing students and practicing psychiatric–mental health nurses. The *Manual* is a learning tool and a reference presenting information, concepts, and principles in a simple and clear format that can be used in a variety of settings. The *Manual* complements theory-based general psychiatric nursing textbooks and provides a solid clinical orientation for students learning to use the nursing process in the clinical psychiatric setting. Its straight-forward presentation and effective use of the nursing process provide students with easily used tools to enhance understanding and support practice.

Too often, students feel ill-prepared for their clinical psychiatric experience, and their anxiety interferes with both their learning and appreciation of psychiatric nursing. The *Manual* can help to diminish this anxiety by its demonstration of the use of the nursing process in psychiatric nursing and its suggestions for specific interventions addressing particular behaviors, together with rationale, giving the student a sound basis on which to build clinical skills.

The continued, widespread, international use of this *Manual* supports our belief in the enduring need for a practical guide to nursing care planning for clients with emotional or psychiatric problems. However, the care plans in this *Manual* do not replace the nurse's skills in assessment, formulation of specific nursing diagnoses, expected outcomes, nursing interventions, and evaluation of nursing care. Because each client is an individual, he or she needs a plan of nursing care specifically tailored to his or her own needs, problems, and circumstances. The plans in the *Manual* cover a range of problems and a variety of approaches that may be employed in providing nursing care. This information is meant to be adapted and used appropriately in planning nursing care for each client.

TEXT ORGANIZATION

The *Manual* is organized into three parts.

Part One, Using the Manual, provides support for nursing students, instructors, and clinical nursing staff in developing psychiatric nursing skills; provides guidelines for developing interaction skills through the use of case studies, role play, and videotaped interaction; and provides strategies for developing written nursing care plans.

Part Two, Key Considerations in Mental Health Nursing, covers concepts that are considered important underpinnings of psychiatric nursing practice. These include the therapeutic milieu, sexuality, spirituality, culture, complementary and alternative medicine, aging, loneliness, homelessness, stress, crisis intervention, community violence, community grief and disaster response, the nursing process, evidence-based practice, best practices, the interdisciplinary treatment team, nurse–client interactions, and the roles of the psychiatric nurse and of the client.

Part Three, Care Plans, includes 52 care plans organized into 13 sections. The section titles are General Care Plans; Community-Based Care; Disorders Diagnosed in Childhood or Adolescence; Delirium, Dementia, and Head Injury; Substance-Related Disorders; Schizophrenia and Psychotic Disorders/Symptoms; Mood Disorders and Related Behaviors; Anxiety Disorders; Somatoform and Dissociative Disorders; Eating Disorders; Sleep Disorders and Adjustment Disorders; Personality Disorders; and Behavioral and Problem-Based Care Plans.

NURSING PROCESS FRAMEWORK

The *Manual* continues to use the nursing process as a framework for care, and each care plan is organized by nursing diagnoses. The care plans provide an outcomes-focused approach, and therapeutic goals content is included in the basic concepts section and the introductory paragraphs of the care plans.

NEW TO THIS EDITION

- New information on Complementary and Alternative Medicine information and Using the Internet
- All care plans revised and updated
- Expanded outcomes statements with specific timing examples
- Updated Recommended Readings in each section
- Updated Resources for Additional Information for each section; additional information is also available on thePoint
- Updated references throughout the *Manual*
- Rationale for correct responses of the section review questions
- Updated NANDA International 2012–2014 nursing diagnoses included*
- New appendix on Electroconvulsive Therapy
- Expanded, updated, and reformatted Psychopharmacology Appendix
- New appendix on Side Effects of Medications and Related Nursing Interventions
- New appendix on Schizoid, Histrionic, Narcissistic, Avoidant, and Obsessive-Compulsive Personality Disorders

USING THE MANUAL

The *Manual* is an ideal text and reference for mental health and general clinical settings, including community and home care nursing, in addition to its use as a text for students. The *Manual* offers sound guidance to those professionals who have less confidence in dealing with clients who are experiencing emotional difficulties and offers new staff members guidelines for clear and specific approaches to various problems. The *Manual* can be especially helpful in the general medical or continuing care facility, where staff members may encounter a variety of challenging patient behaviors.

We believe that effective care must begin with a holistic view of each client, whose life is composed of a particular complex of physical, emotional, spiritual, interpersonal, cultural, socioeconomic, and environmental factors. We sincerely hope that *Lippincott's Manual of Psychiatric Nursing Care Plans*, in its ninth edition, continues to contribute to the delivery of nonjudgmental, holistic care and to the development of sound psychiatric nursing knowledge and skills, solidly based in a sound nursing framework.

RESOURCES FOR STUDENTS, INSTRUCTORS, AND PRACTICING NURSES

Visit thePoint at http://thePoint.lww.com/Schultz9e for materials to assist students and practicing nurses to write individualized care plans quickly and efficiently (see Part One, Using the Manual). Resources on thePoint include all 52 care plans, the Sample Psychosocial

*From *Nursing Diagnoses: Definitions and Classification 2012–2014*. Copyright © 2012, 1994-2012 by NANDA International. Used by arrangement with Blackwell Publishing Limited, a company of John Wiley & Sons, Inc.

Assessment Tool, and lists of resources for additional information. Individual care plan files can be downloaded onto a personal computer to streamline the student's or nurse's efforts, enhance the care planning process, and facilitate the consistent use of care plans in any setting where mental health clients are encountered. Also included is a sample Watch & Learn video clip from *Lippincott's Video Guide to Psychiatric–Mental Health Nursing Assessment,* as well as Practice & Learn activities from *Lippincott's Interactive Case Studies in Psychiatric–Mental Health Nursing.*

ACKNOWLEDGMENTS

We wish to express our appreciation to all of those we have encountered, who have helped our learning and growth, and enabled us to write all the editions of this manual. We are truly grateful for the opportunity to know and work with them and to benefit from their experiences and their work. We also offer our heartfelt thanks to all those in our personal lives who have been supportive of us and of this work since the *Manual's* inception over 35 years ago!

Judith M. Schultz, MS, RN
Sheila L. Videbeck, PhD, RN

CONTENTS

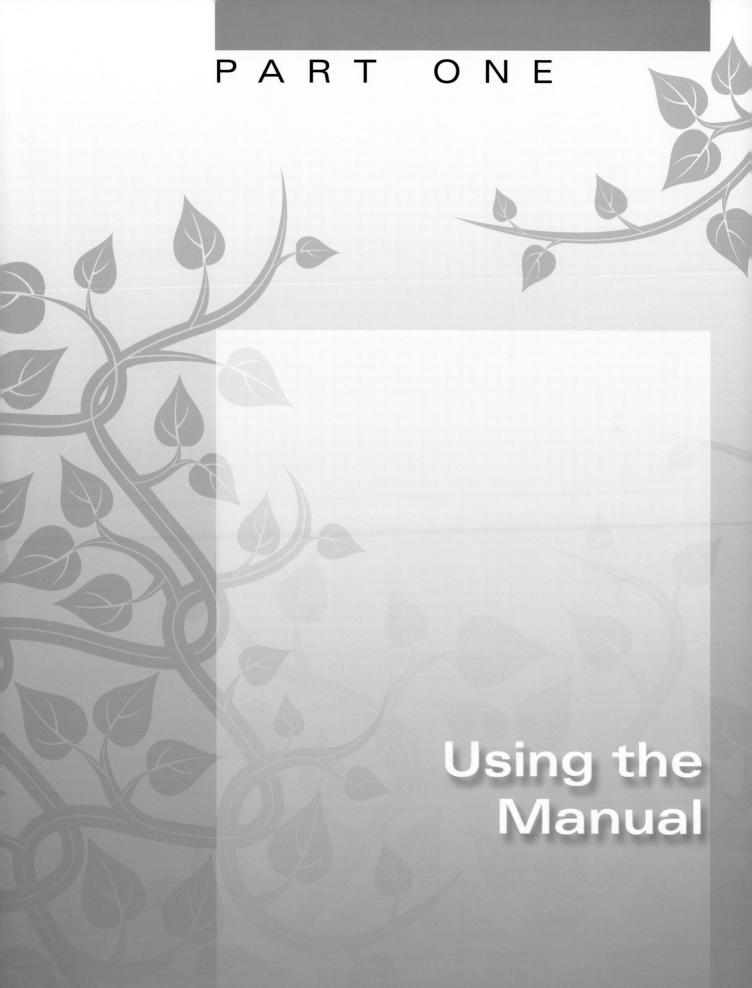

PART ONE

Using the
Manual

The *Manual of Psychiatric Nursing Care Plans* is designed for both educational and clinical nursing situations. Because the care plans are organized according to the nursing process within each nursing diagnosis addressed, the *Manual* can effectively complement any psychiatric nursing text and can be used within any theoretical framework. Because the plans are based on psychiatric disorders, client behaviors, and clinical problems, the *Manual* is appropriate for both undergraduate and graduate levels of nursing education.

In the clinical realm, the *Manual* is useful in any nursing setting. The *Manual* can be used to help formulate individual nursing care plans in inpatient, partial hospitalization, and outpatient situations; in psychiatric settings, including residential and acute care units, locked and open units, and with adolescent and adult client populations; in community-based programs, including individual and group situations; in general medical settings, for work with clients who have psychiatric diagnoses as well as those whose behavior or problems are addressed in the *Manual*; and in skilled nursing facilities and long-term residential, day treatment, and outpatient settings.

NURSING STUDENTS AND INSTRUCTORS

Development of Psychiatric Nursing Skills in Students

For a student, developing nursing skills and comfort with clients with psychiatric problems is a complex process of integrating knowledge of human development, psychiatric problems, human relationships, self-awareness, behavior and communication techniques, and the nursing process with clinical experiences in psychiatric nursing situations. This process can be fascinating, stimulating, and satisfying for both students and instructors, or it may be seen as arduous, frustrating, and frightening. We hope that the former is the common experience and that this *Manual* can be used to add to the students' knowledge base, guide their use of the nursing process, and suggest ways to interact with clients that result in positive, effective nursing care and increased confidence and comfort with psychiatric nursing.

Good interaction skills are essential in all types of nursing, and they enhance the student's nursing care in any setting. In addition, skillful communications enhance the enjoyment of working with clients and help avoid burnout later in a nurse's career. Efficient use of the nursing process and skills in writing

and using care plans also help avoid burnout by decreasing frustration and repetition and increasing effective communication among the staff.

An important part of psychiatric nursing skill is conscious awareness of interactions, both verbal and nonverbal. In psychiatric nursing, interactions are primary tools of intervention. Awareness of these interactions is necessary to ensure *therapeutic*, not social, interactions and requires thinking on several levels while the nurse is planning for and engaged in the interaction:

- The nurse must be knowledgeable about the client's present behaviors and problems.
- The interaction should be goal directed: What is the purpose of the interaction in view of the client's nursing diagnosis and expected outcomes?
- The skills or techniques of communication must be identified and the structure of the interaction planned.
- During the interaction itself, the nurse must continually monitor the responses of the client, evaluate the effectiveness of the interaction, and make changes as indicated.

Techniques for Developing Interaction Skills

The *Manual* can be used to facilitate the development of interaction skills and awareness in classes, group clinical settings, and individual faculty–student interaction in conjunction with various teaching methods. Effective techniques include the following:

Case studies: presentation of a case (an actual client, hypothetical example, or paradigm case) by the instructor or student. The case may be written, presented by role-playing, or verbally described. Students (individually or in groups) can perform an assessment, write a care plan for the client, and discuss interventions and related skills, using the *Manual* as a resource.

Role-play and feedback: used in conjunction with a case study or to develop specific communication skills. Interactions with actual clients can be reenacted or the instructor may portray a client with certain behaviors to identify, practice, and evaluate communication techniques; students and instructors can give feedback regarding the interactions.

Videotaped interactions: for case presentations and role-play situations to help the student develop awareness by seeing his or her own behavior and the interaction as a whole from a different, "outside observer" perspective.

Review of the video by both the instructor and the student (and in groups, as students' comfort levels increase) allows feedback, discussion, and identification of alternative techniques.

Written process recordings: used with brief interactions or portions of interactions with or without videotaping. Recalling the interaction in detail sufficient for a written process recording helps the student to develop awareness during the interaction itself and to develop memory skills that are useful in documentation. Process recordings can include identification of goals, evaluation of the effectiveness of skills and techniques or of the client's responses to a statement or behavior, and ways to change the interaction (i.e., as if it could be redone), in addition to the recording of actual words and behaviors of the client and the student.

Written care plans: developed for each client, based on the student's assessment of the client. Before an interaction with the client, the instructor can review the plan with the student, and the student can identify expected outcomes, nursing interventions, and interactions he or she plans to use, and so forth. After the interaction, both the care plan and the specific interaction can be evaluated and revised.

Using the *Manual* in Teaching Psychiatric Nursing

Instructors may find the *Manual* useful in organizing material for teaching classes and for discussion points. The "Key Considerations in Mental Health Nursing" section examines a number of issues germane to the general practice of psychiatric nursing and the delivery of nonjudgmental nursing care. Each group of care plans deals with a set of related problems that students may encounter in the psychiatric setting. These care plans represent the usual assessments and interventions the student or nurse will use in the planning and delivery of care to clients and families. The information in the "Key Considerations in Mental Health Nursing" section regarding sexuality, culture, aging, and so forth provides the context for the student to individualize the planning and delivery of care for each client. A small group of students could be responsible for the presentation of a client's care plan that illustrates one of these topics (e.g., loss or chemical dependence) to the entire class, with subsequent discussion of specific behaviors, problems, nursing diagnoses, interventions, and so forth.

CLINICAL NURSING STAFF

Written individual nursing care plans are necessary in any clinical setting because

- They provide a focus for using the nursing process in a deliberate manner with each client.
- They provide the basis for evaluating the effectiveness of nursing interventions, allowing revisions based on documented plans of care, not unspecified or haphazard nursing interventions.

- They are the only feasible means of effective communication about client care among different members of the nursing staff, who work at different times and who may not be familiar with the client (e.g., float, registry, or part-time nurses).
- They provide a central point of information for coordination of care, identification of goals, and use of consistent limits, interventions, and so forth in the nursing care of a given client.
- They maintain continuity over time when one nurse is working with a client (e.g., in a home health or other community-based setting).
- They are required to meet nursing standards of care and accreditation standards.
- They facilitate efficient care that saves time and avoids burnout among the staff.

However, written care plans often are perceived as troublesome, time consuming, or unrelated to the actual care of the client. This *Manual* was originally conceived to alleviate some of the challenges involved in writing care plans that deal with psychiatric problems. Many nurses felt that they had to "reinvent the wheel" each time they sat down to write a care plan for a client whose behavior was, in fact, similar to the behavior of other clients in their experience, although they recognized differences among individual clients and their needs. The *Manual* was first written to be a source for nurses, from which to choose parts of a comprehensive care plan appropriate to the needs of a unique person and to adapt and specify those parts according to that person's needs. The *Manual* can be seen as a catalog of possibilities for the care of clients with psychiatric problems that contains suggestions of nursing diagnoses, assessment data, expected outcomes, and interventions. (We do not mean to suggest, however, that all possibilities are contained in the *Manual.*) It is also meant to be a catalyst for thought about nursing care, a starting point in planning care for the client, and a structure for using the nursing process to efficiently address the client's needs.

Strategies for Promoting the Use of Written Care Plans

Even with the *Manual* as a resource, nursing staff still may be reluctant to write and use care plans. To encourage the use of written plans, we suggest that nurses identify the barriers to their use and plan and implement strategies to overcome these barriers. It may be helpful to present the use of written plans in a way that they can be easily integrated into the existing routine of the nursing staff and seen as beneficial to the staff itself (not only to clients but also for other purposes, such as accreditation requirements).

Some possible barriers to the use of written plans and suggested strategies to overcome them are as follows:

Barrier: Not enough time allowed to write care plans.
Strategies: When making nursing assignments, consider writing the nursing care plan as a part of the admission process for a newly admitted client and allot time

accordingly. Enlist the support of the nursing administration in recognizing the necessity of allowing time to write nursing care plans when planning staffing needs. Include writing and using care plans in performance review criteria and give positive feedback for nurses' efforts in this area. Nursing supervisors and nursing education personnel also can assist staff nurses in writing plans on a daily basis.

Barrier: Having to "reinvent the wheel" each time a care plan is written.

Strategies: Use the *Manual* as a resource for each client's care plan to suggest assessment parameters, nursing diagnoses, and so forth, and as a way to stimulate thinking about the client's care. If your unit has standard protocols for certain situations (e.g., behavior modification, detoxification), have these printed in your care plan format with blank lines (___) to accommodate individual parameters or expected outcome criteria as appropriate. If your facility uses electronic medical records, you can construct templates using the *Manual*'s care plans and integrate facility-specific information (e.g., levels of suicide precautions, policies regarding restraints, and so forth), and then complete care plans for each client using the appropriate template.

Barrier: Care plans require too much writing, or the format is cumbersome.

Strategies: Streamline care plan formats and design them to be easily used for communication and revision purposes. Write and revise plans in collaboration with other nursing staff, in care planning conferences, or in informal, impromptu sessions. Design systems to address common problems that can be consistently used and adapted to individual needs (e.g., levels of suicide precautions). These can be specifically delineated in a unit reference book and briefly noted in the care plan itself (e.g., "Suicide precautions: Level 1") or integrated into electronic care plan templates.

Barrier: No one uses the care plans once they have been written.

Strategies: Integrate care plans as the basic structure for change of shift report, staffings and case conferences, and documentation. For example, review interventions and expected outcomes for current problems as you review clients in reports, and revise care plans as clients are reviewed. Base problem-oriented charting on nursing diagnoses in care plans; update care plans while charting on clients.

It may be helpful to hold a series of staff meetings and invite the input of all the nursing staff to identify the particular barriers in place on your nursing unit and to work together as a staff to overcome them.

Additional Benefits of Using Written Care Plans

In addition to overcoming resistance such as that noted, presenting the benefits of using care plans may be useful. Because the use of written care plans can enhance the consistency and effectiveness of nursing care, it also can increase the satisfaction of the staff and help avoid burnout. The following are among the benefits of using written care plans:

- Increased communication among nursing staff and other members of the health care team
- Clearly identified expected outcomes and strategies
- Decreased repetition (i.e., each nursing staff member does not need to independently assess, diagnose, and identify outcomes and interventions for each client)
- Routine evaluation and revision of interventions
- Decreased frustration with ineffective intervention strategies: If a nursing intervention is ineffective, it can be revised and a different intervention implemented in a timely manner
- Increased consistency in the delivery of nursing care
- Increased satisfaction in working with clients as a result of coordinated, consistent nursing care
- Efficient, useful structure for change of shift report, staffings or clinical case conferences, and documentation
- More complete documentation with decreased preparation time and effort related to quality assurance, utilization review, accreditation, and reimbursement issues

In addition to the above points, it may be helpful to integrate care plans and their use into other nursing education programs. For example, nursing grand rounds can include a case study presented using the written care plan as a framework. The care plan can also be used as a handout, a slide presentation, or as an exercise for the participants. Videotaped or role-playing sessions for nursing orientation programs or discussion of nursing assessment, planning, and intervention also can use written care plans. The *Manual* can be used as a resource in planning programs like these or used by the participants during the programs. Also, topics discussed in the "Key Considerations in Mental Health Nursing" section, groups of care plans, or specific care plans can be used to plan and implement topical in-service presentations, nursing development, or nursing orientation programs. Finally, the format used for the care plans in the *Manual* can be easily adapted using thePoint (http://thePoint.lww.com/Schultz9e) to construct nursing care plans for use in the clinical setting (e.g., replace "Rationale" column with "Outcome Criteria" column).

USING THE ELECTRONIC CARE PLANS TO WRITE INDIVIDUALIZED PSYCHIATRIC NURSING CARE PLANS

The *Manual* includes electronic files located on thePoint that can be easily used to write individualized nursing care plans. ThePoint contains all of the care plans included in the *Manual*, plus the Sample Psychosocial Assessment Tool (Appendix A). The student or nurse can save the file(s) from thePoint onto the computer and use the information in the care plan as a guide to perform the client's assessment. Based on the assessment of the individual client, the student or nurse can then cut and paste content, delete information not relevant to the client, include additional information related to the specific client, and add modifiers, time factors (deadlines), and so forth to complete the individualized plan. As the client's care progresses, the plan can be further modified and revised, based on the continuing evaluation of the plan and of the client's needs and progress.

USING WRITTEN PSYCHIATRIC CARE PLANS IN NONPSYCHIATRIC SETTINGS

Written care plans to address emotional or psychiatric needs in the nonpsychiatric setting are especially important. In such settings, certain psychiatric problems are rarely encountered, and the nursing staff may lack the confidence and knowledge to readily deal with these problems. Using the *Manual* in this situation can help in planning holistic care by providing concrete suggestions for care as well as background information related to the disorder or problem itself. In addition, the care plans can be used as the basis for a staff review or nursing in-service regarding the problem or behavior soon after it is assessed in the client.

USING THE INTERNET

The *Manual* includes Resources for Additional Information at the end of each section and the resources' Web addresses are located on thePoint to assist the student or nurse in locating further information related to that section on the Internet. Using search engines such as Google, Yahoo!, or others is quite common and can be an efficient means of locating current information, professional organizations, government agencies, and client- or caregiver-sponsored sites. However, the Internet can also be a source of incorrect and outdated information, as well as advertisements, computer viruses, and spyware that can be misleading or damaging. Therefore, it is important to use the Internet carefully and judiciously, particularly in obtaining information for client care or resources to which to refer clients.

In evaluating publications found on the Web, always evaluate at the source. If you find an article or book chapter or excerpt, check the publication date, authors and their credentials and conflict of interest statements, and the publication itself. Many articles are posted to look like professional articles but are in fact opinion or veiled advertisements. Also, check the references to an article, and determine if it is a research-based article or an opinion or editorial. In checking a publication, try to determine if it is peer-reviewed or published by a reputable professional association or government agency.

If you click on a link to a Web site previously unknown to you, be sure to have adequate virus protection on your computer and to enable your computer's pop-up blockers. When you reach a new site, look for information about the site to determine its source; for example, an "About" or "Contact Us" tab or link. An organization may also list a board of directors or advisors; looking at the background or credentials of such groups can be useful in determining credibility. Many sites are sponsored by pharmaceutical companies or other organizations that may have a vested interest in the information provided. Other sites are sponsored by individuals or client groups that also may have a specific point of view or bias toward or against specific types of information or care, or may be seeking donations or support as their primary purpose. Many such sites are valuable and useful, but others can influence clients to engage in nontherapeutic behavior, often under the guise of providing "support." If you are unable to determine the source or sponsor of a site, be especially cautious about using it or relying on information it provides.

In evaluating the quality of a site, check for currency of the site as well as the information provided. Look for a "date last updated" note or the resources posted. If there are links to other sites and many do not work, the site may be outdated. Looking at the site design and the types of links posted can also help determine its credibility. If there is a registration or log-in required, evaluate the type of information required and read the privacy notice or terms and conditions. Many sites rely on obtaining personal information in order to send newsletters or advertisements in the future; there may also be attempts at identity theft or hacking into computers or e-mail systems.

Clients can benefit from your guidance regarding using the Internet also. Teaching clients guidelines such as those noted above will help them find useful and credible information, but also recognize unfounded or dangerous information as well. Many sites promise dramatic results from using particular products or practices; these should be viewed with caution and evaluated according to the parameters above and checking other, nonaffiliated sources for corroboration. Clients need to be especially careful of advice provided by sites on the Internet; they should be cautioned to always check with their treatment team before changing current treatment or starting a new technique or substance (e.g., supplement) they find on the Internet.

There are a number of resources that specifically address using the Internet. Visit thePoint (http://thePoint.lww.com/Schultz9e) for a list of these and other helpful Internet resources. These include Medline Plus, the Medical Library Association, and the American Academy of Family Physicians. In addition, the US federal government has a number of resources that provide excellent information and initial Web searches, including the National Institutes of Health, Health Finder, and the Substance Abuse and Mental Health Services Administration.

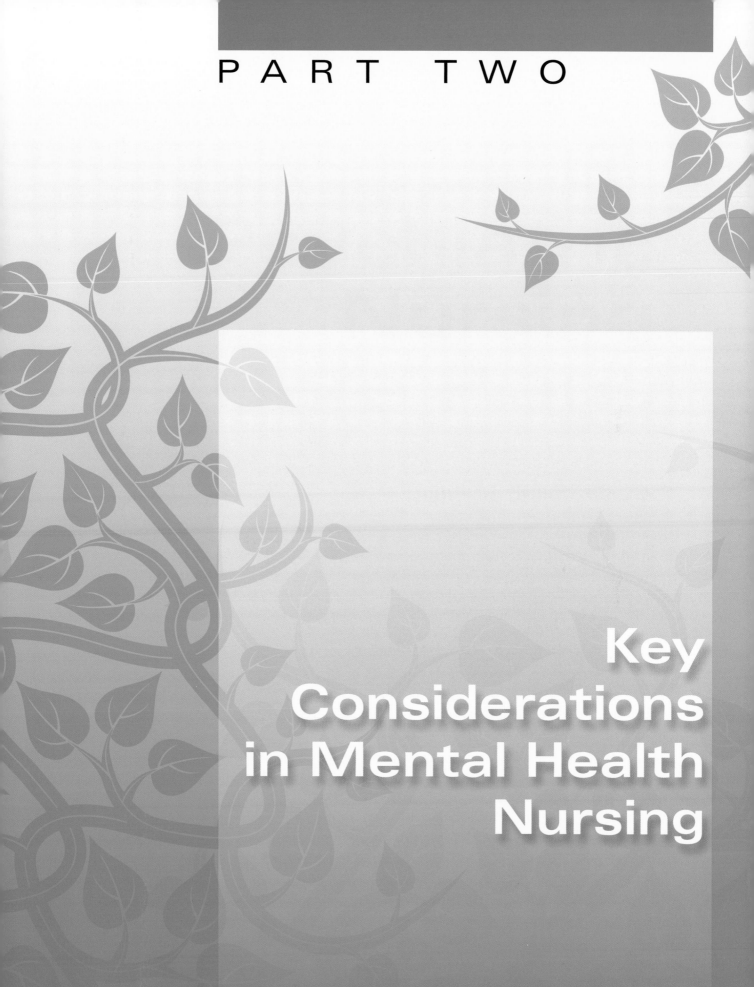

PART TWO

Key Considerations in Mental Health Nursing

The care plans in this book have been created with certain fundamental concepts in mind. These key concepts are critical considerations in planning care and in working with mental health clients. In delineating these concepts and beliefs, we hope to stimulate the reader's thinking about these aspects of working with clients, while providing a solid foundation for mental health nursing practice.

FUNDAMENTAL BELIEFS

1. A nurse provides only the care the client cannot provide for himself or herself at the time.
2. The client basically is responsible for his or her own feelings, actions, and life (see "Client's Responsibilities"), although he or she may be limited in ability or need help.
3. The nurse must approach the client as a whole person with a unique background and environment, possessing strengths, behaviors, and problems, not as a psychiatrically labeled object to be manipulated.
4. The client is not a passive recipient of care. The nurse and the client work together toward mutually determined and desirable goals or outcomes. The client's active participation in all steps of the nursing process should be encouraged within the limits of the client's present level of functioning (see "Client's Responsibilities").
5. The predominant goal is the client's health, not merely the absence or diminution of the disease process. The client's eventual independence from the care setting and the staff must be a focus of care. If this is impossible, the client should reach his or her optimum level of functioning and independence.
6. Given feedback and the identification of alternative ways to meet needs that are acceptable to the client, he or she will choose to progress toward health with more appropriate coping mechanisms if he or she is able to do so.
7. Physical health and emotional health are interconnected, and physical health is a desirable goal in the treatment of emotional problems. Nursing care should include a focus on the client obtaining adequate nutrition, rest, and exercise, and the elimination of chemical dependence (including tobacco, caffeine, alcohol, and over-the-counter medications or other drugs).
8. The nurse works with other health professionals (and nonprofessionals) in an interdisciplinary treatment team; the nurse may function as a team coordinator.

9. The interdisciplinary team works within a milieu that is constructed as a therapeutic environment, with the aims of developing a holistic view of the client and providing effective treatment.

THERAPEUTIC MILIEU

Purpose and Definition

The therapeutic milieu is an environment that is structured and maintained as an ideal, dynamic setting in which to work with clients. This milieu includes safe physical surroundings, all treatment team members, and other clients. It is supported by clear and consistently maintained limits (see "Limit Setting") and behavioral expectations. A therapeutic setting should minimize environmental stress, such as noise and confusion, and physical stress caused by factors, such as lack of sleep and substance abuse.

Removal of the client from a stressful environment to a therapeutic environment provides a chance for rest and nurturance, a time to focus on developing strengths, and an opportunity to learn about the psychodynamics of problems and to identify alternatives or solutions to those problems. This setting also allows clients to participate in an interpersonal community in which they can share feelings and experiences and enjoy social interaction and growth as well as therapeutic interactions. The nurse has a unique opportunity to facilitate (and model) communication and sharing among clients in the creation of a continuing, dynamic, informal group therapy. This may be done by implementing various aspects of a given treatment program (e.g., for chemical dependence), by using therapeutic interactions based on individual clients' care plans, by facilitating structured therapeutic groups, and so forth.

A therapeutic milieu is a "safe space," a nonpunitive atmosphere in which caring is a basic factor. Clients are expected to assume responsibility for themselves within the structure of the milieu as they are able to do so. Feedback from staff and other clients and the sharing of tasks or duties within the treatment program facilitate the client's growth. In this environment, confrontation may be a positive therapeutic tool that can be tolerated by the client. However, nurses and other treatment team members should be aware of their roles in this environment to maintain stability and safety, but they also should minimize authoritarian behavior (e.g., displaying keys as a reminder of status or control; see "Nursing Responsibilities and Functions").

Maintaining a Safe Environment

One important aspect of a therapeutic environment is the exclusion of objects or circumstances that a client may use to harm himself or herself or others. Although this is especially important in a mental health setting, this should be considered in any health care situation. The nursing staff should follow the facility's policies with regard to prevention of routine safety hazards and supplement these policies as necessary, for example:

- Dispose of all needles safely and out of reach of clients.
- Restrict or monitor the use of matches and lighters.
- Do not allow smoking in bedrooms (clients may be drowsy owing to psychotropic drugs).
- Remove mouthwash, cologne, aftershave, and so forth if substance abuse is suspected.

Listed below are *very restrictive* measures for a unit on which clients are present who are exhibiting behavior that is threatening or harmful to themselves or others. These measures may be modified based on assessment of the clients' behaviors.

- Do not have glass containers accessible (e.g., drinking glasses, vases, salt and pepper shakers).
- Be sure mirrors, if glass, are securely fastened and not easily broken.
- Keep sharp objects (e.g., scissors, pocketknives, knitting needles) out of reach of clients and allow their use only with supervision. Use electric shavers when possible (disposable razors are easily broken to access blades).
- Identify potential weapons (e.g., mop handles, hammers, pool cues) and dangerous equipment (e.g., electrical cords, scalpels, Pap smear fixative), and keep them out of the client's reach.
- Do not leave cleaning or maintenance carts, which may contain cleaning fluids, mops, and tools, unattended in client care areas.
- Do not leave medicines unattended or unlocked.
- Keep keys (to unit door and medicines) on your person at all times.
- Be aware of items that are harmful if ingested (e.g., mercury in manometers).
- Immediately on the client's admission to the facility, treatment team members should search the client and all of his or her belongings and remove potentially dangerous items, such as wire clothes hangers, ropes, belts, safety pins, scissors and other sharp objects, weapons, and medications. Keep these belongings in a designated place inaccessible to the client. Also, search any packages brought in by visitors (it may be necessary to search visitors in certain circumstances). Explain the reason for such rules briefly and do not make exceptions.

The Trust Relationship

One key to a therapeutic environment is the establishment of trust. Trust is the foundation of a therapeutic relationship, and limit setting and consistency are its building blocks. Not only must the client come to trust the nurse, but the nurse must trust himself or herself as a therapist and trust the client's motivation and ability to change. Both the client and the nurse must trust that treatment is desirable and productive. A trust relationship between the nurse and the client creates a space in which they can work together, using the nursing process and their best possible efforts toward attaining the goals they have both identified (see Care Plan 1: Building a Trust Relationship).

Building Self-Esteem

Just as a physically healthy body may be better able to withstand stress, a person with adequate self-esteem may be better able to deal with emotional difficulties. Thus, an essential part of a client's care is helping to build the client's self-esteem. However, because each client retains the responsibility for his or her own feelings, and one person cannot *make* another person *feel* a certain way, the nurse cannot increase the client's self-esteem directly.

Strategies to help build or enhance self-esteem must be individualized and built on honesty and the client's strengths. Some general suggestions are as follows:

- Build a trust relationship with the client (see Care Plan 1: Building a Trust Relationship).
- Set and maintain limits (see "Limit Setting").
- Accept the client as a person.
- Be nonjudgmental at all times.
- Provide structure (i.e., help the client structure his or her time and activities).
- Have realistic expectations of the client and make them clear to the client.
- Provide the client with tasks, responsibilities, and activities that can be easily accomplished; advance the client to more difficult tasks as he or she progresses.
- Praise the client for his or her accomplishments, however small, giving sincere appropriate feedback for meeting expectations, completing tasks, fulfilling responsibilities, and so on.
- Be honest; never insincerely flatter the client.
- Minimize negative feedback to the client; enforce the limits that have been set, but withdraw attention from the client if possible rather than chastising the client for exceeding limits.
- Use confrontation judiciously and in a supportive manner; use it only when the client can tolerate it.
- Allow the client to make his or her own decisions whenever possible. If the client is pleased with the outcome of his or her decision, point out that he or she was responsible for the decision and give positive feedback. If the client is not pleased with the outcome, point out that the client, like everyone, can make and survive mistakes; then help the client identify alternative approaches to the problem. Give positive feedback when the client takes responsibility for problem solving and praise his or her efforts.

Limit Setting

Setting and maintaining limits is integral to a trust relationship and to a therapeutic milieu. Effective limits can provide a structure and a sense of caring that words alone cannot. Limits also minimize manipulation by a client and secondary gains such as special attention or relief from responsibilities.

Before stating a limit and its consequence, you may wish to review the reasons for limit setting with the client and involve the client in this part of care planning, possibly working together to decide on specific limits or consequences. However, if this is impossible, briefly explain the limits to the client and do not argue or indulge in lengthy discussions or give undue attention to the consequences of an infraction of a limit. Some basic guidelines for effectively using limits are as follows:

1. State the expectation or the limit as clearly, directly, and simply as possible. The consequence that will follow the client's exceeding the limit also must be clearly stated at the outset.
2. Keep in mind that consequences should be simple and direct, with some bearing on the limit, if possible, and should be something that the client perceives as a negative outcome, not as a reward or producer of secondary gain. For example, if the consequence is not allowing the client to go to an activity it will not be effective if the client did not want to go anyway, or the client is allowed to watch television or receives individual attention from the staff, which the client may prefer.
3. The consequence should immediately follow the client's exceeding the limit and must be used consistently, each time the limit is exceeded and with all staff members. One staff member may be designated to make decisions regarding limits to ensure consistency; however, when this person is not available, another person must take responsibility, rather than deferring the consequences.

Remember, although consequences are essential to setting and maintaining limits, they are not an opportunity to be punitive to a client. The withdrawal of attention is perhaps the best and simplest of consequences to carry out, provided that attention and support are given when the client meets expectations and remains within limits, and that the client's safety is not jeopardized by the withdrawal of staff attention. If the only time the client receives attention and feedback, albeit negative, is when he or she exceeds limits, the client will continue to elicit attention in that way. The client must perceive a positive reason to meet expectations; there must be a reward for staying within limits.

Regarding limits, do not delude yourself in thinking that a client needs the nurse as a friend or sympathetic person who will be "nice" by making exceptions to limits. If you allow a client to exceed limits, you will be giving the client mixed messages and will undermine the other members of the treatment team as well as the client. You will convey to the client that you do not care enough for the client's growth and well-being to enforce a limit, and you will betray a lack of control on your part at a time when the client feels out of control and

expressly needs someone else to be in control (see "Nursing Responsibilities and Functions").

SEXUALITY

Human sexuality is an area in which the feelings of treatment team members are often evoked and must be considered. Because it is basic to everyone, sexuality may be a factor with any client in a number of ways. Too often the discomfort of both the nurse and the client interferes with the client's care; you, the nurse, can significantly overcome this discomfort by dealing with your own feelings and approaching this facet of the client's life in a professional way.

Client problems involving sexual issues or sexuality may be related to the following:

- A change in sexual habits or feelings, such as first sexual activity, marriage, or the loss of a sexual partner (see Care Plan 51: Disturbed Body Image)
- Injury, illness, or disability (see Care Plan 51: Disturbed Body Image)
- Being the victim of a traumatic experience that involved a sexual act, such as incest or rape (see Care Plan 31: Post-Traumatic Stress Disorder and Care Plan 49: Sexual, Emotional, or Physical Abuse)
- Being charged with or convicted of a crime that is associated with sexual activity, such as incest, exhibitionism, or rape (see "Clients With Legal Problems")
- Impotence or menopausal symptoms
- Experiencing sexual feelings that are uncomfortable, confusing, or unacceptable to the client or significant others
- Feeling guilty about masturbation or sexual activity outside of marriage
- Lack of social skills in the area of social and intimate relationships
- Side effects from psychotropic (or other) medications that impair sexual functioning (frank discussion regarding this problem can help prevent noncompliance with medications by possibly identifying alternative medication[s] or helping the client to adapt to the side effects in the interest of treatment goals)

These problems may be difficult for a client to reveal initially or to share with more than one staff person or with other clients. In situations like these, it is often helpful to the client if the nurse asks about problems related to sexuality in the initial nursing assessment and care planning. Be sensitive to the client's feelings, and remember that both male and female clients have a human need for sexual fulfillment. A matter-of-fact approach to sexuality on your part can help to minimize the client's discomfort.

Sexual activity or sexually explicit conversations may occur on the unit, posing another challenge related to sexuality. This may include clients being sexual with one another, a client making sexual advances or displays to others, or a client masturbating openly on the unit. Sexual acting-out on the unit can be effectively managed by setting and maintaining limits (see "Limit Setting"), as with other acting-out situations. Again, a matter-of-fact approach is often most effective.

In residential or long-term care facilities, clients' needs for intimate relationships and sexual activity can pose sensitive, complex issues. It is important to develop policies that incorporate legal considerations regarding clients' rights to sexual relations and obligations to protect clients from harm. These policies may include guidelines for criteria to determine the client's ability to consent to sexual activity and to provide for privacy (e.g., for masturbation or other sexual activity); client education (regarding social skills for developing intimate relationships, saying "no" to unwanted attention or advances, basic anatomy and sexuality, birth control, and prevention of HIV infection and other sexually transmitted diseases); and so forth.

Some aspects of the client's sexuality or lifestyle may be disturbing to treatment team members, even though the client may not be experiencing a problem or believe that the issue is a problem. For example, sexual activity in the young or elderly client, sexual practices that differ from those of the staff member, transvestism, or homosexuality, may evoke uncomfortable, judgmental, or other kinds of feelings in treatment team members. Again, it is important to be aware of and deal with these feelings as a part of your responsibility rather than create a problem or undermine the client's perception of himself or herself by defining something as a problem when it is not. Providing nonjudgmental care to a client is especially important in the area of sexuality because the client may have previously encountered or may expect censure from professionals, which reinforces guilt, shame, and low self-esteem.

Homosexuality is not a mental health disorder. Clients who are gay or lesbian may feel positive about their homosexuality and have no desire to change. If a client who is homosexual seeks treatment for another problem (e.g., depression), do not assume that this problem is related to the client's homosexuality. However, being a homosexual in our society can present a number of significant stresses to an individual, and these may or may not influence the client's problem. Aside from societal censure in general, the client faces possible loss of familial support, employment, housing, or children by revealing his or her homosexuality. A client who is lesbian or gay often must deal with these issues on a daily basis, but even these stresses must not be confused with the client's sexuality per se.

Clients may choose not to reveal their homosexuality or other sexual issues to treatment team members, family members, or others (e.g., employers) in their lives. Confidentiality is an important issue in this situation because of the potential losses to the client should his or her homosexuality become known, and must be respected by the nursing staff. Regardless of whether or not a client's sexual orientation is spoken, his or her primary support persons may be a partner, a lover, a roommate, or friends, rather than family members. It is important to respectfully include this client's significant others in care planning, discharge planning, teaching, and other aspects of care, just as family members are included in the care of clients who are heterosexual. Remain aware of your own feelings about homosexuality and take responsibility for dealing with those feelings so that you are able to provide effective, nonjudgmental nursing care for all clients.

Sexual concerns also may conflict with the religious beliefs and cultural values of both clients and treatment team members. It is important that the nurse is aware of the client's cultural background and its implications for the client's treatment as well as the nurse's own cultural values and how these can influence care provided to the client. It may be helpful to involve a chaplain or other clergy member in the client's treatment. Having respect for the client, examining your own feelings, maintaining a nonjudgmental attitude, encouraging expression of the client's feelings, and allowing the client to make his or her own decisions are the standards for working with clients in situations with a moral or religious dimension, whether the issue is abortion, celibacy, sterilization, impotence, transsexualism, or any other aspect of human sexuality.

SPIRITUALITY

Spirituality can encompass a person's beliefs, values, or philosophy of life. The client may consider spirituality to be extremely important or not at all a part of his or her life. The spiritual realm may be a source of strength, support, security, and well-being in a client's life. However, the client may be experiencing problems that have caused him or her to lose faith, to become disillusioned, or to be in despair. Or, the client's psychiatric symptoms may have a religious focus that may or may not be related to his or her spiritual beliefs, such as religiosity.

Spiritual belief systems differ greatly among people. These systems can range from traditional Western, Eastern, and Middle Eastern religions to alternative, ancient, or New Age beliefs, or they may reflect individual beliefs and philosophy unrelated to a traditional religion or structured set of beliefs. As with other aspects of a client, it is important to assess spirituality in the client's life, particularly as it relates to the client's present problem. It also is important to be respectful of the client's beliefs and feelings in the spiritual realm and to deliver nonjudgmental nursing care regardless of the client's spiritual beliefs. Spiritual issues often are closely linked to the client's cultural background, so you need to be aware of the client's cultural values and of your own feelings in order to avoid giving negative messages about the client's spirituality. Remember that the client has a right to hold his or her own beliefs and it is not appropriate for you to try to convince the client to believe as you do or to proselytize your beliefs in the context of care.

If the client is experiencing spiritual distress, it may be appropriate to contact your facility's chaplain or to refer the client to a leader of his or her faith for guidance. Nursing care can then continue in conjunction with the recommendations of this specialist to meet the client's needs in a respectful manner. The nurse's role is not limited to alleviating spiritual distress, but also includes viewing spirituality as an integral aspect of the client's overall plan of care.

CULTURE

Although many people think of culture in terms of race, ethnicity, ancestry, or country of origin, culture includes other aspects of a person's background and sense of self or identity, including values, practices, and beliefs. Cultural identity is made up of many components related to religion, language, age or peer group, socioeconomic status, community (e.g., urban, suburban, or rural), gender, sexual orientation, social or family situation (e.g., marital status), physical ability or disabilities, political beliefs, work and educational experience, and so forth. Therefore, a person's cultural background can be seen as multidimensional; a person also may belong to several cultural groups. For example, a client may be female, white, agnostic, lesbian, rural, a nurse, a young adult, and so on. In addition, there are differences within cultural groups, including variations among subgroups and among individuals. For example, there is not one Asian culture but many cultures, and within each of these are factors that influence an individual's cultural orientation and the extent to which he or she identifies with traditional cultural values or has adopted other values and beliefs. Some cultural differences are quite obvious, but others are so subtle that they often are overlooked entirely.

Delivering nursing care that is culturally sensitive requires an awareness of both the client and oneself as cultural beings. This awareness should include recognition that while an individual's cultural orientation influences many aspects of life and this influence can be extremely strong, many people do not acknowledge cultural influences as such. Nurses need to maintain their own cultural awareness on a daily basis with all clients because of the multilevel nature of cultural orientation. Maintaining awareness of possible cultural differences and of what the client's culture means to him or her is essential if the nurse is to adequately assess the client and plan care that is culturally appropriate.

Nurses may have different perceptions and expectations of clients and their behavior based on the client's and the nurse's cultural backgrounds, particularly when the differences between them are more pronounced. The greatest danger in this situation is if this occurs without the nurse's awareness. Always evaluate your own attitude toward and expectations of each client, especially if you do not expect full participation or recovery from a particular client.

The client may also have expectations and perceptions of the staff and of health care based on cultural differences and on experiences with health care and providers. For example, the client may be fearful or guarded and may need reassurance, especially if great cultural or language differences exist.

The client's culture may have a strong effect on the client's view of his or her illness, treatment, and expectations for recovery. For example, psychiatric illness may be associated with shame, guilt, or social ostracism in some cultures, or may be accepted fatalistically or with equanimity in other cultures. Similarly, a client from one cultural background may have high expectations of health and may view recovery as a process for which he or she is primarily responsible, whereas a client from a different background may see illness as his or her fate or as being controlled by an external force or being. The latter can lead to clients believing that they will never recover or that they have no influence on their own recovery.

The client's cultural orientation can largely determine what he or she considers "normal" behavior and can provide the framework for interpreting "abnormal" behavior. At times, therapeutic treatment goals (e.g., expressing feelings of anger toward one's parents) are in opposition to cultural norms (e.g., parental authority must always be respected). In addition, clients from different cultural backgrounds may pursue treatments that are quite different from therapeutic interventions of the dominant culture, including consulting alternative health care practitioners and using herbal or traditional medicines. This type of data must be assessed and integrated into the client's plan of care. There are many culturally specific explanations for illness, particularly mental illness (Giger & Davidhizar, 2008). It is important to consider the client's cultural context when assessing behaviors and expecting behavior change and to remember that chances for treatment success are enhanced when expectations and interventions are culturally appropriate.

Remember that members of a dominant culture often expect those from other cultures to adopt the values of the dominant culture, whether consciously or unconsciously. In fact, many people think that their cultural values represent "the right way" to live and feel quite judgmental about others not accepting those values. As in all other aspects of nursing care, this kind of judgment and expectation is inappropriate; nurses need to examine their own thoughts and feelings and provide nonjudgmental care to all clients. You can use the following questions to begin your own self-examination and to make sure your self-awareness continues as you deliver care:

- How do I see this client?
- How is this client different from me?
- How is this client's cultural background different from mine?
- What is the best way to approach this client?
- What do I expect from this client? (*Note:* Ask this question regarding the client's behavior, participation in the treatment plan, expected outcomes, etc.)
- How are my expectations of this client different from my expectations of other clients?
- What am I basing my expectations on?
- Do my values conflict with the client's values and beliefs?
- Does this client seem strange to me?
- Do I have negative feelings about this client?
- Am I frustrated with this client (or with his or her values or beliefs)?
- Am I avoiding this client?
- Do I have adequate knowledge of this client's cultural orientation?
- Are there culturally specific treatment options that may be appropriate or inappropriate in this client's care?

Cultural differences and their effects can be obvious or subtle. In an increasingly multicultural society, a nurse may work with clients from many different cultural groups, and he or she cannot expect to learn enough about each of these cultures to provide culturally competent care for each client. However, the nurse can and should try to learn about the cultures most frequently represented by clients in his or her area. Using that knowledge as a foundation, the nurse can assess each client with regard to his or her cultural background. Remember, however, that it may be falsely reassuring to the nurse to "learn" some aspects of a particular culture; the nurse may then apply that learning to all clients of that culture, which can lead to stereotyping.

Remember also that it is not always desirable to match culturally similar staff with the client (i.e., in making nursing care assignments). Although this may be done with good intentions, the client may feel segregated, devalued, or stereotyped. In addition, both the client and the nurse can benefit from developing cross-cultural relationships.

The greatest obstacles to cross-cultural care are not in what the nurse might not know about the client's culture beforehand, but in the nurse's lack of cultural awareness, assumptions, and prejudices regarding the client; failure to acknowledge the need to learn about the client's culture; or expectation that the client behave in ways that are incompatible with the client's culture. Therefore, the nurse must adopt the practice of learning about each client's unique cultural orientation to provide culturally sensitive care. This learning can be accomplished by gathering information from a variety of sources, including the client and his or her family or significant others. For example, the nurse may want to ask questions regarding the appropriateness or acceptability of certain communication techniques and interventions, or about expectations for recovery and the client's view of his or her behavior or illness.

Good communication skills can help bridge cultural differences. For example, if the client seems uncomfortable with direct questions in certain areas, you might preface your questions by saying, "I know it may feel awkward to talk about these things, but it will help us care for you if you can tell me…," and so forth. In addition, asking the client and the family or significant others about their culture can help to build a trusting relationship by demonstrating respect for and interest in the client and his or her culture. If you are honest about wanting to learn and state your awareness that you do not already know everything, it can help you form a partnership with the client for his or her treatment and encourage the client's participation. It can also reassure a client who may have had negative experiences with health care providers or others from the dominant culture. Then, be sure to share what you learn with other treatment team members and incorporate it in the client's written plan of care.

Nursing interventions also have cultural implications, and these cultural implications need to be considered when writing and implementing a client's care plan. Some interventions may be especially sensitive, such as using touch to comfort a client who is distressed. However, other interventions and communication techniques may be culturally sensitive as well, such as using direct eye contact, speaking directly to the client regarding his or her illness, discussing emotional topics (e.g., sexuality), and so on. Because each nurse cannot have a complete knowledge of all the cultural nuances of all the clients with whom he or she may work, maintaining an awareness that there *may* be cultural implications and evaluating this at each step of the nursing process is the best strategy.

COMPLEMENTARY AND ALTERNATIVE MEDICINE

Complementary and alternative medicine (CAM) is a term that denotes a range of treatments, treatment disciplines, dietary supplements, vitamins, and health practices considered to be alternatives and supplements to conventional medical treatments and medications. There is a wide range of disciplines and substances included under this general term, and there is widespread and increasing use of these practices in the United States and many other countries. CAM services comprise traditional healing methods from many cultures, bodywork and physical activity practices, herbs, vitamins, and other dietary supplements, as well as medical disciplines like chiropractic, holistic, and naturopathic medicine.

Examples of CAM disciplines include acupuncture, chiropractic, osteopathic, Ayurvedic, homeopathic, and holistic practitioners; Tai Chi, Yoga, Pilates physical activity; massage therapies, Rolfing, Feldenkrais bodywork; behavioral feedback, mind/body, guided imagery, relaxation techniques; and herbs, Chinese medicine, dietary supplements, and nutritional therapies.

According to the National Center for Complementary and Alternative Medicine (NCCAM), nearly 40% of adults in the United States and 12% of children reported using CAM treatments or services in 2007 (NCCAM, 2007). Many clients encountered in psychiatric nursing have used, or currently use them, as well. It is important to include CAM treatments, supplements, and so forth, in your assessment of the client, as they may impact his or her condition, behaviors, and recovery. If the client is currently taking or has recently taken herbal or other dietary supplements, it is especially important to determine the details of these and to consult with a pharmacist about their effects and possible interactions with other medications the client may be taking. Because supplements fall under different government regulations than other medications, there may be limited research regarding dosage and efficacy and limited testing for safety and toxicity related to some products. Or, because these substances are sold over the counter, clients may not fully understand their potency and may believe that the suggested use guidelines can be far exceeded without danger. Many of these products are explicitly marketed for mood- or other psychiatrically related problems, such as depression, stress, memory, and insomnia; the client may have used them in an attempt to self-medicate and may believe strongly in their effectiveness or may prefer them to other medications because the client sees these products as more "natural" than traditional pharmaceutical medicines.

The client's culture may influence his or her decision to use CAM resources and may be a strong factor in the client's belief in their efficacy. Because these practices, supplements, and practitioners may be important to and benefit the client, it is important for the nurse to be (or become) familiar with them when a client has used or is thinking of using them. If the client has used CAM resources in the past that have had a positive influence on his or her health, it may be helpful to suggest that the client continue or resume their use. As with other aspects of client care, it is essential to remain nonjudgmental about the client's practices, while assisting the client to evaluate the benefits as well as precautions related to these resources.

There are many Web resources for CAM services and products, including government resources such as the National Center for Complementary and Alternative Medicine and the National Cancer Institute's Office of Complementary and Alternative Medicine; professional associations and foundations, for example, the American Holistic Medicine Association and the Alternative Medicine Foundation; and information on specific disciplines, products, and services. The U.S. Food and Drug Administration provides information on dietary supplements, and the National Library of Medicine provides a Directory of Health Organizations Online (see Web Resources on thePoint).

THE AGING CLIENT

People are aging throughout life; developmental growth, challenges, changes, and concomitant losses occur on a continuum from birth to death. As people go through life stages, they experience changes in many aspects of their daily lives. Some of these changes are gradual and barely noticed; others may be sudden or marked by events that result in profound differences in one's life. Aging necessitates adjustment to different roles, relationships, responsibilities, abilities, work, leisure, and levels of social and economic status; changes in self-image, independence, and dependence; and changes in physical, emotional, mental, and spiritual aspects of life. Adjustment from adolescence into early adulthood entails a major transition in terms of independence, roles, and relationships. Moving from young adulthood into middle age, older age, and becoming elderly results in many changes, some of which affect one's self-esteem and body image, and which may entail significant losses over time. As one becomes increasingly aged, these losses may become major factors in one's life. Loss of physical abilities, altered body image, loss of loved ones, loss of independence, economic security and social status, and the loss of a sense of the future may present significant problems to a client. For example, despair, spiritual disillusionment, depression, or suicidal behavior may occur, to which these life changes are major contributing factors. If the client's presenting problem does not seem to be related to aging or factors associated with aging, developmental or adjustment issues still need to be assessed to gain a holistic view of the client.

Remember that the elderly client is a whole person with individual strengths and needs. Do not assume that a client over a certain age has organic brain pathology, no longer has sexual feelings, or has no need for independence. It is important to promote independence to the client's optimal level of functioning no matter what the client's age and to provide the necessary physical care and assistance without drawing undue attention to the client's needs. An adult or elderly client may never have needed someone to care for him or her and may feel humiliated by being in a dependent position. The client may have previously been proud of his or her independence and may have gained much self-esteem from this. This client may experience both fear and despair at the thought of being a burden. Do not dismiss these feelings as inappropriate because of your own discomfort; instead, encourage the client to express these feelings and give the client support while promoting as much independence as possible (see Care Plan 25: Major Depressive Disorder, Care Plan 50: Grief, and Care Plan 51: Disturbed Body Image).

Feelings about aging can be strongly influenced by cultural backgrounds and spiritual beliefs. In addition, aging is a universal experience that involves multiple losses and grief. Therefore, it can be a difficult issue for treatment team members and can result in uncomfortable feelings, denial, and rejection of the client. With aging or aged clients, as with other difficult issues, discomfort on the part of the nurse influences care given to the client. Respect for the individual and awareness of your feelings and those of the client together contribute to good nursing care that maintains the client's dignity.

LONELINESS

Loneliness is an emotional state of dissatisfaction with the quality or quantity of relationships. It has been described as a painful emotion related to unmet needs for intimacy. Clients who have psychiatric problems may experience loneliness as a result of their psychiatric illness (i.e., if earlier relationships deteriorate because of the client's illness), or loneliness can be a contributing factor to the client's illness. Loneliness also can be a problem for a client's caregiver, especially if he or she is the primary or sole caregiver and if no one else lives with the client.

Feelings of loneliness can result from physically being alone, but they also encompass feelings of emotional isolation or a lack of connection to others. Although social isolation can be a contributing factor to loneliness, they are not the same thing. Loneliness is perceived by the individual as a negative, unpleasant, and undesired state. Social isolation or lack of contact with other people can occur without loneliness and may be a situation preferred and chosen by the client. A client may desire to be alone for a variety of reasons, which may or may not be related to psychiatric problems, yet not feel lonely or desire a change in this situation. Key factors in determining a client's loneliness are that the client is dissatisfied and experiencing discomfort. Finally, a client may choose to be alone, yet also feel lonely; that is, the person may be dissatisfied with the feelings of loneliness that result from choosing to be alone.

The nurse needs to be aware of the risk for and situation of loneliness when working with clients in any setting. Assessment of inpatients should include the client's history of loneliness as well as present feelings of loneliness in the facility. Risk factors for loneliness include mental illness (e.g., depression, schizophrenia), social isolation, certain age groups (e.g., adolescents, the elderly), chronic physical illness or impairment, alcohol or drug abuse, loss of significant other(s), change in residence, and loss of employment. However, loneliness can occur without these risk factors and although assessing risk factors may help identify loneliness, it is the client's perception of his or her feelings that is the key in determining loneliness. Because it is an emotional state, it is not necessarily "rational." That is, a client may appear to have a very supportive familial or social network, yet complain of feeling lonely. Conversely, the client may appear to have virtually no support system or relationships and may be content with that situation. Assessment for loneliness should include the intensity and duration of feelings of loneliness, the client's perception of factors that contribute to the loneliness; the client's perception of the quality of his or her relationships and of himself or herself within those relationships; the client's perception of his or her connection to the community; the client's spiritual beliefs and feelings of support from these beliefs and from the client's relationship to a higher power; actions that the client has taken to relieve loneliness in the past; and the effectiveness of those actions.

A number of nursing interventions can be used in addressing the risk for or situation of loneliness, such as facilitating the client's development of social, relationship, and leisure activity skills; promoting the client's self-esteem; and identifying sources of social contact and support in the client's living situation and community. These include interpersonal relationships, adopting a pet if the client is able to care for an animal, referral to supportive groups, placement in an appropriate group-living situation, identification of continued treatment resources, and so on. In addition, educating the client and significant others about loneliness, and teaching the client how to communicate needs for support and intimacy (e.g., helping the client learn how to tell others when he or she is feeling lonely, and helping the client's significant others learn how to respond by listening or attending to the client) can be effective interventions (see Care Plan 8: Partial Community Support).

HOMELESSNESS

Homelessness represents a significant challenge to nurses and other health care professionals, as well as to society in general, and clients who are homeless may be encountered in any type of health care setting. Homeless persons with mental illness may be found in shelters and jails, as well as living on the streets. An estimated 20% to 40% of the homeless population in the United States have mental illness (American Psychiatric Association, 2010b) and as many as 50% have substance-related problems. Compared with homeless persons without mental illness, the mentally ill homeless are homeless longer, have less family contact, spend more time in shelters or in jail, and face greater barriers (National Coalition for the Homeless, 2009). For this population, professionals replace families as the primary source of help.

Studies have shown that providing housing alone does not significantly change the situation of the mentally ill homeless (Gilmer, Stefancic, Ettner, Manning, & Tsemberis, 2010). Chronically homeless adults with severe mental illness tend to use costly inpatient and emergency services when they become seriously ill, but use few health maintenance services. Projects that provide access to mental health treatment, social services, and rehabilitation services in addition to stable community housing have much greater success in making a significant difference in the lives of this population. One such project in California found that individuals who were engaged in treatment and had financial support in addition to housing had decreased use of inpatient and emergency services, fewer homeless days, less involvement with the justice system, and an improved quality of life compared with persons receiving minimal or traditional, less comprehensive services. Although it is difficult to engage homeless persons in a therapeutic relationship, when that relationship has been established, results can be positive. It is especially important for the nurse to work effectively with the interdisciplinary team to coordinate resources for the client who is homeless and to facilitate planning for the client's future needs.

STRESS

Clients come to a mental health facility with a variety of problems, many of which may be seen as responses to stress or as occurring when the client's usual coping strategies are inadequate in the face of a certain degree of stress. For example, post-traumatic behavior has been identified as a response to a significant stressor that would evoke distress in most people, and grieving is a process that normally occurs in response to a loss or change. A stressor is not necessarily only one major event, however, and some problems may be related to the constant presence of long-term or unrelenting stress, such as poverty or minority status and oppression. Stressors are usually perceived as unpleasant or negative events; however, a significant "happy" event, such as marriage or the birth of a child, also can cause a major change in the client's life and overwhelm his or her usual coping strategies.

Stress may be a significant contributing factor to a client's present problem. For example, psychosomatic illnesses, eating disorders, and suicidal behavior have all been linked to client response to stressors. It is important to assess all clients with regard to the stress in their lives (both perceived and observable) and to their response to stress, regardless of the presenting problem.

There is a danger in labeling a severely stressed client as ill when he or she seeks help. Labeling separates the client from other "normal" people and may lead the nurse to expect illness behavior rather than to continue to see the client as a unique and multifaceted person who possesses strengths and who deals with stress in daily life. It is important to realize that stressors are real and demand responses from everyone: the client, his or her significant others, and treatment team members. Illness and caregiving are themselves stressors (see Care Plan 5: Supporting the Caregiver and "Treatment Team Member Considerations"). One of the most important therapeutic aims in nursing care is to help the client deal with the stress of present problems and to build skills and resources to deal with stress in the future. Teaching stress management skills, including how to identify stress and the problem-solving process, is a critical part of client education (see "Client Teaching").

CRISIS INTERVENTION

Individuals experience a crisis when they are confronted by some life circumstance or stressor that they cannot manage effectively through use of their customary coping skills. Caplan (1964) identified the stages of crisis: (1) the individual is exposed to a stressor, experiences anxiety, and tries to cope in a customary fashion; (2) anxiety increases when the customary coping skills are ineffective; (3) all possible efforts are made to deal with the stressor, including attempts at new methods of coping; and (4) when previous coping attempts fail, the individual experiences disequilibrium and significant distress. Crises may occur as an acute response to an external situation; an anticipated life transition; traumatic stress; maturational or developmental issues; psychopathology, such as a personality disorder; or a psychiatric emergency, such as an overdose or psychosis.

Aguilera (1998) identified three factors that influence whether or not an individual experiences a crisis: the individual's perception of the event, the availability of situational supports, and the availability of adequate coping mechanisms. When the person in crisis seeks assistance, these factors represent a guide for effective intervention. The person can be assisted to view the event or issue from a different perspective, that is, as an opportunity for growth or change rather than a threat. Assisting the person to use existing supports or helping the individual to find new sources of support can decrease the feelings of being alone and overwhelmed. Finally, assisting the person to learn new methods of coping will help resolve the current crisis and give him or her new coping skills to use in the future.

Persons experiencing a crisis are usually distressed and likely to seek help for their distress. They are ready to learn and even eager to try new coping skills as a way to relieve their distress. This is an ideal time for intervention that is likely to be successful.

COMMUNITY VIOLENCE

Violence within a community has been identified as a national health concern and a priority for intervention in the United States, where violent incidents exceed 2 million occurrences per year. Victims of violence or abuse can be any age, from small infants to the elderly; they may be a child, spouse, partner, parent, or acquaintance. Violence is often perpetrated by someone known to the victim. There is also a growing concern for children who witness acts of violence. Results of multiple studies indicate that exposure to violence has a profound negative effect on children's cognitive, social, psychological, and moral development (Gwynne, Blick, & Duffy, 2009).

Nurses working with children and adults who have experienced or witnessed violence in their home or community need to understand and recognize the mental–emotional distress that can result from these experiences. These individuals may be seen in a clinic, doctor's office, or school while being treated for other medical problems. The challenges for the nurse are to recognize when individuals have been affected by violence in their lives, provide support to them, and, through collaboration with other disciplines, make referrals to address the resulting emotional issues.

COMMUNITY GRIEF AND DISASTER RESPONSE

Terrorism, large-scale violence, and disaster are severely disturbing problems that engender feelings of profound grief, anxiety, vulnerability, and loss of control throughout the communities that they affect, whether local or worldwide. Incidents like the terrorist attacks on the World Trade Center in New York City, the shootings at Columbine High School in Colorado, the Oklahoma City bombing, Pearl Harbor, and the assassinations of political leaders have triggered *national grief*. Awareness of these issues has increased profoundly in the United States and around the world. Workplace violence, threats of biological and chemical weapons attacks, and major accidents or natural disasters, like Hurricane Katrina and its aftermath also trigger this type of response, which has been called *critical incident stress* or *disaster response*, though deliberate human attacks generally result in more severe stress (Eisenman et al., 2009). Traumatic events such as these are expected to produce significant distress in any person, including the distress of surviving such an event when others did not (see Care Plan 31: Post-Traumatic Stress Disorder). Previously healthy, fully functional people would be expected to need support from others to deal with their response to the event, and the effects of such events extend well beyond those directly harmed—including significant others and people in the local community, in the nation, and throughout the world.

Terrorism, a disaster, or a violent event in one's community can be seen as a life-changing event, both in terms of actual changes (e.g., the loss of a family member) and less-concrete changes (e.g., seeing the world differently or the loss of feeling safe). Grief resulting from such an event can last months or years, although the intensity of feelings is expected to diminish over time. Many people, however, expect that they "should get over" their grief in a much shorter time, and the nurse's knowledge of the grief process can validate their continued feelings and reassure them. In fact, certain circumstances can trigger a renewed intensity of grief-related feelings many years after the event, such as sensory experiences (sights, smells, and songs), anniversary dates (of the event, of a loved one's birthday, or of major holidays or experiences shared with the community), or similar disastrous events seen in the media.

Although grief can be expected to be prolonged after a major disaster, individuals may need more intensive therapeutic intervention if disabling grief persists beyond several months' duration. For individuals with mental illness, poor coping skills, or inadequate social support, traumatic events of this nature can be overwhelming and result in exacerbation of illness or symptoms, loss of functional abilities, and need for hospitalization or increased community-based treatment (see Care Plan 50: Grief and Care Plan 31: Post-Traumatic Stress Disorder).

Optimal community response to this type of event includes making resources available to offer support and assist with the grief and post-trauma response. Crisis intervention techniques, such as individual or group counseling to acknowledge the event and associated feelings and to facilitate the individual's expression of feelings in a safe environment, can be effective in working with those directly or indirectly affected. Community responses, such as mourning or honoring rituals (e.g., memorial services) or a geographic location where people can go to express grief and leave tokens, flowers, and so forth in honor or memory, can help people find community support in sharing their grief. Media programming that acknowledges the event and people's responses can help community members to process their feelings related to the event, even if they are housebound or distant from the rest of the affected community.

Several phases have been identified in a community's response to disaster: *heroic, honeymoon, inventory, disillusionment,* and *reconstruction.* Similar to the stages of the grief process, these phases represent the collective feelings and responses of the community to a significant loss or change. The first, or *heroic,* phase includes the immediate response to the event, when people perform acts of courage to save others. The *honeymoon* phase describes the period of longer-term rescue and relief efforts, when people are relieved, grateful, and receiving the tangible support of others. During the *inventory* phase, people become stressed and fatigued from dealing with the increased efforts of recovery and the limits of available assistance. The *disillusionment* phase often begins when relief teams withdraw from the community and community members are expected to resume independent functioning; feelings of anger and resentment surface, as they do in the normal grief process. The *reconstruction* phase represents the community's return to functioning and integrating the event and associated losses. As in the grief process, these phases vary in length and progression among individuals and communities.

It is important for nurses and other mental health professionals to remember that many people lack earlier exposure to significant grief and do not have the knowledge or skills to identify, express, and accept feelings they experience in response to an overwhelming event. Nurses can play a significant role in helping their communities deal with traumatic events by joining in *disaster nursing* efforts, direct involvement in crisis intervention and community response, and also by educating individuals and the community about such events and their sequelae. For example, nurses can speak to community groups to help people understand that a normal response to traumatic events includes deep and prolonged feelings of grief, anxiety, and so forth. Nurses can also help people less directly affected by the event to understand the needs of those more directly affected, and help to minimize any negative impact of others' reactions, media coverage, and so forth, on those most affected. There are many resources available that can help prepare nurses to assist their communities and clients in dealing with terrorism, disaster, or other traumatic events, in nursing and other mental health–related literature. A number of government agencies and professional and community organizations also have Web-based resources, such as the following:

- National Association of School Psychologists: Crisis Resources
- American Psychiatric Association Healthy Minds.org
- American Psychological Association Help Center
- Center for Mental Health Services National Mental Health Information Center
- U.S. Department of Veterans Affairs National Center for PTSD
- National Institute of Mental Health Post-Traumatic Stress Disorder Health Information
- National Partnership for Workplace Mental Health
- International Council of Nurses

Using resources like these, nurses can learn more about *disaster nursing,* educate their communities, and help enable effective responses to future events.

THE NURSING PROCESS

The nursing process is a dynamic and continuing activity that includes nurse–client interaction and the problem-solving process. Because the client is an integral part of this process, client input in terms of information, decision making, and evaluation is important; the client should participate as a team member as much as possible. The client's family or significant others also may be included in the nursing process, as the client may be seen as part of an interactive system of people. Contracting with the client and his or her significant others can be a useful, direct way of facilitating this participation and may help the client and the family to see themselves as actively involved in this process of change.

The nursing process includes the following steps:

1. Assessment of data about the client, including identification of his or her personal strengths and resources
2. Formulation of nursing diagnoses

3. Identification of expected outcomes, *Problem, Etiology, Symptoms* (PES) statement, including establishing timing and specific client-centered goals
4. Identification of therapeutic goals, or nursing objectives
5. Identification and implementation of nursing interventions and solutions to possible problems
6. Evaluation and revision of all steps of the process (ongoing)

Because every client is in a unique situation, each care plan must be individualized. The care plans in this *Manual* consist of background information related to a behavior or problem and one or more nursing diagnoses that are likely to be appropriate to clients experiencing the problem. Other related diagnoses also are suggested, but the care plans in the *Manual* are written using the primary diagnoses given as the basis for the nursing process. Within each of these diagnoses are assessment data commonly encountered with the particular behavior being addressed, suggestions of expected outcome statements appropriate to the diagnosis, and interventions (with rationale) that may be effective for clients with that nursing diagnosis. All of this is meant to be used to construct individualized care plans that are based on nursing diagnoses, using specific data, outcomes, and interventions for each client.

Assessment

The first step in the nursing process—the assessment of the client—is crucial. The following factors are important in assessing a client to formulate nursing diagnoses and to plan and implement care in mental health nursing (see Appendix A: Sample Psychosocial Assessment Tool):

1. *Client participation.* Ask for the client's perceptions regarding the following:
   • The client's expectations of hospitalization and the staff
   • What would the client like to change?
   • How can this happen?
   • What is the client most concerned about right now?
2. *Client's strengths.*
   • What are the client's strengths as perceived by the client?
   • As perceived by the nurse?
3. *Client's coping strategies.*
   • How does the client usually deal with problems?
   • What problem-solving techniques have been successful for the client in the past?
   • How is the client attempting to deal with the present situation?
4. *The client's family or significant others.*
   • Note family patterns and history of behaviors.
   • How are other people's behaviors or problems affecting the client?
   • How is the client affecting others?
   • What are the perceptions of the client's family or significant others regarding the client's illness, hospitalization, and hopes for recovery?
5. *Primary language.*
   • What is the client's primary language?
   • Does the client read in this primary language?
   • Is the client able to speak and read English?
   • Is an interpreter needed for teaching and interactions with the client and significant others?
6. *Cultural considerations.* (Remember that cultural background extends beyond race or ethnicity; see "Culture")
   • What is the client's cultural background?
   • In what kind of cultural environment is the client living (or was the client raised)?
   • What is the client's group identification?
   • What influence does the client's cultural background have on his or her expectations (and the expectations of the client's significant others) for treatment and recovery?
   • What are the client's culturally related health beliefs and health practices?
   • Are there culturally related sources of support for the client?
   • Are there culturally based health practices that the client has used or is using now (in connection with the current problem or other issues)?
7. *Appearance.* Describe the client's general appearance, clothing, and hygiene.
8. *Substance use or dependence.* Include the client's use of the following:
   • Caffeine (symptoms of anxiety and high caffeine intake can be similar)
   • Tobacco
   • Alcohol
   • Illicit drugs
   • Prescription drugs
   • Over-the-counter drugs (e.g., bromide poisoning can occur with abuse of some over-the-counter medications)
   • Vitamins, herbs, and dietary supplements (see "Complementary and Alternative Medicine")
9. *Orientation and memory.* Check for
   • Recent and remote memory
   • Orientation to person, place, and time
10. *Allergies to both food and medication.* It may be necessary to ask the client's significant others for reliable information or to check the client's past records if possible.
11. *Complete physical systems review.* The client may minimize, maximize, or be unaware of physical problems.
12. *Dentures and dentition.* These may be a factor in nutritional problems.
13. *Physical disabilities, prostheses.* Does the client need assistance in ambulation or other activities of daily living?
14. *Medications.* Include questions about
    • The client's knowledge of current medication regimen, effects, and adverse effects—include complementary and alternative medicines (see "Complementary and Alternative Medicine")
    • When the last dose of medication was taken
    • Psychotropic medications the client has taken in the past
    • Whether the client has been prescribed medications that he or she is not taking now

15. *Suicidal ideation.* Include questions regarding
    • Suicidal ideas
    • Plan for suicide
    • History of suicidal behavior
16. *Perceptions, presence of hallucinations or delusions.*
    • The nature and frequency of delusions or hallucinations
    • How does the client feel about the delusions or hallucinations?
17. *Aggression.* Does the client have
    • A history or a present problem of aggression toward others?
    • Homicidal thoughts or plans?
    • Possession of weapons?
18. *Family history.* Have there been mental health problems in the client's family?
19. *Present living situation.*
    • Describe the client's living situation.
    • How does the client feel about it?
20. *Relationships with others.*
    • How does the client see others?
    • Are present relationships helpful to the client or stressful?
    • Does the client have anyone to talk with?
    • Does the client trust anyone?
    • Are relationships dependent or abusive?
21. *Sexuality.* Are any aspects of sexuality causing problems for the client?
22. *Behavior and activity level.* Describe the client's general behavior during the assessment.
    • What is the client's psychomotor activity level?
    • What can the client do for himself or herself?
23. *Eye contact.*
    • Does the client make eye contact with treatment team members or significant others?
    • What is the frequency and duration of eye contact?
24. *Affect and mood.* Describe the client's general mood, facial expressions, and demeanor.
25. *Ability to communicate.*
    • Include the nature and extent of both verbal and non-verbal communication.
    • Does the client's significant other speak for him or her?
26. *Tremors or fidgeting.* Describe the nature, extent, and frequency of repetitive movements.
27. *Daily living habits.*
    • What does the client do all day?
    • How do the client's habits differ now from before the client's present problems began?
28. *Health practices.*
    • Does the client get adequate nutrition?
    • Adequate sleep?
    • Regular exercise?
    • General medical care?
29. *Cognition and intellectual functioning.* Include the client's
    • Present level of functioning, judgment, and insight
    • Educational level
    • Prior abilities and achievements

30. *Employment.* Include the client's
    • Present job
    • History of employment
    • Perception of his or her work
31. *Level of income.*
    • Is the client's income level adequate for his or her needs?
    • Is it a stressful factor in the client's life?
32. *Spirituality.*
    • Is spirituality important to the client?
    • Does it serve as a supportive factor in the client's life?
    • Does the client have culturally specific spiritual beliefs or practices that you need to be aware of?
    • Is there a religious aspect to the client's illness?
33. *Value system and personal standards.*
    • Does the client have very high standards for himself or herself or others?
    • Does the client manifest a sense of personal responsibility?
34. *Interests and hobbies.* Include the client's hobbies, both before the present problems began and those of continuing interest to the client.
35. *Previous hospitalizations, treatment history.* Include both medical and psychiatric hospitalizations and significant treatment history (e.g., significant outpatient therapy or other treatment). Note length of stay and reason for hospitalization. Include complementary and alternative medicine treatment (see "Complementary and Alternative Medicine").

Assess the client in a holistic way, integrating any relevant information about the client's life, behavior, and feelings as the initial steps of implementing the nursing process. Remember that the focus of care, beginning with the initial assessment, is toward the client's optimum level of health and independence from the hospital.

Nursing Diagnosis

The second step of the nursing process is to formulate nursing diagnoses. The nursing diagnosis is a statement of an actual or potential problem or situation amenable to nursing interventions. It is based on the nurse's judgment of the client's situation following a nursing assessment. It provides information and a focus for the planning, implementation, and evaluation of nursing care and communicates that information to the nursing staff.

The nursing diagnosis is not a medical diagnosis. Medical psychiatric diagnoses are used to categorize and describe mental disorders. The *Diagnostic and Statistical Manual of Mental Disorders Text Revision* (*DSM-IV-TR*) (American Psychiatric Association, 2000) is a taxonomy that describes all recognized mental disorders with specific diagnostic criteria. For each disorder, the *DSM-IV-TR* also provides information about symptoms; associated features; laboratory findings; prevalence; etiology; course of the disorder; and relevant age, gender, and cultural features. The manual is used by all mental health disciplines for the diagnosis of psychiatric disorders.

A multiaxial classification system that involves assessment on five axes, or domains of information, allows the practitioner to identify factors that relate to or influence the person's condition.

- Axis I identifies all major psychiatric disorders (except mental retardation and personality disorders), such as major depressive disorder, schizophrenia, bipolar disorder, anxiety, and so forth.
- Axis II lists mental retardation, personality disorders, and any prominent maladaptive personality characteristics and defense mechanisms.
- Axis III identifies current medical conditions that are potentially relevant to the understanding or management of the person and his or her mental disorder.
- Axis IV lists psychosocial and environmental problems that may affect the diagnosis, treatment, and prognosis of the mental disorder. Included are problems with primary support group, social environment, education, occupation, housing, economics, and access to health care and legal systems.
- Axis V reports the clinician's rating of the person's overall psychological functioning using the Global Assessment of Functioning (GAF), which rates functioning on a scale from 0 to 100. A score is given for the person's current functioning, and a score may also be given for earlier functioning (e.g., highest GAF in the past year, or GAF 6 months ago) when that information is available.

Although nursing students or staff nurses do not use the *DSM-IV-TR* to diagnose clients, it can be a helpful resource to describe the characteristics of the various disorders and to understand other aspects of psychiatric care.

Nursing diagnoses differ from medical psychiatric diagnoses in that it is the client's *response* to that medical problem, or how that problem affects the client's daily functioning, which is the concern of the nursing diagnosis. Only those problems that lend themselves to nursing's focus and intervention can be addressed by nursing diagnoses. And, like other parts of the nursing process, the nursing diagnosis is client-centered; the focus of the nursing diagnosis is the client's problem or situation rather than, for example, a problem the staff may have with a client.

A nursing diagnosis statement consists of the *problem* or client *response* and one or more *related factors* that influence or contribute to the client's problem or response. The phrase *related to* reflects the relationship of problem to factor rather than stating cause and effect per se. If the relationship of these contributing factors is unknown at the time the nursing diagnosis is formulated, the problem statement may be written without them. In the *Manual*, the problem statement or diagnostic category is addressed, leaving the "related to" phrase to be written by the nurse working with the individual client. Signs and symptoms, or defining characteristics, are the subjective and objective assessment data that support the nursing diagnosis, and they may be noted "as evidenced by specific symptoms" in the diagnostic statement. This second part of the diagnostic statement is written to communicate the nurse's perception of the factors related to the problem or contributing to its *etiology*.

NANDA International is developing a taxonomy of officially recognized nursing diagnoses. The organization reviews proposed nursing diagnoses according to certain criteria to ensure clear, consistent, and complete statements. The list of official diagnoses is organized into 13 domains, including Health Promotion, Nutrition, Elimination, Activity/Rest, Perception/Cognition, Self-Perception, Role Relationships, Sexuality, Coping/Stress Tolerance, Life Principles, Safety/Protection, Comfort, and Growth/Development (NANDA International, 2009). Nurses are encouraged to develop, use, and submit other nursing diagnoses to NANDA International for approval.

Each care plan in this *Manual* is written using nursing diagnoses frequently identified with the disorder, behavior, or problem addressed in the care plan. In addition, related nursing diagnoses are identified that are often associated with the problems addressed in that care plan; interventions for these related diagnoses can be found in other care plans in the *Manual*. The specific diagnoses in the individualized nursing care plan for a given client will be based on the actual data collected in the nursing assessment of that client.

Expected Outcomes

The next step is the identification of expected outcomes, which gives direction and focus to the nursing process and provides the basis for evaluating the effectiveness of the nursing interventions used. Expected outcomes are client-centered; they are statements that reflect the client's progress toward resolving the problem or nursing diagnosis or preventing problems identified as potential or high risk. Expected outcomes also are called *outcome criteria* or *goals*, and they contain specific information (*modifiers*) and time factors (*deadlines*) so that they are measurable and can be evaluated and revised as the client progresses. The expected outcomes in this *Manual* have been written as general statements to be used in writing specific expected outcomes for an individual client. For an individualized care plan, specific modifiers and timing must be added for outcome criteria.

The general outcome statements in the *Manual* are identified as immediate, stabilization, or community outcomes to suggest time frames, but specific timing must be written in the individual nursing care plan. In the care plans that follow, examples of timing have been provided as suggestions for immediate outcomes, but they are intended to be modified by the nurse as the individual client's care plan is being written and revised. Other examples of individualized outcomes are as follows:

- The client will talk with a staff member (modifier) about loss (modifier) for 10 minutes (modifier) each day by 11/18/13 (time factor).
- The client will eat at least 50% (modifier) of all meals each day by 1/6/14 (time factor).
- The client will sleep at least 6 hours per night (modifier) by 9/16/12 (time factor).

- The client will initiate verbal interaction with another client (modifier) at least twice a day (modifier) by 6/12/13 (time factor).

The specific criterion may be an amount of food, fluid, or time, an activity or behavior, a topic of conversation, a certain person or group, and so forth. Expected outcomes should be stated in behavioral or measurable terms and should be reasonable and attainable within the deadlines stated. The suggested outcomes in the *Manual* are not written in any particular order to denote priority; in a specific plan of care, the nurse will designate priorities. The community outcomes noted in the *Manual* can be seen as discharge criteria and viewed as the goals of the nursing process for the hospitalized client.

Implementation

The identification of nursing interventions and their implementation are the next steps in the nursing process. Here, the nurse can choose and implement specific measures to achieve the expected outcomes identified. Nursing interventions may be called *actions*, *approaches*, *nursing orders*, or *nursing prescriptions*. They must be individualized to include modifiers that specify parameters, for example,

- Walk with the client for at least 15 minutes each shift (days, evenings)
- Approach the client for verbal interaction at least three times per day
- Weigh the client at 8:00 AM daily prior to breakfast in hospital gown only

Interventions address specific problems and suggest possible solutions or alternatives that nurses use to meet client needs or to assist the client toward expected outcomes. Writing specific nursing interventions in the client's care plan helps ensure consistency among treatment team members in their approaches to the client and aids in the evaluation of the client's care. In addition to specific problem-solving measures, nursing interventions include additional data gathering or assessment, health promotion and disease prevention activities, nursing treatments, referrals, and educating the client and family or significant others.

Evaluation and Revision

The final steps in the nursing process are not termination steps but ongoing activities incorporated into the entire process to evaluate and revise all other steps. As new information is discovered throughout the client's care, it must be added to the original assessment. Evaluation and revision are necessitated as the client reveals additional (or different) information and as the client's behavior changes over time. Evaluation and revision include the following:

- Nursing diagnoses: Are the diagnoses accurate? Are there different, or additional, related factors that will change the diagnostic statements?
- Expected outcomes, modifiers, and time factors: Have these been achieved? Do they need to be revised? Are they still reasonable?

- Nursing interventions and modifiers: Are they effective? Should a different approach be used? Are additional interventions needed?
- The extent of the client's participation and assumption of self-responsibility (as the client progresses, he or she may be able to participate and take more responsibility in both treatment and care planning)
- Staff consistency (Is the staff implementing the specified interventions consistently?)

Ideally, evaluation and revision should be integrated into the client's daily care; each observation or nurse–client interaction provides an opportunity to evaluate and revise the components of the client's care plan. Nursing report (change of shift) meetings are an ideal time to evaluate the plan's effectiveness and revise interventions and expected outcome criteria. Client care conferences or nurse–client sessions also may be used to discuss revisions. The nursing staff may want to schedule time to evaluate and discuss care planning at each shift, several times per week, or on whatever timetable is appropriate for the unit. Regardless of how it is scheduled, however, it is essential to incorporate evaluation and revision into care planning for each client and to view nursing care as the flexible, dynamic, change-oriented, thoughtful process that it can and should be.

Therapeutic Goals

Therapeutic goals, also known as nursing objectives, help guide the nurse's thinking about the therapeutic process of working with the client. As the nurse chooses specific interventions designed to resolve the problem stated in the nursing diagnosis or to improve the client's health, an awareness of the therapeutic framework of the nurse's role in working with the client can be helpful, especially to nursing students learning this process. General nursing objectives can apply to the care of clients with many different problems or behaviors. Some of these objectives include the following:

- Prevent harm to the client or others
- Protect the client and others from injury
- Provide a safe, supportive, nonthreatening, therapeutic environment for the client and others
- Establish rapport with the client
- Build a trusting relationship with the client
- Diminish or eliminate psychotic symptoms and suicidal or aggressive behavior
- Facilitate the client's participation in the treatment program
- Facilitate treatment for associated or other problems
- Assist the client in meeting basic needs and self-care activities only as necessary to meet needs and promote the client's independence in self-care
- Promote adequate nutrition, hydration, elimination, rest, and activity
- Teach the client and significant others about the client's illness, treatment, and medications
- Promote self-esteem
- Facilitate the client's appropriate expression of feelings

- Facilitate the client's insight into illness and situation
- Facilitate the client's development of coping skills
- Promote the client's problem-solving and decision-making abilities
- Provide emotional support to the client and significant others
- Prepare the client for discharge from the acute setting or to a greater level of independence

To maintain a client-centered care planning focus with a direct connection between expected outcomes and interventions, the *Manual* does not include a separate section delineating therapeutic goals for each nursing diagnosis. Instead, specific therapeutic goals (in addition to those listed above) that are particularly important to consider in working with clients with specific problems or behaviors are included in the introduction sections of the care plans.

Documentation

Another aspect of nursing and interdisciplinary team care is documentation. Written records of client care are important in several ways.

1. Written care plans serve to coordinate and communicate the plan of nursing care for each client to all team members. Using a written plan of care maximizes the opportunity for all team members to be consistent and comprehensive in the care of a particular client. Ongoing evaluation and revision of the care plan reflect changes in the client's needs and corresponding changes in care.
2. A written care plan is an effective, efficient means of communication among team members who cannot all meet as a group (i.e., who work on different shifts, float staff, supervisors, etc.).
3. Nursing documentation or charting in the client's medical record serves to clearly communicate nursing observations and interventions to other members of the interdisciplinary treatment team (e.g., physicians, social workers, discharge planners, etc.). Information in the chart is also available as a record in the event of transfer to another facility, follow-up care, or future admissions.
4. The chart is a legal document, and the written record of nursing care may be instrumental in legal proceedings involving the client.
5. The documentation of care is important for accreditation and reimbursement purposes. Quality assurance and utilization review departments, accreditation bodies, and third-party payers depend on adequate documentation to review quality of care and determine appropriate reimbursement.

EVIDENCE-BASED PRACTICE

The term *evidence-based practice* is used to describe care planning and treatment decisions that are based on research or expert opinion, which supports the efficacy of the intervention. Often, evidence-based practice refers to using *standards of practice*, *practice guidelines*, *practice parameters*, *treatment* or *medication protocols*, or *algorithms* recommended for use in treating patients with acute or chronic disease. There are many examples of such standards or protocols in the medical literature, such as the American Diabetes Association's (ADA) *Clinical Practice Guidelines* (ADA, 2011), and an increasing number of guidelines in the psychiatric and nursing literature, such as the American Psychiatric Association's (APA) *Practice Guidelines* (APA, 2011). Organizations may also publish *position papers*, which represent the official view of the organization and may be based on research or on expert opinion.

Levels of evidence or *evidence-grading systems* often are used in evidence-based documents to refer to the sources of information supporting the recommendations. For example, *levels of evidence* may be defined as follows:

- Level 1: evidence from meta-analysis or well-conducted, generalizable, randomized controlled trials
- Level 2: evidence from well-conducted cohort or case–control studies
- Level 3: evidence from observational or poorly controlled studies or conflicting evidence
- Level 4: evidence from expert consensus or clinical experience (ADA, 2011)

The authors of guidelines may also distinguish supportive evidence sources as *scientific* or *research-based* recommendations and *clinical* recommendations. Such clinical recommendations are not supported by scientific (i.e., randomized, controlled) research, but are based on clinical studies, recommendations found in the literature, or from the authors' clinical experience.

Standards and guidelines may be issued by governmental, professional, or academic organizations, and generally are revised by the organization from time to time or as indicated by new evidence that comes to light. For example, the Agency for Healthcare Research and Quality (AHRQ), part of the U.S. Department of Health and Human Services, issues information and recommendations related to a number of conditions and medications. The National Guideline Clearinghouse publishes evidence-based clinical practice guidelines and related information documents produced by the AHRQ and many other organizations, and the National Mental Health Information Center has published a number of Evidence-Based Practice KITs (Knowledge Informing Transformation) (see Web Resources on thePoint). The American Psychiatric Nurses Association (APNA) has published a series of position articles that include *Standards of Practice* related to seclusion and restraint (APNA, 2010). The University of Iowa Gerontological Nursing Interventions Research Center has published evidence-based guidelines that address many aspects of nursing, including a number of guidelines related to the care of elderly clients; clients with dementia; caregiving; abuse; and suicide (University of Iowa College of Nursing, 2010).

Evidence-based practice documents can be invaluable to nurses and nursing students in planning care for clients in mental health nursing. Nurses can consult these documents in the literature or on the Internet (see Web Resources on thePoint) and use them to learn about a condition, related research and treatment recommendations, and other considerations. Nurses can incorporate this information in building care plans and in developing *best practices* in their own practice area.

BEST PRACTICES

The terms *best practice*, *clinical pathway*, *critical pathway*, *care path*, *multidisciplinary action plan (MAP)*, and *integrated care pathway* refer to documents written to guide care for clients with a specific diagnosis or situation. This type of document may be developed and published by an individual or group in a specific clinical practice or academic setting and proposed or described as a best practice. Or, it may be the result of a collaborative effort or generated by an organization or based on research, as in evidence-based practice. Authors who develop and propose best practices contribute to the body of nursing knowledge by carefully documenting the nursing care process and practices, including the evaluation of the practice and suggestions for adaptation or future research by others. When a specific situation has not yet been addressed by evidence-based practice recommendations, best practices are an effective way to share clinical information and experiences.

Best practice documents usually are specific and detailed in their approach to care. They may include detailed information regarding the problem addressed, assessment data, tests or monitoring, medical and nursing diagnoses, roles of the interdisciplinary team members, equipment, timing, expected outcomes, interventions, sequences for treatment decisions or medications and dosages, evaluation criteria, client and family education, special considerations, exceptions or variances, complications, documentation requirements, and references. These documents may include flow charts, algorithms, decision trees, matrices, or fill-in-the-blank formats and may include physician and nursing orders, procedure-specific instructions, and information sheets for client or staff education. These documents may guide care over a continuum, beginning prior to admission to a facility and continuing through community-based care. They also can be integrated with the documentation system in a practice setting to streamline charting by the nursing staff and other disciplines. Best practices can help ensure positive outcomes for clients, a consistent approach to care, increased collaboration among members of the interdisciplinary team, routine evaluation of care, enhanced nursing satisfaction, compliance with accreditation standards, and efficient use of resources.

Although best practices are not equivalent to standards of care and may not necessarily be based on scientific research, they can be extremely valuable to nurses and nursing students in care planning. By learning from the documented approach of others, nurses can avoid "reinventing the wheel" in their own clinical practice and setting in much the same way as they might use this *Manual* as a starting point for written care plans. Within a practice setting, nurses can collaborate to adapt published best practices or design best practices for the types of clients usually seen, incorporating specific factors such as age or other demographic groups, cultural characteristics, institutional policies (such as suicide or seizure precautions), expected time frames, outcome criteria, and so forth. In fact, nurses can use the care plans in the *Manual* to begin to explore potential best practice areas for the situations most commonly encountered in their setting, and use the care plan as a starting point in drafting a best practice.

Nurses can work effectively in their respective practice settings with the other members of the interdisciplinary team (see below) to develop or adapt best practices. Steps in developing and implementing best practices include the following:

• Educate others (administration and the rest of the interdisciplinary treatment team) about best practices and the proposed effort
• Define the behavior, problem, diagnosis, or situation to be addressed
• Gain support for the project from administrators
• Search the literature (and the Internet) for existing evidence-based or best practice information and related research
• Evaluate existing information and its applicability to the situation
• Adapt or write the document, making it as specific as possible to the practice setting (e.g., clients, institution, outcome criteria) and considering how it can be integrated into existing practices at the setting
• Educate the interdisciplinary team to be involved in piloting the best practice
• Pilot the best practice in the setting, noting outcomes, variances, client and staff responses, and so forth
• Evaluate the outcomes and revise the document
• Educate the full interdisciplinary team regarding implementation
• Implement the best practice
• Evaluate and revise on a continuing basis (or integrate with the practice setting's quality improvement process)
• Share the best practice document with others and submit it for publication

INTERDISCIPLINARY TREATMENT TEAM

In all treatment and rehabilitation settings or programs, the concept of the interdisciplinary treatment team approach is most effective in dealing with the multifaceted problems of persons with mental illness. Team members have expertise in their specific areas, and through their collaborative efforts, they can better meet the client's needs. Members of the interdisciplinary treatment team can include the psychiatrist, psychologist, psychiatric nurse, psychiatric social worker, occupational therapist, recreation therapist, vocational rehabilitation specialist, and other professional and paraprofessional staff. Depending on the client's needs, a dietitian, pharmacist, physical or speech therapist, pastoral care counselor, or member of the clergy may be consulted. Not all settings have a full-time member from each discipline on their team; the program and services offered in any given setting will determine the composition of the team. The treatment team may also extend across settings to include other professionals involved in the client's care, for example, a community-based case manager or home health nurse.

The role of case manager has become increasingly important in the current managed care environment and clients' needs for a variety of services that may involve various resources in order to coordinate care. Although individuals may become certified as case managers, there is not a standard educational preparation for this role. People from different backgrounds (e.g., social work, nursing, psychology) may fill this role by virtue of their skills and experience. The psychiatric nurse is in an ideal position to fulfill the role of case manager for clients with mental health problems, with knowledge and skills in psychopharmacology, client and family education, and medical as well as psychiatric disorders. Whether or not you function as a case manager, it is essential to be an integral part of the interdisciplinary team, bringing nursing expertise and clinical perspective to the team. Each team member can benefit from the expertise and clinical perspectives of the other disciplines as well as access more information and resources on behalf of the client.

NURSE–CLIENT INTERACTIONS

Communication Skills

Effective therapeutic communication between a nurse and a client is a conscious, goal-directed process that differs greatly from a casual or social interaction. Therapeutic communication is grounded in the purposeful, caring nature of nursing care. It is a tool with which to

• Develop trust
• Effect change
• Promote health
• Provide limits
• Reinforce
• Orient
• Convey caring
• Identify and work toward goals
• Teach
• Provide other types of nursing care.

The nurse must be aware of the client and his or her needs when communicating with the client; as with all nursing care, it is the client's needs that must be met, not the nurse's needs.

Therapeutic conversations are goal-oriented, used as nursing interventions to meet therapeutic goals. However, therapeutic communication is not a stiff, rote recitation of predetermined phrases used to manipulate the client. Rather,

it is a part of the art and science of nursing, a blend of conversation and caring, of limits and reinforcement, of communication techniques and one's own words. Communicating with a client can range from sitting with a client in silence to speaking in a structured, carefully chosen way (e.g., in behavior modification techniques). Or an interaction may be in the context of a social or recreational activity, in which the nurse teaches or models social skills through his or her own conscious "social" conversations. Regardless of the situation, remember that every interaction with a client is part of your professional role and therefore must be respectful of the client and his or her needs.

A number of communication skills, or techniques, have been found to be effective in therapeutic interactions with clients (see Appendix D: Communication Techniques). These techniques, or communication tools, are meant to be specifically chosen to meet the needs of particular clients and modified to be used most effectively. It is important for you to be comfortable as well as effective in therapeutic communication: use your own words; integrate purposeful communication techniques into conversations; following an interaction, evaluate its effectiveness and your own feelings, and then modify your techniques in subsequent interactions. Like other aspects of nursing care, communication is dynamic, and should be evaluated and revised. The following are suggestions, or guidelines, to improve therapeutic communication:

• Offer yourself to the client for a specific time period for the purpose of communication. Tell the client that you would like to talk with him or her.
• Call the client by name and identify yourself by name. The use of given (first) names may be decided by the facility or the individual unit philosophies or may depend on the comfort of the client and the nurse or the nature of the client's problem.
• Make eye contact with the client as he or she tolerates. Do not stare at the client.
• Listen to the client. Pay attention to what the client is communicating, both verbally and nonverbally.
• Be comfortable using silence as a communication tool.
• Talk with the client about the client's feelings, not about yourself, other treatment team members, or other clients.
• Ask open-ended questions. Avoid questions that can have one-word answers.
• Allow the client enough time to talk.
• Be honest with the client.
• Be nonjudgmental. If necessary, directly reassure the client of your nonjudgmental attitude.
• Know your own feelings and do not let them prejudice your interaction with the client.
• Encourage the client to express his or her feelings.
• Reflect what the client is saying back to him or her. In simple reflection, repeat the client's statement with an upward inflection in your voice to indicate questioning. In more complex reflection, rephrase the client's statement to reflect the feeling the client seems to be expressing. This will allow the client to validate your perception of what he

or she is trying to say, or to correct it. You also can point out seemingly contradictory statements and ask for clarification (this may or may not be confrontational). Do not simply describe what you think the client is feeling in your own terms; instead, use such phrases as "I hear you saying … Is that what you are feeling? Is that what you mean?"

- Tell the client if you do not understand what he or she means; take the responsibility yourself for not understanding and ask the client to clarify. This gives the client the responsibility for explaining his or her meaning.
- Do not use pat phrases or platitudes in response to the client's expression of feelings. This devalues the client's feelings, undermines trust, and may discourage further communication.
- Do not give your personal opinions, beliefs, or experiences in relation to the client's problems.
- Do not give advice or make decisions for the client. If you advise a client and your advice is "good" (i.e., the proposed solution is successful), the client has not had the opportunity to solve the problem, to take responsibility or credit for a good decision, and to enjoy the increased self-esteem that comes from a successful action. If your advice is "bad," the client has missed a chance to learn from making a mistake and to realize that he or she can survive making a mistake. In effect, the client has evaded responsibility for making a decision and instead may blame the staff member for whatever consequences ensue from that decision.
- Help the client to identify and explore alternatives and use the problem-solving process (see "Client Teaching").
- Give the client honest, nonpunitive feedback based on your observations.
- Do not try to fool or manipulate the client.
- Do not argue with the client or get involved in a power struggle.
- Do not take the client's anger or negative expressions personally.
- Use humor judiciously. Never tease a client or use humor pejoratively. Clients with certain problems will not understand abstractions such as humor. Remember to evaluate the use of humor with each individual client.

Expression of Feelings

A significant part of therapy is the client's expression of feelings. It is important for the nurse to encourage the client to ventilate feelings in ways that are nondestructive and acceptable to the client, such as writing, talking, drawing, or physical activity. The client's cultural background may significantly influence his or her expression of feelings and the acceptability of various means of expression. Asking the client what he or she has done in the past and what methods of expression are used in the family, peer group, or cultural group(s) may help you identify effective and culturally acceptable ways in which the client can express and work through various feelings.

It also may be desirable to encourage expressions, such as crying, with which the client (or the nurse) may not feel entirely comfortable. You can facilitate the expression of emotions by giving the client direct verbal support, by using silence, by handing the client tissues, and by allowing the client time to ventilate (without probing for information or interrupting the client with pat remarks).

The goal in working with a client is not to avoid painful feelings but to have the client express, work through, and come to accept even "negative" emotions, such as hatred, despair, and rage. In accepting the client's emotions, you need not agree with or give approval to everything the client says—you can support the client by acknowledging that he or she is experiencing the emotion expressed without agreeing with or sharing those feelings. If you are uncomfortable with the client's ventilation of feelings, it is important that you examine your own emotions and talk with another staff member about them, or that you provide the client with a staff member who is more comfortable with expression of those feelings.

Teaching the Client and Significant Others

Client teaching is an essential component of nursing care. In mental health nursing, client teaching can take many forms and address many content areas. It is important to consider the learning needs of the client and significant others when performing an initial assessment, when planning for discharge, and throughout the client's treatment. The assessment of a client (or significant others) with regard to teaching includes consideration of the following:

- Level of present knowledge or understanding
- Present primary concern (you may need to address the client's major emotional concerns before he or she can attend to learning information)
- Client's perceived educational needs
- Level of consciousness, orientation, attention span, and concentration span
- Hallucinations or other psychotic or neurologic symptoms
- Effects of medications
- Short-term and long-term memory
- Primary language, ability to read primary language, and to read or comprehend English
- Literacy and educational level
- Visual, hearing, or other sensory impairment
- Client's preferred learning methods
- Cultural factors
- Learning disabilities
- Motivation for learning
- Barriers to learning (e.g., denial or shame related to mental illness)

Optimal conditions for client teaching and learning may not exist during an inpatient stay; many factors may be present that diminish the effectiveness of teaching. However, the client's hospital stay may be the only opportunity for teaching, and certain information (especially regarding medications and self-care activities) must be conveyed before discharge. In addition, follow-up appointments may be scheduled for continued teaching after discharge, if indicated. Significant others can assist in reinforcing teaching, and home care with continued instruction may be possible.

Choosing the mode of education best suited to the client and the situation is also important. A variety of teaching techniques and tools can be integrated into the teaching plan according to the client's needs, the clinical setting, available resources, and the nurse's expertise. Effective teaching tools include the following:

Presentation of information to a group or an individual: lecture, discussion, and question and answer sessions; verbal, written, or audiovisual materials

Simple written instructions, drawings or photographs, or both (especially for clients with low literacy or language differences)

Repetition, reinforcement, and restatement of the same material in different ways

Group discussions to teach common topics, such as safe use of medications, and to promote compliance with medication regimens by encouraging peer support

Social or recreational activities to teach social and leisure skills

Role-playing to provide practice of skills and constructive feedback in a supportive milieu

Role-modeling or demonstration of skills, appropriate behaviors, and effective communication

Interpreters or translated materials for clients whose primary language is different from your own

Return demonstrations or explanations: Asking for the client's perception of the information presented is crucial. Clients may indicate understanding because they want to please, because they are embarrassed about low literacy levels, or because they think they "should" understand. Remember, learning does not necessarily occur because teaching is done.

Remember that educational materials will be most effective when they match the client's culture, language, and learning abilities. If culturally specific materials are not available, be sure to choose or develop materials that are culturally sensitive and reflect some acknowledgment of diversity. Use pictorial materials if written materials are unavailable for a given language or if the client's reading skills are limited.

If you need to use a translator for teaching or other interactions, remember that family members or others significant to the client may not be the best people to translate for the client. The client may be reluctant to talk about certain things with family or significant others present, or the family members or significant others may not be accurate in translating because of their own feelings about the client, the illness, and so on. If you must use a client's significant others to translate because a staff member or volunteer is not available, be aware of these issues and try to discuss them with the client and translator, as appropriate. Ideally, a translator would be available who is a health care worker accustomed to translating in mental health interactions and education.

Several considerations are important for translated sessions even with an experienced translator:

- Allow adequate time so that information can be relayed to the client through the translator; the client should demonstrate understanding by verbalizing the information back to the translator, who can then relay it to the nurse, to ensure accuracy of communication.
- Be sure to speak to the client, not to the translator. Although you also may need to talk with the translator at some points, it is important to address the client directly when giving information, asking questions, and listening to the client's responses. Speaking directly to the client allows you to make eye contact, to demonstrate your awareness of the client as a person, to use your tone of voice and facial expression to convey interest and caring, and so forth.
- Remember that abstract concepts and examples are difficult to convey through a third person and another language. Be as simple and as direct as possible when using a translator.
- Use gestures, pictures, actual equipment (e.g., the medication cup that the client will use to measure the medication dose at home), or other simple materials (e.g., a calendar to record medication doses, which you then give to the client).
- Encourage the client to take notes in his or her language that the translator can review with you and the client for accuracy.
- Try to have at least two translated sessions with the client so that you have an opportunity to follow up to assess the learning and accuracy that occurred in the first session.

Examples of topics appropriate for nurse–client teaching include the following:

General health, wellness, health promotion: basic information regarding nutrition, exercise, rest, hygiene, and the relationship between physical and emotional health

Emotional health: ways to increase emotional outlets, expression of feelings, and increasing self-esteem

Stress management: identifying stressors, recognizing one's own response to stress, and making choices about stress, relaxation techniques, and relationships between stress and illness

Problem-solving and decision-making skills: the use of the problem-solving process, including assessment of the situation, identification of problems, identification of goals, identification and exploration of possible solutions, choice of a possible solution, evaluation, and revision

Communication skills: effective communication techniques, expressing one's needs, listening skills, and assertiveness training

Social skills: developing trust, fundamentals of social interactions, appropriate behavior in public and in social situations, eating with others, eating in restaurants, intimate relationships, saying "no" to unwanted attention or advances

Leisure activities: identification of leisure interests, how to access community recreation resources, and use of libraries

Community resources: identification and use of social services, support groups, transportation, churches, social or volunteer groups

Vocational skills: basic responsibilities of employment, interviewing skills, and appropriate behavior in a work setting

Daily living skills: basic money management (e.g., bank accounts, rent, utility bills), use of the telephone and Internet, and grocery shopping

Specific psychodynamic processes: grieving, developmental stages, interpersonal relationships, secondary gain, and so forth

Specific mental health problems: eating disorders, schizophrenia, suicidal behavior, and so forth

Specific physical illness pathophysiology and related self-care: HIV/AIDS, diabetes mellitus, Parkinson's disease, and so forth

Prevention of illness: prevention of HIV and other communicable disease transmission, tobacco cessation, and so forth

Relationship dynamics: healthy relationships, secondary gains, and abusive relationships

Self-care or caregiver responsibilities: how to change dressings, range of motion exercises, and safety and supervision concerns for neurologic illness

Medications: purpose, action, side effects (what to expect, how to minimize, if possible, when to call a health professional), dosage, strategies for compliance, special information (e.g., monitoring blood levels), and signs and symptoms of overdose or toxicity

ROLE OF THE PSYCHIATRIC NURSE

Nursing Responsibilities and Functions

As a nurse in a therapeutic relationship with a client, you have certain responsibilities. These include the following:

- Recognizing and accepting the client as an individual
- Advocating on behalf of the client (see "Client Advocacy")
- Assessing the client and planning nursing care
- Involving the client and the client's significant others in the nursing process
- Accepting the client's perceptions and expression of discomfort (i.e., do not require the client to prove distress or illness to you)
- Respecting the client's stated needs, desires, and goals (within the limits of safety, ethics, and good nursing care)
- Identifying the client's optimum level of health and functioning and making that level the goal of the nursing process
- Providing a safe and therapeutic environment, including protecting the client and others from injury
- Providing external controls for the client until such time as the client can maintain self-control
- Recognizing and examining your own feelings and being willing to work through those feelings

- Cooperating with other professionals in an interdisciplinary approach to care
- Accurately observing and documenting the client's behavior
- Maintaining awareness of and respect for the client's cultural values and practices, especially if they differ from your own
- Providing safe nursing care, including medication administration, individual interactions (verbal and nonverbal), formal and informal group situations, activities, role-playing, and so forth
- Forming expectations of the client that are realistic and clearly stated
- Teaching the client and significant others
- Providing opportunities for the client to make his or her own decisions or mistakes and to assume responsibility for his or her emotions and life
- Providing feedback to the client based on observations of the client's behavior
- Maintaining honesty and a nonjudgmental attitude at all times
- Maintaining a professional role with regard to the client (see "Professional Role")
- Continuing nursing education and the exploration of new ideas, theories, and research

Professional Role

Maintaining a professional role is essential in working with clients. A client comes to a treatment setting for help, not to engage in social relationships, and needs a nurse, not a friend. It is neither necessary nor desirable for the client to like you personally (nor for you to like the client) in a therapeutic situation.

Because the therapeutic milieu is not a social environment, interactions with clients should be directed only toward therapeutic goals, teaching interaction skills, and facilitating the client's abilities to engage in relationships. The nurse must not offer personal information or beliefs to the client, nor should the nurse attempt to meet his or her own needs in the nurse–client relationship. Although this may seem severe, its importance extends beyond the establishment and maintenance of a therapeutic milieu. For example, a client who is considering an abortion but who has not yet revealed this may ask the nurse if he or she is Catholic. If the response is, "Yes," the client may assume that the nurse is therefore opposed to abortion, and may be even more reluctant to discuss the problem. The point is that the client must feel that the nurse will accept him or her as a person and his or her feelings and needs. If the nurse reveals personal information, the client may make assumptions about the nurse that preclude such acceptance or that confuse the nature and purpose of the therapeutic relationship.

Because a therapeutic relationship is not social, there is no reason for the nurse to discuss his or her marital status or to give his or her home address or telephone number to the client. Giving the client information of a personal nature may encourage a social relationship outside the health care setting, foster dependence on a staff member after termination of the professional relationship, or endanger the nurse if the client is or becomes aggressive or hostile. If information of a personal nature like this is requested by the client, it is appropriate for the nurse to respond by stating that such information is not necessary to the client and is inappropriate to the therapeutic relationship. The nurse can use this opportunity to teach the client about the nature and importance of the therapeutic relationship (as opposed to a social relationship), as the client may not have experience with this type of relationship.

Treatment Team Member Considerations

This *Manual* often refers to the identification, awareness, and expression of feelings treatment team members have when working with clients. It is essential that you recognize that you have an emotional response to clients. Many situations arise that may evoke an emotional response in you (e.g., issues of sexuality or religion) or that prompt you to remember similar experiences of your own (present or past). Your response may be painful or uncomfortable, may involve fear or judgment, or may be something of which you are hardly aware. The importance of recognizing and working through these emotions lies in the fact that if you do not do this, you will respond nevertheless but in a way that may adversely affect both you and the client. For example, you may unconsciously convey disapproval to the client, or you may avoid interacting with the client on certain topics or problems. You may deny your feelings and project them onto the client, or your frustration tolerance with the client may be very low. If the client's problems remind you of an experience that was painful in your own life, which you may or may not remember (such as abuse or incest), then you may minimize the client's feelings or distance yourself from the client. Finally, working with clients may become so stressful to you that you may suffer from burnout and may even leave nursing. Not only do attempts to ignore such emotions often lead to a decreased awareness of the client's feelings and interference with the therapeutic relationship, they also take an emotional toll on the nurse and increase the stress involved in interpersonal work.

Remember that emotional responses to clients are to be expected and are not unprofessional. It is indeed not professional to act these out with the client, but it is part of the nurse's professional role to acknowledge and accept responsibility for them. A good way to increase awareness of staff feelings is to hold client care conferences and staff meetings. At least a part of these meetings can be devoted to the staff's feelings regarding the client. For example, treatment team members may be frustrated about a client's lack of response to treatment. At a client care conference, these feelings can be explored and the nursing care plan evaluated and revised, thus improving the client's care as well as dealing with the staff's feelings of hopelessness and averting apathy regarding the client. Staff meetings can provide support for the feelings of treatment team members and assure staff members that they are not alone in their reactions toward a client. Meetings with the nursing supervisor or a psychiatric nurse consultant or specialist to discuss emotions and plan nursing care also can be used in this way.

Treatment team members may find themselves becoming angry with a client who is manipulative, hostile, or aggressive. It is important in an acute situation to identify your own emotions and deliberately withdraw from the client (if safety considerations allow) if those feelings are interfering with your care of the client. If you find yourself reacting in an angry or punitive way, for example, it is best to ask another staff member to deal with the client. If a client has become aggressive, requiring interventions such as restraint or seclusion, treatment team members may meet for a brief conference after an event to discuss the interventions as well as emotions generated by the client's behavior and the measures taken to provide safety. Sometimes a client's behavior is simply difficult to tolerate or work with for extended periods (as with manic behavior); nursing care assignments can be discussed and structured to limit individual staff contacts with this client to brief periods (maybe 1 or 2 hours at a time).

Remember, however, that expression of emotions by treatment team members is not to pass judgment on the client or the client's behavior. Rather, such discussions are held to avoid being judgmental or passive–aggressive in the client's care. Other ways to deal with staff considerations include scheduling and encouraging breaks from the unit, making nursing assignments that vary treatment team members' experiences and client interactions, supporting educational activities and other professional growth opportunities for staff members, and using support groups for nursing staff that include peers from other units.

Client Advocacy

The nurse in the mental health care setting has a unique and vital role as a client advocate. Clients who are experiencing emotional problems are often unaware of their rights or unable to act in their own interest. Some clients (those hospitalized or restrained against their will) are almost completely dependent on the staff to safeguard their legal rights. Also, the trauma and confusion of entering a mental health facility may be so overwhelming to the client and his or her significant others that they may become extremely passive in this regard. In addition to planning and implementing individualized nursing care in the best interest of the client, the nurse should be familiar with the rights of hospitalized clients and should monitor all aspects of client care with these in mind. As a client advocate, the nurse can offer to help the client and his or her family or significant others.

Client's Rights

In any nursing practice in which mental health problems are encountered, the nurse must be aware of the state and federal laws regarding the client's rights and certain aspects of client care. Anything that is deemed part of treatment but against the client's will must be examined by the nurse with respect to the law as well as to the client's well-being and the nurse's conscience. Do not assume that someone else on the treatment team or in the facility has taken or will take responsibility for treating the client within legal or ethical limits. Your role as client advocate is especially important here. Commitment of a client to a treatment facility, the use of physical restraints, and the use of medication and electroconvulsive or other invasive therapies against the client's will must be scrutinized and handled carefully by the nurse.

In any situation that might have legal ramifications, the nurse must know the law, must acutely observe the client, and must document those observations accurately. Good documentation is essential and should be specific in all respects. For example, if a client is physically restrained, the nurse must chart the following:

- Precipitating factors, situation, behaviors, and reason for restraints
- The time and way in which the client was restrained
- Actions taken to meet the client's basic needs and rights while he or she was restrained (e.g., removing one limb restraint at a time and performing range of motion exercises; offering liquids, food, and commode)
- Frequent individual observations of the client for the duration of the restraint, including observations and determinations related to the continued need for restraints
- The time the client was released from restraints
- The client's behavior on release
- Any other pertinent information

Difficult situations may arise when the nurse and another member of the treatment team (such as a physician) disagree regarding the treatment of a client when legal considerations may be a factor. For example, the nurse may believe that a client is actively suicidal, whereas the other members of the treatment team feel that the client is ready for a weekend at home. In this kind of situation, the nurse must document all observations that led to this judgment and should seek help from nursing or other administrators at the facility.

Clients with Legal Problems

Another potentially difficult situation is the treatment of a client who has been charged with or convicted of a violent crime (such as rape, child abuse, murder, or arson) or who talks about these behaviors while in the hospital. Again, it is essential to be aware of legal factors pertinent to the client's treatment, for example:

- Why is the client in the treatment setting?
- Has a court-ordered observation to establish competence or insanity?
- Is treatment ordered by the court instead of or as part of a sentence for a crime?
- Is the client being treated for another problem and during treatment confesses a crime to the staff?

If a client is at the facility for observation, it must be determined if there will be any treatment given (beyond safety considerations) or if the staff will only observe the client and document those observations. In any case, this observation must be accurate and thoroughly documented in the client's chart because the chart is a legal document and may be presented as evidence in court.

Examination of your own feelings about the client is crucial in situations in which criminal activity is involved. You must become and remain aware of your feelings to work effectively with the client and remain nonjudgmental. For instance, whether you feel that the client "could not possibly be guilty" or "is absolutely despicable," you will not be treating the client objectively. And yet it is realistic to expect that anyone working with the client will have feelings about a crime. Use staff conferences and interactions to ventilate, explore, and deal with emotions so that you can remain objective in your nursing care of the client.

ROLE OF THE CLIENT

The client plays an active role in the therapeutic relationship. It is important to engage the client in as much of his or her care planning and treatment as possible. Encouraging the client to identify treatment goals will help the client see his or her role as an active one and be more invested in the outcome of the strategies used. Asking the client to help evaluate the effectiveness of nursing interventions can promote the client's sense of control and responsibility and can aid in learning to evaluate his or her condition over time. In addition, it will maintain a focus on expected results from treatment, progress, and eventual discharge from the facility.

Client's Responsibilities

A client has certain responsibilities within the therapeutic relationship. The client's ability to accept or fulfill some of these responsibilities may vary according to his or her mental state or problems. As the client progresses, the degree of self-responsibility he or she assumes should increase. Client responsibilities include the following:

- Recognizing and accepting hospitalization or treatment as a positive step toward the goal of optimum health
- Recognizing and accepting the nurse as a therapist
- Recognizing and accepting his or her emotional problems
- Accepting responsibility for his or her own feelings, even though that may be difficult
- Accepting an active role in his or her own treatment
- Being motivated toward pursuing the goal of optimum health
- Actively participating in care planning and implementation as soon and as much as possible
- Recognizing and accepting that there is a relationship between physical and mental health
- Reporting honest information, even if it is perceived as undesirable, to form an accurate database on which to plan and evaluate care

PART 2 Recommended Readings

Ali, A., Hawkins, R. L., & Chambers, D. A. (2010). Recovery from depression among clients transitioning out of poverty. *American Journal of Orthopsychiatry, 80*(1), 26–33.

Fukui, S., Davidson, L. J., Holter, M. C., & Rapp, C. (2010). Pathways to recovery (PTR): Impact of peer-led group participation on mental health recovery outcomes. *Psychiatric Rehabilitation Journal, 34*(1), 42–48.

Russinova, Z., Cash, D., & Wewiorski, N. J. (2009). Toward understanding the usefulness of complementary and alternative medicine for individuals with serious mental illnesses: Classification of perceived benefits. *Journal of Nervous and Mental Disease, 197*(1), 69–73.

Webster, D. A. (2009). Addressing nursing students' stigmatizing beliefs toward mental illness. *Journal of Psychosocial Nursing and Mental Health Services, 47*(10), 34–42.

PART 2 Resources for Additional Information

Visit thePoint (http://thePoint.lww.com/Schultz9e) for a list of these and other helpful Internet resources.

Agency for Healthcare Research and Quality

Alternative Medicine Foundation

American Association for Geriatric Psychiatry

American Counseling Association

American Psychiatric Association

American Psychiatric Nurses Association

American Psychological Association

American Red Cross

BMC (BioMed Central) Complementary and Alternative Medicine Journal

Center for Mental Health Services National Mental Health Information Center

Centers for Disease Control Division of Violence Prevention

Department of Homeland Security disaster response

Disaster Center disaster response agency listing

Food and Drug Administration dietary supplement information

Institute of Medicine of the National Academies

International Critical Incident Stress Foundation

International Society of Psychiatric-Mental Health Nurses

Mental Health America

National Center for Complementary and Alternative Medicine

National Guideline Clearinghouse

National Institute of Mental Health

National Institute on Aging

National Library of Medicine Directory of Health Organizations

National Mental Health Association

National Mental Health Information Center—Substance Abuse and Mental Health Services (SAMHSA)

National Mental Health Information Center—Evidence-Based Practice KITs

National MultiCultural Institute

Office of Cancer Complementary and Alternative Medicine

University of Iowa College of Nursing Centers Gerontological Nursing Interventions Research Center

PART THREE

Care Plans

The *Manual of Psychiatric Nursing Care Plans* is intended as a resource in planning for each client's care. Because each client is a person with a unique background and a particular set of behaviors, problems, strengths, needs, and goals, each client needs an individual plan of nursing care. The care plans that follow provide information concerning clients' behaviors and suggestions regarding nursing care, including nursing diagnoses, that are most likely to be used in writing an individual client's care plan.

For each diagnosis addressed in the following care plans, suggestions are given for the following:

- Assessment data commonly encountered with behaviors or problems addressed in the care plan.
- Expected outcomes for three time frames: immediate (as early as possible in the client's stay); stabilization (to be achieved before discharge from an acute care setting); and community (following discharge, when the client remains stable with the support of the community). Immediate time frames are provided in the care plans as examples only; actual time frames need to be determined by the nurse as he or she performs nursing assessment and ongoing evaluation of care.
- Nursing interventions often effective in addressing the nursing diagnosis, to be selected for implementation as appropriate for a given client's situation. Care plans may contain more interventions than needed for a particular client's situation or alternative approaches; alternatively, the individual client's plan of care may need additional interventions as is developed.
- Rationale for each intervention, provided as a learning tool to help in understanding the intervention and as an aid in selecting the appropriate interventions for an individual care plan.

Because of individual differences and because the care plans in this *Manual* are based primarily on behaviors (as opposed to psychiatric diagnoses), a plan from this *Manual* should not be copied verbatim for an individual client's plan of care. Some care plans contain seemingly contradictory problems that call for different approaches or suggest different possible approaches for the same problem. Remember that the plans in the *Manual* are intended as resources from which to glean appropriate information and suggestions for use in each client's case.

This *Manual* focuses primarily on the client's behavior, which enables the nurse to plan care using nursing diagnoses formulated on the basis of nursing assessment, rather than depending on a psychiatric diagnosis, or in the absence of a specified psychiatric diagnosis. This is important for several reasons: not all clients with emotional problems are found in psychiatric settings or carry a psychiatric diagnosis; psychiatric diagnoses are not always immediately determined; and most important, good nursing care must involve seeing the client holistically, using a nursing framework, rather than solely in terms of a psychiatric diagnosis.

The nursing process includes assessment, formulation of nursing diagnoses, determination of expected outcomes, identification of nursing interventions that may lead to expected outcomes, establishment of a timetable to evaluate all parts of the process, and revision of each step when appropriate. Each part of this dynamic and continuing process is specific to the person—it must be determined for each client. The sections included in each plan in this *Manual* are intended to be used as resources and references; in planning care for a client, the nurse must select appropriate items from these care plans or use them as a framework from which to write others more appropriate for the individual client and then supply timing, evaluation, and revision specific to the situation.

The following is a brief explanation of each section found in each of the care plans in the *Manual:*

- The section that begins each care plan contains information about the diagnosis, behaviors, or problems addressed in the care plan. This information may include a basic description of the problem(s), key definitions, etiology, epidemiology, course of the disorder, and general interventions.
- *Nursing Diagnoses*: The nursing diagnoses most likely to be formulated from the assessment of clients exhibiting the behaviors or problems to be addressed in the care plan are presented, followed by a list of other nursing diagnoses addressed elsewhere in the *Manual* that may be useful in planning care for some clients with these behaviors or problems. Neither list is intended as a complete list of all nursing diagnoses that may be generated; rather, the diagnoses presented address problems that commonly occur and are to be used as guides in formulating diagnoses appropriate for individual clients.

For each nursing diagnosis addressed in the care plan, the following elements of care planning are given:

- *Assessment Data*: Information likely to be assessed with regard to the client's appearance, behavior, and situation.

35

- *Expected Outcomes*: Outcomes or outcome criteria that the nurse and the client may identify as a focus for nursing care, for the client's progress, and for evaluating the effectiveness of the care plan. The outcome criteria, or goals, are written in terms of the client's behavior. The nurse should write these outcomes in very specific terms so that they can be used as a basis for evaluation and revision. Deadlines or other timing criteria need to be included in the individual client's care plan for each outcome. Other specifications (or modifiers), such as the amount of interaction, specific people or types of people involved (e.g., staff members, other clients), amounts of food or fluids, and so forth also should be included. An example of an expected outcome written for a client's care plan is, "The client will talk with a staff member about loss for 10 minutes each day by 3/6/15" (see "Key Considerations in Mental Health Nursing: The Nursing Process").
- *Implementation (Nursing Interventions* and *Rationale)*: This section presents choices and alternatives that the nurse can select (with the client, if possible) as a means of achieving the expected outcomes. Interventions, also called nursing orders or nursing prescriptions, are given as specific practical suggestions, and, often, details are given for more than one approach so that care can be tailored to individual differences within a given behavior or problem. Nurses are an integral part of the interdisciplinary treatment team and they collaborate in providing care and supporting common goals, outcomes, and interventions with other health professionals, the client, and the client's significant others. Interventions in the text that are especially collaborative in nature are indicated by an asterisk. When writing interventions for an individual's care plan, the nurse should add modifiers similar to those for expected outcomes. Rationale for nursing interventions is an important part of the nursing process, although it is seldom written out in an individual client's care plan. It has been included in this *Manual* as a means of communicating the principles on which the suggested interventions are based and to show that nursing interventions are to be written based on rationale. That is, rationale exists whether it is explicitly written or is only implicit in the construction of each care plan. As nursing research expands the body of nursing knowledge, rationale for nursing interventions will become more distinct and specific.

General Care Plans

The first two care plans in this section should be used in every client's care because they address two of the most important facets of treatment: establishing the therapeutic relationship and planning for the client's independence from treatment. For work with any client to be most effective, it must be soundly based in a trusting relationship. The client and the nurse must see each other and their work as valuable, strive toward mutually agreed-on goals, and enter into the problem-solving process together as described in Care Plan 1: Building a Trust Relationship.

Equally important is the client's discharge from treatment or from the therapeutic relationship. Discharge planning should begin immediately when therapy begins, providing a focus for goals and an orientation toward as much independence as possible for the client. Discussing discharge plans with the client from the outset will help minimize the client's fears of discharge and will facilitate goal identification and an active role for the client in therapy. By using Care Plan 2: Discharge Planning, the nurse may anticipate the client's optimum level of functioning, the quality of the client's home situation and relationships with significant others, and the need for client teaching throughout nursing care planning and implementation.

Care Plan 3: Deficient Knowledge speaks to the situation in which clients and their significant others may lack knowledge or understanding of their condition, treatment, safe use of medications, and other care-related needs. Clients who are unable or unwilling to adhere to their treatment plans, regardless of their primary problems or behaviors, are addressed in Care Plan 4: Nonadherence. The nursing diagnoses and care planning found in these plans may be appropriate for use in clients with any of the behaviors addressed elsewhere in the *Manual*.

Many times clients are cared for at home by a family member, partner, or friend. Caregivers often undertake the care of a client with little preparation or knowledge and with little attention to their own needs. Care Plan 5: Supporting the Caregiver examines some of the considerations related to caregiving and the needs of caregivers. Using it will help the nurse in planning care for the client after discharge and in addressing the needs of caregivers to ensure continued success.

CARE PLAN 1

Building a Trust Relationship

The nurse–client relationship is an interpersonal process in which mutual learning occurs and in which the nurse supports the client's growth in insight and changing behavior. The therapeutic relationship is built on trust between the nurse and the client, and, in contrast to personal or social relationships, has specific goals and expectations; it is a professional relationship that is time limited and focused on the client in terms of learning, meeting needs, and growing. The nurse is responsible for facilitating and guiding the relationship to achieve these goals.

Phases of the Relationship

The trust relationship between client and nurse can be viewed in four phases or stages. Each phase has primary tasks and characteristics, but transition from one phase to the next is gradual and is not always clearly delineated. These phases are as follows:

1. *Introductory or orientation phase.* This phase is the foundation of the relationship. The nurse becomes acquainted with the client and begins to establish rapport and mutual trust. The purpose, goals, limits, and expectations of the relationship are established.
2. *Testing phase.* The nurse's truthfulness, sincerity, and reliability are tested in this phase. The client may say or do things to shock the nurse to see if he or she will reject the client. The client may become manipulative in an attempt to discover the limits of the relationship or test the nurse's sincerity and dependability. The client's attitude and behavior may vary a great deal, for example, from pleasant and eager to please to uncooperative and angry. This phase can be extremely trying and frustrating for the nurse, but provides an opportunity for the nurse to demonstrate respect, consistency, and effective limit setting.
3. *Working phase.* Transition to this phase is accompanied by the client's willingness to assume a more active role in the relationship. This usually is the longest phase of a trust relationship and the most overtly productive. The client begins to trust the nurse and starts to focus on problems or behaviors that need to be changed. During times of frustration, the client may revert to testing behaviors. The nurse should anticipate this and avoid becoming discouraged or giving up on the relationship.
4. *Termination phase.* This phase provides closure to the relationship. Ideally, planning for termination of the relationship begins during the orientation phase or as soon as the client is able to comprehend it. As the client begins to rely more on himself or herself, plans for the client to return home, to the community, or to a more permanent placement can be made (see Care Plan 2: Discharge Planning). When the client leaves the relationship (or agency) for unanticipated reasons, termination is less organized and usually more difficult. In that situation, it is important to try to talk with the client, even briefly, to achieve some closure to the relationship.

General Interventions

The nurse needs to be aware of a number of factors as he or she begins a relationship with a new client, including the client's presenting problems and relationship behavior, the client's experiences with nurses and other (mental) health professionals, and the client's cultural background and its implications for the client's perceptions of and participation in a therapeutic relationship. Many clients are unaware of the characteristics of a therapeutic relationship, and the nurse may need to help the client learn to participate to the greatest benefit.

NURSING DIAGNOSIS ADDRESSED IN THIS CARE PLAN
Impaired Social Interaction

RELATED NURSING DIAGNOSES ADDRESSED IN THE MANUAL
Ineffective Coping
Ineffective Role Performance
Anxiety

Nursing Diagnosis

Impaired Social Interaction
Insufficient or excessive quantity or ineffective quality of social exchange.

ASSESSMENT DATA

* Difficulty trusting others
* Difficulties in relationships with significant others
* Difficulties with others in school or work environment
* Discomfort in social or interactive situations
* Poor social skills
* Feelings of anxiety, fear, hostility, sadness, guilt, or inadequacy

EXPECTED OUTCOMES

Immediate

The client will

* Demonstrate the ability to interact with staff and other clients within the therapeutic milieu (e.g., make eye contact, verbally respond to others) within 24 hours
* Participate in interactions with staff and in building the trust relationship within 48 hours

Stabilization

The client will

* Assume increasing responsibility for interactions and own behavior within the context of the therapeutic relationship
* Identify relationships and resources outside the hospital environment to be used as support system
* Terminate the nurse–client relationship successfully

Community

The client will

* Use community support system successfully
* Participate in follow-up or outpatient therapy as indicated

IMPLEMENTATION

Nursing Interventions *denotes collaborative interventions	Rationale
Introduce yourself to the client. Explain your role on the unit or within the treatment team.	An introduction and explanation will help the client know what to expect from you, other staff, and the hospitalization.
Assess the client's behavior, attitudes, problems, and needs.	Baseline data are essential for developing a plan of nursing care.
Obtain the client's perception of his or her problems and what the client expects to gain from the relationship or hospitalization.	The client's actions are based on his or her perceptions, which may or may not be the same as other people's perceptions or objective reality.
Make your expectations for the relationship clear to the client.	Defining your expectations helps the client identify his or her role and understand what is expected of him or her.
Be honest in all interactions with the client. Avoid glossing over any unpleasant topics or circumstances. Take a	Honesty is essential if a trusting relationship is to develop. You are not doing the client a favor by avoiding unpleasant

(continued on page 40)

IMPLEMENTATION (continued)

Nursing Interventions *denotes collaborative interventions	Rationale
matter-of-fact approach to such problems as commitment, legal difficulties, and so forth.	areas; the client will need to deal with these problems. You show that you are trustworthy by discussing these issues without judging or rejecting the client.
Let the client know that you will work with him or her for a specified period of time and that the relationship will end when the client is no longer in treatment.	Explaining the time limitations helps to set the limits of the professional relationship. It also conveys your positive expectation that the client will improve and leave the hospital.
Show the client you accept him or her as a person by initiating interactions, remaining with the client in silence, using active listening, and so forth.	Conveying acceptance can help the client feel worthwhile. It is possible to accept the client yet not accept "negative" or undesirable behaviors.
Encourage the client to interact with other staff and clients. Avoid becoming the only one the client can talk to about his or her feelings and problems.	Becoming the sole confidant of the client may seem flattering, but it may be manipulative on the part of the client, and it inhibits the client's ability to form relationships with others.
Let the client know that pertinent information will be communicated to other staff members. Do not promise to keep secrets (e.g., from other staff) as a way of obtaining information from the client.	A promise of keeping secrets is not one you can keep. The client has a right to know how information is communicated and used in his or her treatment.
Be consistent with the client at all times.	Your consistency demonstrates that you are trustworthy, and it reinforces limits.
Set and maintain limits on the client's "negative" or unacceptable behavior; withdraw your attention from the client if necessary when it is safe to do so.	Lack of attention can help extinguish unacceptable behavior. The client's safety and the safety of others are priorities.
Do not allow the client to bargain to obtain special favors, avoid responsibilities, gain privileges, or otherwise subvert limits.	Allowing bargaining permits the client to be manipulative and undermines limits and trust.
Give attention and positive feedback for acceptable or positive behavior.	Desirable behaviors increase when they are positively reinforced.
When limiting the client's behaviors, offer acceptable alternatives (e.g., "Don't try to hit someone when you're angry—try punching your pillow instead."). See "Key Considerations in Mental Health Nursing: Limit-Setting."	By offering alternative ways to express feelings, you teach acceptable as well as unacceptable behavior. The client is more likely to abandon old behaviors if new ones are available.
Establish a regular schedule for interacting with the client (such as 1 hour each day or 10 minutes every hour), whatever fits your schedule and the client is able to tolerate.	Regular schedules provide consistency, which enhances trust. The client also can see that your interest in him or her continues.
At the beginning of your interaction with the client, inform him or her of how much time you have to spend. If you must interrupt the interaction, tell the client when you expect to return.	Discussing your schedule conveys your respect for the client and lets the client know what to expect from you.
Do whatever you say you will do, and, conversely, do not make promises you cannot keep. If extenuating circumstances prevent you from following through, apologize and honestly explain this to the client. Expect the client to be disappointed or angry; help him or her to express these feelings appropriately, and give support for doing so.	The client must know what to expect and will trust you more when you follow through. Extenuating circumstances that necessitate a change of plans happen in everyday life; the client has the opportunity to deal with the frustration or disappointment that may ensue in an acceptable manner.
Teach the client social skills. Describe and demonstrate specific skills, such as eye contact, attentive listening, nodding, and so forth. Discuss the types of topics that are appropriate for social conversation, such as the weather, news, local events, and so forth.	The client may never have learned basic social skills and how to use them appropriately.

IMPLEMENTATION (continued)

Nursing Interventions *denotes collaborative interventions	Rationale
Help the client identify and implement ways of expressing emotions and communicating with others.	The client's ability to identify and express feelings and to communicate with others is impaired.
Assist the client in identifying personal behaviors or problem areas in his or her life situation that interfere with relationships or interactions with others.	The client must identify what behaviors or problems need modification before change can occur.
Teach the client a step-by-step approach to solving problems: identifying the problem, exploring alternatives, evaluating the possible consequences of the alternative solutions, making a decision, and implementing the solution.	The client may be unaware of a logical process for examining and resolving problems.
Assist the client in identifying more effective methods of dealing with stress. Teach the client basic stress management techniques, such as conscious breathing and relaxation, moderate physical activity, and so forth.	The client may be dealing with stress in the most effective way he or she can and may need to learn new skills and behaviors.
Anticipate the client's anxiety or insecurity about being discharged from the hospital and terminating the therapeutic relationship, including the possibility that the client may revert to manipulative behavior or his or her presenting problem behavior as termination approaches. Remember: The termination phase of the therapeutic relationship should begin in the introductory or orientation phase and should be reinforced as a goal and as a positive outcome throughout the entire therapeutic relationship.	Once the client is comfortable in the relationship, you may expect that he or she will perceive the end of the relationship as threatening and the beginning of other relationships as entailing risk. In addition, the termination of the relationship is a loss for the client (and for the staff).
Point out to the client that his or her success in relationships in the hospital can serve as learning experiences to be used in establishing and maintaining other types of relationships after discharge.	The client may not be aware of the steps in building relationships; you can help the client learn about relationships and build social skills by using the client's current relationships and interactions as examples. Recognizing the client's successes can help build confidence.
*Assist the client in identifying sources of support outside the hospital, including agencies or individuals in the community and on the Internet, if appropriate, as well as significant others in his or her personal life.	Community support may help the client deal with future stress and avoid hospitalization.
*Assist the client in making plans for discharge (returning home, employment, and so on). See Care Plan 2: Discharge Planning.	Making specific discharge plans enhances the client's chances for success in the community.

CARE PLAN 2

Discharge Planning

Discharge planning is a process that should begin on the client's admission to the treatment setting and should be addressed in the initial care plan. Planning for eventual discharge should underlie the client's plan of care throughout a hospital stay in recognition of the temporary nature of hospitalization.

When a client has been in an inpatient setting, discharge from that setting does not necessarily mean that no further assistance is needed. It is important to assess the client's need for services along a continuum of care, for example, in-home services, formalized community activities or programs, or an agency-based outpatient or partial hospitalization program. When clients are discharged from the hospital with significant needs, it is particularly important to provide thorough discharge planning and emotional support to enhance the client's likelihood of successful transition to the community.

Discharge planning is a dynamic process and must undergo evaluation and change throughout the client's care. If the client needs continued care, the following alternatives may need to be evaluated:

* Transfer to another hospital or institution
* Discharge to a sheltered or transitional setting
* Discharge with other supportive services in the community
* Relocation to a living situation other than the client's prehospitalization situation

The basic goal related to discharge from any treatment setting is that the client will reach his or her optimal level of wellness and independence. Such an approach will encourage goal-oriented planning and discourage the client and the staff from seeing hospitalization as an end in itself or a panacea. The client should work with the staff as soon as possible to develop an ongoing plan of care that is oriented toward discharge. In assessing the client with regard to discharge plans, it is important to obtain the following information:

* The client's ability to function independently before hospitalization
* The client's home environment
* The type of situation to which the client will be discharged
* The client's optimal level of functioning outside the hospital
* The client's own support system outside the hospital
* The client's need for follow-up care, including frequency, type, location, or specific therapist or program

It also is important to assess the client's feelings about hospitalization and discharge and the client's motivations to remain hospitalized or in treatment, to be discharged, and to change his or her former situation to prevent readmission. The nurse should remain aware of any secondary gains the client obtains from being hospitalized or in treatment.

NURSING DIAGNOSES ADDRESSED IN THIS CARE PLAN
Impaired Home Maintenance
Anxiety

RELATED NURSING DIAGNOSES ADDRESSED IN THE MANUAL
Ineffective Coping
Ineffective Health Maintenance
Risk for Loneliness

Nursing Diagnosis

Impaired Home Maintenance
Inability to independently maintain a safe growth-promoting immediate environment.

ASSESSMENT DATA

- Lack of skills with which to function independently outside the hospital
- Lack of confidence
- Dependence on hospital or treatment team
- Perceived helplessness
- Nonexistent or unrealistic goals and plans
- Lack of knowledge
- Inadequate support system
- Inadequate financial resources
- Disorganized or dysfunctional living environment

EXPECTED OUTCOMES

Immediate

The client will

- Verbalize concrete realistic plans within 2 to 5 days, regarding:
- Meeting essential physical needs (housing, employment, financial resources, transportation, and physical care, if needed)
- Meeting emotional needs through significant relationships, social activities, a general support system, and so forth
- Dealing with stress or problems
- Dealing with other facets of living specific to the client (legal problems, physical or health limitations, etc.)

Stabilization

The client will

- Demonstrate the ability to meet essential needs (self-reliance when possible)
- Verbally identify and contact resource people in the community for various needs
- Identify needed services or resources to use after discharge
- Express willingness to follow through with identified plans

Community

The client will

- Participate in follow-up care
- Implement plans to maintain community functioning

IMPLEMENTATION

Nursing Interventions *denotes collaborative interventions	Rationale
On admission, ask the client about his or her expectations for hospitalization and plans for discharge. Attempt to keep discharge plans as a focus for discussion throughout the client's hospitalization.	Discussing discharge plans will reinforce the idea that the client's hospitalization is temporary and that discharge is the eventual goal.
Encourage the client to identify his or her goals and expectations after discharge.	Focusing on the client's life outside the hospital may help to diminish fears of discharge.
Help the client assess personal needs for specificity and structure. If it is indicated, assist the client in making a time schedule or other structure for activities (work, study, recreation, solitude, social activities, and significant relationships).	The client may be overwhelmed by the lack of structure in the home environment after a stay in an institution, which often is very structured and in which the client's choices and need for decision making are limited.
Use role-playing and setting up hypothetical situations with the client when discussing discharge plans.	Anticipatory guidance can be effective in preparing the client for future situations. Role-playing and hypothetical

(continued on page 44)

IMPLEMENTATION (continued)

Nursing Interventions *denotes collaborative interventions	Rationale
	situations allow the client to practice new behaviors in a nonthreatening environment and to receive feedback on new skills.
Teach the client about his or her illness, medications (action, toxic symptoms, and side effects), nutrition, exercise, and medical conditions requiring physical care, if needed.	The client needs health information to participate effectively in his or her own care and to achieve independence and optimal health outside the hospital.
Talk with the client regarding medication or other treatment schedules and reasons for continuing therapy. Attempt to involve the client in treatment decisions, especially regarding therapies after discharge.	The client's participation in decisions may increase his or her motivation to continue therapies.
Talk with the client about ways to meet personal needs after discharge (e.g., obtaining food, money, shelter, clothing, transportation, and a job).	The client may need direction or assistance in making these plans.
*Assess the client's skills related to meeting the above needs (e.g., using a telephone and directory, managing a checkbook and bank accounts, contacting other community resources, arranging job interviews). Work with the client and obtain help from other disciplines if indicated, such as vocational rehabilitation, therapeutic education, and so forth.	The client may lack daily living skills and may need to develop and practice them before discharge.
*Before discharge, encourage the client to make arrangements as independently as possible (e.g., find housing, open bank accounts, obtain a job). Give support for these activities. Work with other members of the treatment team to identify resources if additional assistance is needed.	The client will be leaving the support of the hospital and staff and needs to be as independent as possible.
Encourage the client to continue working toward goals that have been identified but not yet realized (e.g., obtaining a high school diploma or graduate equivalent, vocational plans, divorce). Give positive support for goal identification and work that has begun.	The client is leaving a supportive environment and may need encouragement to continue working toward goals outside the hospital.
If the client is transferring to another facility, give the client factual feedback regarding his or her progress, and discuss the need for further treatment. Point out the reasons for the transfer, if possible, such as the need for longer-term or another type of care, different treatment structure, or another location. Involve the client in the decision-making process and offer the client choices as much as possible.	It is important that the client understand the reasons for continued treatment, transfer decisions, and so forth, as much as possible. Giving the client choices or input will help diminish feelings of helplessness and frustration.
Stress that transfer to another care setting is not a punishment.	The client may see the need for continued care as a failure on his or her part.
*Attempt to give the client information about this new environment; arrange a visit before the transfer, if possible, or provide the name of a contact person at the new facility.	Information about the new environment will help diminish the client's anxiety.

Nursing Diagnosis

Anxiety

Vague uneasy feeling of discomfort or dread accompanied by an autonomic response (the source often nonspecific or unknown to the individual); a feeling of apprehension caused by anticipation of danger. It is an alerting signal that warns of impending danger and enables the individual to take measures to deal with threat.

ASSESSMENT DATA

- Verbalized nervousness, apprehension
- Fear of failure
- Withdrawn behavior
- Reappearance of symptoms as discharge is near
- Refusal to discuss future plans
- Lack of confidence in own skills and abilities

EXPECTED OUTCOMES

Immediate

The client will

- Discuss termination of staff–client relationships within 2 to 3 days
- Verbally acknowledge eventual discharge within 2 to 3 days
- Verbalize feelings about hospitalization, discharge, and follow-up services within 4 to 5 days

Stabilization

The client will

- Participate actively in discharge planning
- Identify and demonstrate alternative ways to deal with stress or problems (e.g., demonstrate the problem-solving process, discuss feelings with staff rather than acting out hostile behavior)
- Realistically evaluate own skills related to proposed discharge plans and posttreatment situation
- Terminate staff–client relationships

Community

The client will

- Solve problems and make decisions independently
- Manage anxiety, stress, or life events effectively

IMPLEMENTATION

Nursing Interventions *denotes collaborative interventions	Rationale
Help the client identify factors in his or her life that have contributed to need for treatment (e.g., living situation, relationships, drug or alcohol use, inadequate coping mechanisms). Discuss each contributing factor, how the client sees these now, what can be changed, what the client is motivated to change, and how the client will deal differently with these things to prevent rehospitalization.	The client's therapy and work inside the hospital must be integrated with his or her life outside the hospital to remain effective. Outside influences or situations may need to be changed to promote the client's well-being. Anticipatory guidance can be effective in helping the client prepare for future situations.
Always orient discussions with the client toward his or her eventual discharge.	Providing a focus on discharge will minimize the client's focusing only on the hospitalization and will promote the client's acceptance of discharge plans as discharge nears.
Support the client and give positive feedback when the client plans for discharge or talks positively about discharge.	Your support for the client's active progress toward and acceptance of discharge may enhance the client's positive anticipation of discharge.

(continued on page 46)

IMPLEMENTATION (continued)

Nursing Interventions *denotes collaborative interventions	Rationale
Encourage the client to view discharge as a positive step or sign of growth, not as being forced to leave the hospital. Try to convey this in your attitude toward the client.	The client may see discharge as punishment or rejection. Your conveyance of the client's discharge and independence as positive may help the client view discharge in a more positive light.
Encourage the client to express feelings about leaving the hospital, including anticipated problems, fears, and ways to deal with the outside world.	The client may be fearful of being outside a structured, supportive environment; may fear a return of symptoms; or may be anxious about dealing with significant others, his or her job, and so forth.
Encourage the client to express his or her feelings regarding termination of therapeutic relationships and the loss of hospitalization.	Discharge from the safety, security, and structure of the hospital environment represents a real loss to the client for which grief is an expected and appropriate response. Encouraging the client to work through his or her feelings regarding this loss will foster acceptance and growth.
*Use formal and informal group settings for discussions. A discharge group that includes all clients who are near discharge may be helpful.	Groups allow clients to offer support for the feelings of others in similar situations, and they provide a nonthreatening environment in which to explore new behaviors.
Talk with the client about the feelings he or she may experience after discharge (such as loneliness) and how the client will deal with those feelings.	Identifying feelings and exploring ways to deal with them can help diminish the client's fears and help the client learn effective ways of coping with them.
*Give the client a telephone number and name (if possible) to call in case of a crisis or situation in which the client feels overwhelmed.	Tangible information can help decrease the client's fears and prepare for dealing with crises in ways other than returning to the hospital.
Deliberately terminate your relationship with the client, and talk with him or her about this. Acknowledge and deal with your own feelings about the client and the client's discharge before talking with the client; try not to merely withdraw attention from or avoid the client because he or she will be leaving.	Your relationship with the client is a professional one and must be terminated at the time hospitalization ends. The client needs to develop and maintain optimal independence. Your own feelings of discomfort or loss must not prevent you from helping the client acknowledge and work through termination of the relationship.
*Do not encourage the client's dependence on the staff members or hospital by suggesting the client pay casual visits to the unit or by giving the client home addresses or telephone numbers of staff members. It may be necessary to establish a policy that clients may not visit the unit socially after being discharged.	It is not desirable or therapeutic for clients to become friends with staff members or to engage in social relationships with them after discharge.

CARE PLAN 3

Deficient Knowledge

Deficient knowledge, or the lack of specific information, in the client or significant others or caregiver(s) is a common finding when assessing clients with psychiatric problems. This care plan has been included in the *Manual* to address the situation in which the client or the significant others lack the information necessary to regain, maintain, or improve health. Many nursing and other health care organizations have mandated client teaching as a basic part of the rights of all clients to health care.

A specific knowledge deficit may be in relation to the client's specific problem, medical diagnosis, or health state; treatment plan or regimen; safe use of medications, self-care needs, social skills, problem solving, or other general daily living activities; prevention of future problems; or resources related to any of the above. Knowledge deficits may be related to a wide range of factors, including cognitive or skill deficits, cultural factors, physical limitations, or psychiatric problems such as denial of problems, lack of motivation, or feelings of being overwhelmed.

Nursing goals in addressing deficient knowledge include accurately assessing the deficit and the ability of the client and his or her significant others to learn and promoting the integration of the needed information and skills (not just conveying information).

Specific techniques regarding assessment, content areas, and methods of client teaching are found in the "Key Considerations in Mental Health Nursing: Client Teaching" section in this *Manual*. In creating a client's individual care plan, the nurse can integrate the information included here into the nursing diagnoses most appropriate to that client's care, as the nursing interventions for virtually all nursing diagnoses can include teaching the client and his or her significant others.

NURSING DIAGNOSIS ADDRESSED IN THIS CARE PLAN
Deficient Knowledge (Specify)

Nursing Diagnosis

Deficient Knowledge (Specify)

Absence or deficiency of cognitive information related to a specific topic.

ASSESSMENT DATA

> **Note:** The following steps of the nursing process are written in terms of the client but may be equally or more appropriate for the client's significant others and caregivers.

- Verbalization of knowledge deficit or need for learning
- Incorrect or inadequate demonstration of self-care skills
- Incorrect verbal feedback regarding self-care information
- Inappropriate behavior related to self-care

EXPECTED OUTCOMES

Immediate   The client will

- Demonstrate decreased denial within 24 to 48 hours
- Demonstrate decreased problems that impair learning ability (such as altered thought processes, sensory-perceptual alterations, etc.) within 2 to 4 days
- Verbalize interest in learning within 2 to 4 days
- Participate in learning about self-care needs; behaviors, problems, or illness; treatment program; or safe use of medications within 2 to 4 days

Stabilization   The client will

- Verbalize accurate information related to self-care needs (such as safe use of medications)
- Demonstrate adequate skills related to self-care needs (such as basic money management and vocational skills)
- Verbalize knowledge of resources and their use for anticipated needs (such as social services and support groups)

Community   The client will

- Meet own self-care needs independently
- Use community resources to meet own needs

IMPLEMENTATION

Nursing Interventions *denotes collaborative interventions	Rationale
Assess the client's current level of knowledge, misconceptions, ability to learn, readiness to learn, knowledge needs, level of anxiety, and perceptions of greatest needs and priorities.	To be effective in meeting the client's needs, your teaching plan must be based on an accurate assessment of the client's knowledge deficit and ability to learn. In addition, if the client is anxious, his or her ability to learn will be impaired until the level of anxiety decreases. Interventions will be most effective if you focus first on meeting the client's perceived needs and priorities, and then progress to other necessary teaching.
Provide information and teach skills as appropriate to the specific knowledge deficit. In the individual care plan, write a formal teaching plan with specific information, techniques, timing, and outcome criteria appropriate to the	Different clients may have very different learning needs, abilities, and situations. It is just as important to individualize a client's teaching plan as it is to write an individual nursing care plan for each client. A written, formal teaching plan will

IMPLEMENTATION (continued)

Nursing Interventions *denotes collaborative interventions	Rationale
individual client (see "Key Considerations in Mental Health Nursing: Client Teaching").	help ensure consistency among nursing staff and a method of evaluating progress.
Provide written information or other supporting materials as appropriate.	Informational materials or sample products support and reinforce learning and recall, especially after the client is discharged.
Provide information in a matter-of-fact, nonjudgmental, reassuring manner.	Information concerning psychiatric problems or illnesses can be threatening or have negative connotations to a client, especially in some cultures. The client may have misconceptions or internalized judgment, humiliation, shame, and so forth, related to his or her behaviors, experiences, or psychiatric diagnoses. Conveying information in a nonjudgmental manner can reassure the client and help with his or her acceptance of the condition or situation.
Provide information at a pace at which the client can learn effectively. Do not try to teach all necessary information at one time. Use as many teaching sessions as the client needs to learn, if at all possible.	The client's ability to learn may be impaired.
Ask the client to verbalize or demonstrate understanding of the information or skill. Ask the client directly if he or she has any questions; assure the client that asking questions or asking for clarification is an important part of the learning process. Allow the client sufficient time to formulate and ask questions.	The client may feel inadequate or intimidated in a learning situation and may indicate understanding (e.g., by nodding his or her head or answering "yes" to the question, "Do you understand?") when he or she actually does not understand or has not learned the information or skill. Adequate assessment of learning requires verbalization or active demonstration of learning.
Give the client positive feedback for asking questions, verbalizing information, demonstrating skills, and otherwise participating in the teaching–learning process.	Recognition and positive support will reinforce the client's efforts and encourage further participation.
Document teaching, the client's response to teaching, and indications of understanding verbalized or demonstrated by the client.	It is important to document teaching and learning both for successful implementation of the teaching plan and to protect the nurse from later claims that such teaching and learning did not occur.
Repeat your assessment of the client's learning and understanding at another time (i.e., after the instructional episode) before the client's discharge.	Repeated assessment of learning is essential to ensure that the client has retained the information.
If possible, allow and encourage the client to assume increasing responsibility in performing his or her own self-care before discharge.	Learning is most effective when the client actually practices and integrates new information and skills. Encouraging the client to integrate and demonstrate new information and skills in a protected environment allows the client to ask questions, clarify understanding, and build confidence in his or her self-care abilities.

CARE PLAN 4

Nonadherence

Nonadherence, or failure to accurately follow a therapeutic regimen, is a common phenomenon in health care. In this care plan, two approaches to nonadherent behavior are presented. The first approach, using the nursing diagnosis "Noncompliance," is designed for use with clients who refuse to comply or who make a specific decision to be noncompliant. The second approach uses the nursing diagnosis "Ineffective Self-Health Management" for the client who is unable to follow the therapeutic regimen.

Initially, neither the nurse nor the client may be aware of the reasons for noncompliance. It is essential to explore the factors underlying noncompliant behavior to determine whether the client is unable or unwilling to follow his or her treatment regimen and to assist the client to make positive changes. Factors related to noncompliance include the following (Kneisl & Trigoboff, 2009):

Psychologic factors, including lack of knowledge; clients' attitudes, values, and beliefs; denial of the illness or other defense mechanisms; personality type; and anxiety levels

Environmental and social factors, including lack of support system, finances, transportation, and housing, and other problems that may distract from health needs

Characteristics of the regimen, such as not enough benefit perceived by the client, demands too much change from the client, too difficult or complicated, distressing side effects, leads to social isolation or stigma

Characteristics of the nurse–client (or other health care personnel) relationship, such as faulty communication in which the client perceives the nurse as cold, uncaring, or authoritative; the client feels discouraged or treated as an object; or the client and the nurse are engaged in a struggle for control

It is estimated that up to 50% of all clients fail to follow their prescribed regimen correctly. These clients are often able to verbalize their understanding of the therapeutic regimen, but their behavior (noncompliance) indicates a problem. In mental health clients, noncompliance regarding prescribed medications is a significant problem that often leads to rehospitalization. Noncompliance with medication can take many forms, including complete refusal to take any medications, taking a larger or smaller dose than prescribed, erratic or sporadic ingestion of the medication, or taking the medication of others.

Working with the noncompliant client can be frustrating. The nurse may feel angry or impatient when the client fails to follow the prescribed regimen, which can damage the therapeutic relationship. It is important for the nurse to recognize and deal with his or her own feelings regarding the client's noncompliant behavior to remain effective in the nurse–client relationship, and to help the client achieve the goal of maximizing the effectiveness of the therapeutic regimen.

If the client is willing but unable to follow his or her regimen, it is important to assess the causes of his or her inability to adequately care for himself or herself. These factors may include lack of knowledge, complexity of therapeutic regimen, unpleasant effects of medications, financial or other resources, relationships with significant others, living situation, and so forth. Using this information, the nurse can collaborate with the interdisciplinary team to make changes to the regimen or identify ways to impact other aspects of the client's situation to enhance his or her ability to provide self-care.

NURSING DIAGNOSES ADDRESSED IN THIS CARE PLAN
Noncompliance
Ineffective Self-Health Management

Nursing Diagnosis

Noncompliance

Behavior of a person and/or caregiver that fails to coincide with a health-promoting or therapeutic plan agreed upon by the person (and/or family and/or community) and health care professional. In the presence of an agreed-on, health-promoting, or therapeutic plan, person's or caregiver's behavior is fully or partially nonadherent and may lead to clinically ineffective or partially ineffective outcomes.

ASSESSMENT DATA

- Objective tests indicating noncompliance, such as low neuroleptic blood levels
- Statements from the client or significant others describing noncompliant behavior
- Exacerbation of symptoms
- Appearance of side effects or complications
- Failure to keep appointments
- Failure to follow through with referrals

EXPECTED OUTCOMES

Immediate

The client will

- Recognize the relationship between noncompliance and undesirable consequences (i.e., increased symptoms, and hospitalization) within 24 to 48 hours
- Express feelings about therapeutic regimen within 2 to 3 days
- Identify barriers to compliance within 2 to 4 days

Stabilization

The client will

- Verbalize acceptance of illness
- Identify risks of noncompliance (e.g., exacerbation of symptoms related to not taking medication)
- Negotiate acceptable changes in the therapeutic regimen that the client is willing to follow (e.g., change in medication to alleviate unpleasant side effects)

Community

The client will

- Adhere to therapeutic recommendations independently
- Inform care provider of need for changes in therapeutic recommendations

IMPLEMENTATION

Nursing Interventions *denotes collaborative interventions	Rationale
Observe the client closely to ensure that medications are ingested. Remain with the client long enough to see that the medication was swallowed.	The client must ingest medications because he or she is being evaluated for the drug's effectiveness, side effects, or any problems associated with the prescribed medication.
Explain the need for medications honestly and directly. Give the client full explanations (e.g., "This is an antidepressant to improve your mood so you'll feel less suicidal").	Honest and complete explanations foster trust. The client may be more likely to comply if he or she feels fully informed.
Help the client to draw a connection between noncompliance and the exacerbation of symptoms.	The client may not have made this connection previously. The client is more likely to comply if he or she can see the benefits of compliance.
Encourage the client to express his or her feelings about having a chronic illness and the continued need for medication.	The client may be hesitant to express feelings, especially negative ones, without explicit permission from the nurse. Discussing feelings about chronic illness and the continued

(continued on page 52)

IMPLEMENTATION (continued)

Nursing Interventions *denotes collaborative interventions	Rationale
	need for medication can be an initial step toward the client's acceptance of his or her health status. The client may begin to see long-term medication as a positive way to remain more healthy rather than a negative indication of an illness.
If the client expresses feelings of being stigmatized (i.e., being observed taking medications by friends or coworkers), assist the client to arrange dosage schedules so that he or she can take medications unobserved.	Taking medications regularly in the presence of others may have elicited unwanted questions about the client's illness, need for medications, and so forth.
If the client has stopped taking medications when he or she "feels better," discuss the role of the medication in keeping the client free of symptoms.	Many people believe that people take medications when they are sick and should not have to take them when they are not sick or feel better. The client on long-term or maintenance therapy needs a different perspective to remain compliant.
If the client is noncompliant because he or she feels "dependent" on the medication, assist the client to gain a sense of control over the medication regimen. This may include supervised self-administration of medication, selecting convenient and acceptable times to take the medication, or setting limits on essentials and allowing control of nonessentials (e.g., "You may take the medication before or after breakfast, but you must take it before 10:00 AM").	Allowing the client to make choices or decisions about some aspects of the therapeutic regimen enhances a sense of personal control, thus decreasing feelings of helplessness and dependency.
If the client is experiencing distressing side effects, encourage him or her to report them rather than stopping medication entirely.	A negotiated change of dosage or medication may alleviate side effects and eliminate noncompliance.
If the client still refuses to be compliant, encourage him or her to report this decision accurately. Remain matter-of-fact and nonjudgmental in your approach to the client when he or she is discussing this decision. Give positive feedback for honest reporting.	If the client perceives a greater reward for honesty than for strict compliance, he or she is more likely to report accurately. It is essential to have accurate information before decisions regarding changes in medication or dosages are made; therefore, it is necessary to know whether the client is taking the medication. If the client refuses to comply and subsequently experiences the return of symptoms or rehospitalization, you can use these data for future discussions about compliance.
*Teach the client and the family or significant others about the client's illness, treatment plan, medications, and so forth.	The client and the significant others may have incomplete or inaccurate information that is contributing to the client's noncompliance.

Nursing Diagnosis

Ineffective Self-Health Management
Pattern of regulating and integrating into daily living a therapeutic regimen for the treatment of illness and its sequelae that is unsatisfactory for meeting specific health goals.

ASSESSMENT DATA

- Verbalized desire to comply with therapeutic regimen
- Objective tests indicating ineffective regimen management, for example, neuroleptic blood levels outside therapeutic range

- Exacerbation of symptoms
- Appearance of side effects, toxic effects, or complications
- Difficulty integrating therapeutic regimen into daily life

EXPECTED OUTCOMES

Immediate   The client will

- Learn skills needed for effective regimen management (such as taking medications as prescribed) within 48 hours
- Verbalize knowledge of illness and therapeutic regimen within 3 to 4 days
- Identify barriers to compliance for effective regimen management within 3 to 4 days
- Identify resources needed to ensure effective regimen management within 4 to 5 days

Stabilization   The client will

- Demonstrate skills or knowledge needed to ensure effective regimen management
- Arrange needed services or resources in the community

Community   The client will

- Follow through with discharge plans, including evaluation of adherence to and effectiveness of therapeutic regimen

IMPLEMENTATION

Nursing Interventions *denotes collaborative interventions	Rationale
*Teach the client and the family or significant others about the client's illness and therapeutic regimen.	The client and significant others may have incomplete or inaccurate information about the client's illness or therapeutic regimen.
Explore reasons for ineffective regimen management with the client. For example, can the client perform needed skills for compliance? Can the client afford the medication? Does he or she forget to take medicines? Does he or she forget that medicine was taken and repeat doses? Can the client find transportation to appointments to get refills or new prescriptions?	Identifying barriers to effective management will determine the interventions needed.
If the client does not have appropriate skills, teach him or her the skills required for effective management. Break skills into small steps, and proceed at a pace with which the client is comfortable. Give positive feedback for the client's efforts and progress.	The client must know the needed skills before he or she can become independent in performing them and remain compliant. Positive feedback will enhance the client's confidence and thus will enhance chances for success.
Do not limit skill teaching and evaluation of the client's mastery of skills to one session. Evaluate the client on several occasions if necessary to determine confidence and mastery of the skill (see Care Plan 3: Deficient Knowledge).	The client may be able to perform the skill once adequately if it has just been demonstrated. That does not mean the client knows all he or she needs to know to comply at home.
*If the client cannot afford medicines, refer him or her to social services or discuss possible alternative, less expensive medications with the physician.	The client may need financial assistance if that is the only barrier to compliance. A less expensive medication that would meet the client's therapeutic needs may be available.
If the client cannot remember to take medicines or forgets he or she has already taken medicines and repeats doses, set up a concrete system to eliminate this type of problem. For example, help the client make a chart on which the client can cross off doses as they are taken, or use a pill box with separate compartments for each dose that the client can have filled at the pharmacy.	A concrete system for taking medicines eliminates the client's problems with trying to remember dosages and schedules.

(continued on page 54)

IMPLEMENTATION (continued)

Nursing Interventions *denotes collaborative interventions	Rationale
*If the client is taking a medication that is available as a long-acting intramuscular preparation, such as fluphenazine (Prolixin) or haloperidol (Haldol), investigate the possibility of its use with the client and his or her physician.	Many clients prefer receiving injections once every 2 to 4 weeks to taking oral medications on a daily or more frequent basis.
*If the client has difficulty finding transportation to appointments or to the pharmacy for new prescriptions or refills, help the client identify resources in this area. If public transportation is available, teach the client the specific routes he or she will need to take and procedures necessary to access public transportation (e.g., if exact change is required). If the client forgets appointments, arrange to have someone at the client's clinic and call to remind him or her of the appointment.	Once a specific barrier has been identified, plans can be made to eliminate that barrier, resulting in the client's compliance. The client may be able to order prescription refills by telephone or online and receive by mail, and may be able to use a reminder service through this type of provider.
If the client has areas of nonadherence other than medication, such as a prescribed or restricted diet, use the interventions described previously to resolve that area of noncompliance.	Exploring reasons for noncompliance, teaching, validating needed skills, and arranging needed resources are effective methods of dealing with many types of nonadherent behavior.

CARE PLAN 5

Supporting the Caregiver

In the past, many clients with debilitating or terminal neurologic or psychiatric illnesses were placed in institutional facilities, particularly in the later stages of the illness, often because of inappropriate behaviors and inability to manage self-care. Today an increasing number of these individuals receive home care. This trend toward caring for family members at home is related to the high costs of institutional care, dissatisfaction with care in long-term settings, and rejection of some clients by institutions because of the nature of their illness or the behaviors that result from the illnesses. In addition, many clients and their families want to draw closer together, rather than experience the isolation that may occur when the client is in an institutional setting. Because of their increasing role in health care, family caregivers require special attention and support from nurses. This care plan is designed to include the caregiver as a team member, identifying the special needs of the caregiver in this dual role of both providing and needing care.

The effect on the family unit of caring for a client is profound, and it has given rise to the phrase, *caregiver's syndrome.* Family caregivers need an ongoing relationship with a knowledgeable health professional in the community who can provide information, support, and assistance (Videbeck, 2011). Adequate support in these areas promotes the well-being of caregivers and maximizes quality of life for the client.

The rise in the number of reported incidents of *elder abuse* or *dependent adult abuse* (emotional or physical abuse of an adult who is dependent on others for his or her care for financial, physical, or mental health reasons) is a major cause for concern. Inadequate knowledge, meager financial resources, and inadequate training or support for caregivers are some of the factors thought to influence this alarming trend.

If home care is being considered following an inpatient stay, the caregiver must be involved in the client's hospital treatment: this enables the caregiver to gain experience in providing care in a supportive environment and allows the nurse to assess the abilities and behaviors of the caregiver. The caregiver may show signs of emotional wear and tear, such as frustration, resentment, apathy, and inattention to personal needs. In a long-term home care situation, a frustrated caregiver may say, "No one asks how *I* am. He or she (the client) is the center of attention—what about me and my needs?" Primary nursing goals in working with caregivers include providing information, emotional support, and referrals for continued support in the community.

NURSING DIAGNOSES ADDRESSED IN THIS CARE PLAN
Caregiver Role Strain
Social Isolation

RELATED NURSING DIAGNOSES ADDRESSED IN THE MANUAL
Ineffective Role Performance
Interrupted Family Processes
Insomnia
Deficient Diversional Activity
Risk for Suicide
Risk for Other-Directed Violence
Deficit Knowledge

Nursing Diagnosis

Caregiver Role Strain
Difficulty in performing family/significant other caregiver role.

ASSESSMENT DATA

- Change in role or responsibility
- Lack of knowledge or needed skills in providing the client's care
- Intermittent apathy toward the client
- Ambivalence (feelings of resentment and guilt, as well as concern and care) toward the client
- Inattention to own needs
- Fatigue
- Conflict between caregiver role and other roles, for example, spouse or parent

EXPECTED OUTCOMES

Immediate

The caregiver will

- Participate in the care of the client within 2 to 4 days
- Verbalize knowledge of the client's treatment plan within 2 to 4 days
- Learn interactive and psychomotor skills needed for the client's care (e.g., identifying client needs, setting limits, feeding the client) within 4 to 5 days

Stabilization

The caregiver will

- Identify community and agency resources for assistance, if indicated
- Verbalize knowledge of the client's illness, care requirements, safe use of medications, and so forth

Community

The caregiver will

- Demonstrate needed psychomotor skills independently
- Follow through with plans for support after discharge

IMPLEMENTATION

Nursing Interventions *denotes collaborative interventions	Rationale
*Teach the caregiver and other family members or significant others about the client's illness, treatment, and medications. Discuss a care plan for home use that clearly defines the client's responsibilities and the caregiver's responsibilities.	Giving the caregiver(s) specific information will help clarify expectations of the client, caregiver(s), and others.
*Allow the caregiver to observe you working with the client during meals and other activities of daily living. Give the caregiver the rationale for the type and manner of assistance you provide the client.	The caregiver can learn techniques by watching you and practicing them with supervision. Understanding the rationale for care techniques can enhance the caregiver's success in providing effective care.
*Gradually increase the caregiver's responsibility for mealtimes and other activities of daily living until he or she is ready for the primary role in each area.	Gradual assumption of responsibility will enable the caregiver to feel less overwhelmed and to move at his or her own pace, which will enhance success.
*Help the caregiver identify potential hazards in the home.	The home situation must be physically safe for the client.
*If the client requires constant supervision at home, help the caregiver plan to do daily chores, errands, and recreational activities when someone else is available to stay with the client.	The caregiver must be able to manage the home and do necessary chores. Also, the caregiver needs periods of relief from constant involvement with the client.

IMPLEMENTATION (continued)

Nursing Interventions *denotes collaborative interventions	Rationale
*Discuss the client's safety needs with the caregiver. If possible, arrange a home care nurse visit to evaluate the home environment and make recommendations. Encourage the caregiver to remain aware of safety considerations as the client's condition changes.	The client's safety and the safety of others is a priority. The home environment may need to be altered for safety and the caregiver may need to learn to recognize the need for further changes or placing the client outside the home.
*Discourage the caregiver from making unnecessary changes in the client's immediate environment. Encourage the development of a routine for the client's activities at home. (This routine does not have to be strictly rigid, but it should have some structure.)	Familiar activities help the client to maintain reality orientation, which also helps the caregiver. The caregiver, however, needs to feel that some flexibility is acceptable so that he or she does not feel like a slave to the client and his or her routine.
*Encourage structure in care, hygiene, sleep, and activity. Caution the caregiver to avoid letting the client sleep whenever he or she desires, such as all day.	An established regular routine also allows the caregiver to meet his or her own need to sleep at night, which is important for the caregiver's health.
*Ask the caregiver about the client's previous bedtime routines, and encourage adherence to prior routines.	The client may be unable to provide this information. Replicating prior habits will enhance successful adherence in the future.
*Help the caregiver plan how to manage visitors at home (not too many in 1 day, preferably 1 or 2 people at a time, etc.).	The client will be less confused and be able to enjoy visitors more if he or she is not too fatigued by too many people at once. Too much stimulation can increase confusion or acting-out behavior.
*Remind the caregiver that the client's memory may be very poor and that this is out of the client's control.	Recognition of the client's memory impairment can help the caregiver avoid the frustration of repeated explanations and avoid expecting the client to work harder to remember.
*Remind the caregiver that the client is not a child. In fact, a child can be expected to learn to provide self-care independently—the client may not be able to do so.	When seeing childlike behaviors (such as the inability to dress oneself), it is easy to begin treating the client like a child. This must be avoided to preserve the client's dignity.
*Encourage the caregiver to discuss any feelings he or she may have about meeting the client's personal needs.	The caregiver may be repulsed or upset by the idea of an adult parent or family member needing help with bathing, dressing, and so forth.
*Encourage the caregiver to discuss feelings associated with role reversal. ("My mother used to help me dress when I was a child, and now I'm helping her get dressed.")	It may be difficult for the caregiver to see a parent, spouse, or partner (on whom the caregiver used to depend) become dependent on the caregiver.
*Assist the caregiver in identifying supportive resources in the community and on the Internet.	Resources can provide tangible support (e.g., respite care, meals, transportation) as well as emotional and informational support (e.g., caregiver Web sites).

Nursing Diagnosis

Social Isolation
Aloneness experienced by the individual and perceived as imposed by others and as a negative or threatening state.

ASSESSMENT DATA

- Disinterest in previous hobbies or other pleasurable activities
- Refusal to leave the client in the care of someone else
- Feelings of helplessness
- Feelings of frustration

- Absence of other support people
- Failure to use available resources
- Inadequate or ineffective coping skills

EXPECTED OUTCOMES

Immediate

The caregiver will

- Acknowledge his or her personal health needs (e.g., physical activity, social needs, rest, sleep) within 24 to 48 hours or one to three interactions with nursing staff
- Verbalize plans to meet his or her own needs independent of the caregiving situation within 3 to 4 days or three to four interactions with nursing staff
- Express feelings related to his or her unmet needs within 3 to 4 days or three to four interactions with nursing staff

Stabilization

The caregiver will

- Implement plans for using resources to help care for the client (e.g., contact agencies identified for services)
- Manage his or her own feelings regarding the client's behavior

Community

The caregiver will

- Implement plans to meet his or her own needs independent of the caregiving situation
- Use coping strategies to deal with stress without abusing alcohol or drugs (e.g., participate in a support group, express feelings to supportive friend or family member, increase physical activity)

IMPLEMENTATION

Nursing Interventions *denotes collaborative interventions	Rationale
*Encourage the caregiver to continue any activities in which the client can engage and feel successful and that the client and caregiver enjoy.	Enjoyable activities between the client and caregiver can enhance their relationship. Not all of the interactions between the client and the caregiver have to be centered on care and physical or emotional dependence.
*Remind the caregiver that inappropriate behaviors such as indiscriminate undressing and profanity are not within the client's conscious control; they are part of the illness.	Out of frustration, the caregiver may become angry with the client about his or her behavior. It is important that the caregiver make a distinction between the client and his or her behavior and deal with behaviors without punishing the client. The caregiver can then express anger to others and not become angry with the client.
*Encourage the caregiver to discuss his or her feelings of embarrassment related to the client's inappropriate social behavior.	The caregiver can use you as a sounding board—he or she may not be able to share these feelings with the client or other family members.
*Role-play with the caregiver to help him or her have a short explanation to give visitors or others regarding the client's behavior.	If the caregiver practices what to say and how to prepare others for the client's behavior, he or she can alleviate some of the shock or discomfort experienced when the client displays such behavior. The caregiver is less likely to become isolated if feelings of guilt or embarrassment are minimized.
*Encourage the caregiver to plan time away from home regularly to meet his or her own needs. The caregiver should not wait until the client is better or until the caregiver "can't take any more."	The caregiver needs to spend personal time away from the client regularly. Burnout can occur quickly if the caregiver has no relief.
Encourage the caregiver to engage in regular physical activity, outside or inside the home.	Physical activity will promote the caregiver's health and well-being. Simple home exercise equipment or video resources (e.g., interactive video exercise programs) can be used when the caregiver is unable to leave the client. When possible, walking with a neighbor or friend provides both physical activity and social contact.

IMPLEMENTATION (continued)

Nursing Interventions *denotes collaborative interventions	Rationale
*Teach the caregiver stress management principles and techniques.	The caregiver may be unaware of effective stress management techniques. Managing stress will enhance the caregiver's well-being and ability to care for the client.
*Refer the caregiver or family members to community or Internet resources as indicated by the client's problems or the caregiver's needs.	Community and Internet resources can offer support, information, and tangible help (e.g., respite care, meals, transportation).

SECTION 1 REVIEW QUESTIONS

1. During an admission interview the nurse learns that the client hasn't taken any medication for 3 weeks. Which of the following is the best initial response by the nurse?

   a. Don't you know your symptoms will return if you don't take your medication?

   b. Taking medication is a very important part of your treatment.

   c. Tell me what was happening when you stopped taking medication.

   d. Why would you stop taking your medication?

2. Which of the following is essential for successful discharge planning?

   a. Adequate client income

   b. Client participation in planning

   c. Follow-up medical appointments

   d. Support of family for the plan

3. Which of the following behaviors by the nurse would undermine building a trust relationship?

   a. Avoid giving feedback on negative behavior

   b. Being honest with the client at all times

   c. Meeting with the client on a regular schedule

   d. Setting limits on unacceptable behavior

4. Which of the following statements most likely indicates a Caregiver Role Strain?

   a. "It's difficult to see my mother's health going downhill."

   b. "No one else can care for my mother the way I do."

   c. "Sometimes I need to get away from caring for my father."

   d. "Taking care of my son is a tremendous responsibility."

SECTION 1 Recommended Readings

Buila, S. M., & Swanke, J. R. (2010). Patient-centered mental health care: Encouraging caregiver participation. *Care Management Journal, 11*(3), 146–150.

Gray, R., White, J., Schulz, M., & Abderhalden, C. (2010). Enhancing medication adherence in people with schizophrenia: An international programme of research. *International Journal of Mental Health Nursing, 19*(1), 36–44.

Jespersen, S., Chong, T., Donegan, T., Gray, K., Kudinoff, T., McGain, L., & Gant, D. (2009). Reflections on facilitated discharge from a mental health service. *Australasian Psychiatry, 17*(3), 195–201.

Stamino, V. R., Mariscal, S., Holter, M. C., Davidson, L. J., Cook, K. S., Fukui, S., & Rapp, C. A. (2010). Outcomes of an illness self-management group using wellness recovery action planning. *Psychiatric Rehabilitation Journal, 34*(1), 57–60.

SECTION 1 Resources for Additional Information

Visit thePoint (http://thePoint.lww.com/Schultz9e) for a list of these and other helpful Internet resources.

Family Caregiver Alliance
National Center on Elder Abuse
National Family Caregivers Association

SECTION TWO

Community-Based Care

For many years, the majority of mental health care was provided in the hospital setting. Since the 1970s, many clients have been treated in less restrictive or community-based settings. Although this trend has had many positive aspects, adequate funding for community programs as an alternative to inpatient care has not kept pace with the need. In addition, some clients with mental illness are reluctant to use community services, which adds to the number of people whose needs are not adequately met.

Individuals who enter inpatient treatment settings now are often acutely ill when they are admitted and have a relatively short length of stay. Inpatient care is primarily focused on stabilization of the client's symptoms or behavior, early and effective discharge planning, specific treatment planning with achievable, short-term goals, and referral to follow-up care in the community. Clients who are chronically mentally ill have a broad range of problems. Some clients have been discharged from a long-term hospital setting and may have been hospitalized as adults, with problems such as schizophrenia or bipolar disorder. Others may have been institutionalized in facilities for the developmentally disabled when they were children and have been discharged into the community as adults. In addition to the difficulties encountered because of a developmental disability or a major psychiatric illness, these clients may have special needs as a result of having lived in a long-term facility. Their basic needs may have been met by the staff of the institution, sometimes for many years; consequently, they have become very dependent. Often, they have minimal skills in meeting their own needs independently. These are skills that the community assumes that any adult can do, such as using the telephone or public transportation, buying groceries, preparing meals, doing laundry, and so forth. The inability of such clients to care for themselves in these ways may have nothing to do with their psychiatric illness or other disability, but may be the result of long-term institutional living without learning or practicing these skills.

Another segment of the chronically ill population, one that is rapidly expanding, includes clients who have not been in long-term care facilities for extended periods. Instead, they have lived in the community, either on their own or in an environment that is structured or supervised to some degree. Such clients often are intermittently admitted to acute care facilities and discharged to a community setting. They may or may not receive care on an outpatient basis between hospital admissions. Lacking adequate skills or abilities to live in the community, they often have costly rehospitalizations.

The care plans in this section are designed to assist nurses in providing care for chronically mentally ill clients in the hospital, during an acute episode of illness, and in the community setting between episodes of acute care, or addressing problems after long-term institutionalization.

CARE PLAN 6

Serious and Persistent Mental Illness

In the United States, more clients with serious and persistent mental illness (SPMI) are receiving care in the community than at any other time. This is related to the cost of hospitalization and to medications that control symptoms, enabling clients to return to the community setting earlier and remain in the community for longer periods.

People with SPMI are found across the adult life span, usually from 20 to 60 years of age. They experience "positive" symptoms of illness, such as delusions and hallucinations, which frequently determine the criterion for admission and discharge in the acute setting and usually respond in some degree to psychopharmacology. "Negative" symptoms, such as social withdrawal, anhedonia (inability to experience pleasure), anergy (lack of energy), and apathy, unfortunately often persist over time and do not necessarily respond to medications. The ongoing presence of these negative symptoms presents a major barrier to the client's recovery and improved functioning in the community.

Traditional methods of treatment often are unsuccessful with clients who are functionally impaired because these methods do not address the primary problems of this group. Clients with SPMI often lack skills for successful community living and typically are readmitted to hospitals because of frustration, stress, loneliness, and the poor quality of their lives, rather than the reemergence of positive psychiatric symptoms.

Skills needed for community living fall into five categories:

1. *Activities of daily living*: This includes personal hygiene, grooming, room care, laundry, restaurant use, cooking, shopping, budgeting, public transportation, telephone use, and procurement of needed services, and financial support. Clients may have difficulty in any or all of these areas, related to lack of knowledge, skill, experience, or support.
2. *Vocational skills*: This includes paid employment in a competitive or sheltered work setting, volunteer work, or any productive, useful service that the client perceives as making a contribution. Clients may lack specific work skills or good work habits, job-seeking or job-keeping skills, interest, or motivation.
3. *Leisure skills*: This includes the ability to choose, plan, and follow through with pleasurable activities during unstructured time. Clients may lack the interest or skills to fill their free time or may lack leisure habit patterns, such as taking a walk, reading the newspaper, and so forth.
4. *Health maintenance*: This includes managing medications, keeping appointments, preventing or treating physical illnesses, and crisis management. Clients with SPMI frequently use medications inappropriately or trade them with friends, use chemicals, or drink alcohol. These clients often do not recognize or seek treatment for physical illness, and they are reluctant to keep appointments due to denial of illness, lack of control over their lives, fear of hospitals and physicians, and so forth.
5. *Social skills*: This includes social conversation, dealing with landlords and service providers, talking about feelings and problems, and so forth. When clients have severe social skill deficits, they have increased difficulties in the other four areas, as well as the inability to maintain a state of well-being.

The ability to generalize knowledge frequently is impaired in clients with SPMI; learning skills in their own homes or communities eliminates that very difficult step. Outreach programs, in which practitioners go to the clients' own environments, have been most successful in helping clients develop needed skills. Settings like community support services and drop-in centers also have been more successful than traditional outpatient or hospital-based day programs. This also may be due to a "less clinical" approach and a lack of association with inpatient treatment.

In the community, people with SPMI usually have a case manager. It is important to communicate closely with the case manager during the client's hospital stay to facilitate achievement of treatment goals and to make the client's transition into the hospital and back to the community as smooth and "seamless" as possible.

NURSING DIAGNOSES ADDRESSED IN THIS CARE PLAN
Ineffective Health Maintenance
Impaired Social Interaction
Deficient Diversional Activity

RELATED NURSING DIAGNOSES ADDRESSED IN THE MANUAL
Chronic Low Self-Esteem
Impaired Home Maintenance
Disturbed Thought Processes
Ineffective Coping
Risk for Loneliness

Nursing Diagnosis

Ineffective Health Maintenance
Inability to identify, manage, and/or seek out help to maintain health.

ASSESSMENT DATA

* Lack of daily living skills
* Difficulty making choices
* Deficient problem-solving skills
* Apathy
* Anergy
* Low frustration tolerance

EXPECTED OUTCOMES

Immediate

The client will

* Communicate accurate information regarding symptoms, medication compliance, eating habits, and so forth within 24 hours
* Maintain contact with community professionals throughout hospitalization

Stabilization

The client will

* Participate in planning self-care
* Verbalize knowledge of illness, treatment, safe use of medications, and independent living skills

Community

The client will

* Seek medical treatment for health-related needs
* Demonstrate maintenance of safe home environment
* Demonstrate adherence to established daily routine
* Demonstrate adequate independence in activities of daily living

IMPLEMENTATION

Nursing Interventions *denotes collaborative interventions	Rationale
Review with the client the events that have led to increases in psychiatric symptoms or hospitalizations.	The client may not recognize the relationship between the need for hospitalization, particular health behaviors, and recurrence of the illness.
*Engage the client in mutual goal-setting, such as avoiding hospitalization, becoming more satisfied with his or her life, meeting needs, and so forth.	The client's willingness to participate is increased if he or she values the reasons for doing so.
Use an assertive approach when attempting to engage the client in a particular activity.	A positive attitude is conveyed with this approach. The client may respond to a tentative approach with a negative answer, and there will be no opportunity to proceed.
Be directive with the client, and do not ask "yes/no" questions or questions that require a choice. For example, say "It is time for group," rather than "Do you want to go to group?"	The client is likely to respond "no" to "yes/no" questions because of the negativism he or she feels, or it may simply seem easier not to do something.
Use a behavioral approach when teaching skills.	A behavioral approach decreases reliance on the client's verbal skills and ability to think abstractly and provides the client with the experience of doing the skill rather than simply hearing about how to do the skill.
Model the skill or behavior for the client.	Modeling provides a clear, concrete example of what is expected.
Coach the client to replicate the skill or behavior.	Coaching allows *shaping*—a behavioral procedure in which successive approximations of a desired behavior are positively reinforced—toward successful completion of the target behavior.
Prompt the client to continue practicing the skill or behavior. Reinforce success with verbal praise and tangible rewards, such as a soda, a snack, and so forth.	The client may need reminders because of a lack of interest or initiative. Coupling verbal praise with tangible rewards is the most successful means of reinforcement. It helps the client perpetuate the behavior or skill until it becomes part of his or her daily routine.
Teach the client a basic problem-solving sequence. It may help to write the steps.	Problem solving in a methodical fashion may be a skill the client has never had, or it may have been impaired by the illness.
Help the client establish a daily schedule. Writing on a daily or weekly calendar is usually helpful. Once the client agrees to a particular appointment or activity, instruct the client to write it on the calendar.	A written schedule provides a visual aid to which the client can refer. Once the client has written it on the calendar, it is more likely that he or she will follow through, much as with a written contract.
Assess the client for living skills that are absent or need improvement. Include hygiene, grooming, shopping, obtaining housing, budgeting, using telephones and transportation, cooking, and ability to call a doctor or other agencies for service.	A variety of skills are needed for independent living. It is imperative to identify deficient areas as the initial step of the learning process.
*Teach the client about cooking and requirements for adequate nutrition. Referral to a dietitian may be indicated.	The client may have little or no knowledge of nutritional needs or food preparation skills.
Have the client demonstrate skills if possible. If skills are assessed verbally, avoid asking "Do you know how to...?" Rather, say "Tell me how you...?"	Areas such as hygiene or grooming are easily assessed by the client's appearance, but skill demonstration may be necessary in areas such as use of telephone or transportation. If you ask the client if he or she has a particular skill, the response may be "yes" because the client is embarrassed at not having the skill or because the client mistakenly believes that he or she has the skill.

IMPLEMENTATION (continued)

Nursing Interventions *denotes collaborative interventions	Rationale
Teach skills in the client's own environment when possible. For example, if you are teaching how to do laundry, use the laundromat the client will use regularly.	Transferring or generalizing knowledge from one situation to another may be difficult for the client.
Instruct the client about signs of physical illness that require medical attention. Give specific parameters, such as a "fever of 102° F."	Specific indicators are easier for the client to recognize because the client's judgment often is ineffective.
*Assist the client to identify the clinic or physician services that he or she will contact if physical illness occurs.	It is easier to choose health care providers when the client is well, before an urgent situation develops. Knowing who to call when a need arises will help the client follow through.
*Encourage the client to discuss with his or her physician any difficulties with medications or needs for changes before the client initiates changes on his or her own.	This strategy allows the client to participate in managing his or her health and to meet perceived needs regarding medication changes.
Tell the client that if he or she does alter the pattern of medications without professional help, you would like him or her to report this honestly.	It is more important to have accurate information on which to base decisions than to create the illusion of a "good" patient.
Give the client positive feedback for attempts in the self-care area and for honesty in reporting.	Even if attempts at self-care are unsuccessful initially, it is important to reinforce the client's sense of personal control over his or her life and honesty in relationships with health care providers.
*Teach the client and the family and significant others, if any, about the client's illness, treatment, and safe use of medications.	The client and significant others may have little or no knowledge of the client's illness, treatment, or medications.

Nursing Diagnosis

Impaired Social Interaction
Insufficient or excessive quantity or ineffective quality of social exchange.

ASSESSMENT DATA

- Feelings of worthlessness
- Difficulty initiating interaction
- Lack of social skills
- Social withdrawal
- Low self-esteem
- Absence of available significant others

EXPECTED OUTCOMES

Immediate The client will

- Engage in social interactions with nursing assistance within 24 hours
- Demonstrate acceptance of feedback from others within 24 to 48 hours

Stabilization The client will

- Continue to participate in social activities
- Verbalize decreased anxiety during social interactions

Community The client will

- Communicate with others in sufficient quantity to meet basic needs
- Verbalize increased feelings of self-worth

IMPLEMENTATION

Nursing Interventions *denotes collaborative interventions	Rationale
Teach the client appropriate interactive and social skills. Describe and demonstrate specific skills, such as eye contact, attentive listening, nodding, and so forth. Discuss basic manners (please, thank you), especially in making requests. Discuss topics appropriate for casual social conversation, such as the weather, local events, news, and so forth.	The client may have little or no knowledge of social interaction skills. Use of basic manners will result in more successful interactions for the client. Modeling provides a concrete example of the desired skills.
*Assist the client to approach someone and ask a question or make a request. Use real-life situations, such as seeking assistance in a store, asking directions, or renting an apartment.	Asking questions is an essential skill in daily life. Using real situations makes the exercise more meaningful for the client.
*Role-play situations in which the client must accept "no" to a request and in which the client must appropriately refuse a request from someone else.	Low frustration tolerance makes hearing a negative answer difficult for the client. Clients frequently comply with requests from others, and then regret doing so because they are unable to refuse in a socially appropriate manner.
Practice giving and receiving compliments with the client. Make sure compliments are sincere.	Chronically mentally ill clients rarely notice things about other people without practicing that skill. Receiving compliments can be awkward due to low self-esteem.
Facilitate the client's practicing interactions, requests, and conversations with other clients as well as staff.	Varying the client's exposure to others in social situations can help build the client's confidence and comfort level in approaching and dealing with other people.

Nursing Diagnosis

Deficient Diversional Activity

Decreased stimulation from (or interest or engagement in) recreational or leisure activities.

ASSESSMENT DATA

- Anhedonia
- Inattentiveness
- Feelings of boredom
- Expressed desire for purposeful activity
- Lack of leisure skills
- Inability to manage unstructured time

EXPECTED OUTCOMES

Immediate   The client will

- Participate in leisure activities organized by others within 24 to 48 hours
- Express feelings of satisfaction with a leisure activity within 2 to 3 days

Stabilization   The client will

- Prepare a list of activities to pursue in the community, such as taking walks, going to a library, and so forth
- Develop a schedule that includes leisure activities

Community   The client will

- Engage in leisure activities independently
- Participate in productive activities

IMPLEMENTATION

Nursing Interventions *denotes collaborative interventions	Rationale
Encourage the client to develop leisure habits, such as reading the newspaper or watching television at a certain time each day. It may be beneficial for the client to write these activities on a daily schedule.	Lack of interest or past pleasure experiences causes clients to be reluctant to try activities. Establishing habits or a schedule eliminates the need to make a decision about whether or not to pursue an activity each day.
Introduce the client to activities that are suitable for one person, such as drawing, solitaire, reading, writing, or sketching in a journal.	The client needs to have some leisure activities to pursue independently for those times when other people are not available.
Assist the client in identifying and trying activities that are free or low cost, such as taking walks, attending free concerts, and so forth.	Chronically mentally ill clients usually have limited financial resources. The cost of movies, bowling, or independent transportation can be prohibitive.
Facilitate client's interactions and relationships with other clients as well as staff.	Varying the client's exposure to others in social situations can help build the client's confidence and comfort level in approaching and dealing with other people.
*Facilitate the client's interactions with others outside the hospital setting. If a drop-in center or other service is available, accompany the client to acquaint him or her with others. Plan a group activity that three or four clients attend.	It is important for the client to establish a social network because professionals cannot meet all of the person's needs. The client is not likely to form relationships independently.
*Assist the client in finding a suitable volunteer activity or an activity involving helping other people, animals, or the environment. Refer to vocational services as appropriate.	Many clients resist doing things just for fun because these activities do not provide a sense of productivity or making a contribution. Feeling useful or needed enhances self-esteem and provides an opportunity for praise or recognition from others.

CARE PLAN 7

Acute Episode Care

Clients with SPMI living in the community may need periodic short-term hospitalizations or extended supervision in a sheltered setting due to an exacerbation of psychiatric symptoms or a lack of success in community living. This is often related to failure to take medication as prescribed or to disordered water balance (DWB). DWB, also called psychogenic polydipsia, can lead to water intoxication and has become a major management problem for many clients with SPMI. The types of services the client needs for success may not exist in the community or may have waiting lists, and financial difficulties due to lack of successful employment or limited governmental support usually complicate the client's problems.

Psychiatric treatment and nursing care of clients with SPMI usually focus on minimizing inpatient hospitalization, maximizing client self-reliance, decreasing dependence on institutions and services, and placing the client in the community in the least restrictive environment.

Research has shown that interventions designed to promote social support improve the quality of life in the community and improve the functional abilities of the client are strongly correlated with a decreased need for rehospitalization. Different groups of clients have varying needs, and one of the challenges in community care is identifying the interventions associated with success for a particular group. Socialization, housing, crisis intervention, integrated medical services, vocational rehabilitation, and individually tailored plans have been successful (Bartels & Pratt, 2009; Mohamed, Neale, & Rosenheck, 2009) Nurses must work closely with the client's case manager, community agencies, and other community resources to achieve these objectives.

It can be frustrating to see the client return to the hospital setting repeatedly after careful planning for follow-up or placement. Although it may be challenging, it is necessary to take a "fresh look" at the client's behavior, problems, and situation with each admission to provide effective care and promote the client's chances for future success. The nurse must be aware of his or her attitudes toward the client with SPMI. One pitfall in working with these clients is failing to view the client as an adult, especially if the client exhibits immature or attention-seeking behavior. It also is important not to see the client's readmissions as failures of the staff or of the client.

NURSING DIAGNOSES ADDRESSED IN THIS CARE PLAN
Risk-Prone Health Behavior
Ineffective Self-Health Management
Ineffective Health Maintenance

RELATED NURSING DIAGNOSES ADDRESSED IN THE MANUAL
Disturbed Thought Processes
Disturbed Sensory Perception (Specify: Visual, Auditory, Kinesthetic, Gustatory, Tactile, Olfactory)
Risk for Injury

Nursing Diagnosis

Risk-Prone Health Behavior

Impaired ability to modify lifestyle/behaviors in a manner that improves health status.

ASSESSMENT DATA

- Poor impulse control
- Difficulty making decisions and choices
- Limited ability to deal with stress or changes
- Feelings of fear, hopelessness, and inadequacy
- Low self-esteem
- Anxiety

EXPECTED OUTCOMES

Immediate

The client will

- Be free of injury throughout hospitalization
- Demonstrate decreased acting-out behavior within 24 to 48 hours
- Verbally express feelings of fear, hopelessness, inadequacy, if present, with nursing assistance, within 24 to 48 hours

Stabilization

The client will

- Return to the community to the least restrictive environment that is safe
- Establish supportive relationships in the community setting

Community

The client will

- Use relationships in the community to meet needs
- Maintain community placement or move to a more independent setting

IMPLEMENTATION

Nursing Interventions *denotes collaborative interventions	Rationale
Ask the client about any ideas or plans for suicide.	The client's safety is a priority.
Remove any potentially harmful objects from the client's possession (razor, nail file, etc.).	These items may be used for self-destructive actions or acting out toward others.
Remove the client to a quiet area or seclusion if he or she is acting out.	Acting-out behavior usually decreases when the client is alone or has no one to pay attention to the behavior.
Withdraw your attention when the client is acting out if it is safe to do so. Tell the client that you will return when he or she is more in control.	Your inattention to the client's behavior will facilitate the extinction of the behavior. Your stated intent to return conveys your acceptance of the client.
Encourage the client to talk about his or her feelings when the client is not upset or acting out.	The client will be better able to verbalize feelings when he or she is in control of his or her behavior.
As the client gains skill in discussing feelings, encourage the client to talk with someone when he or she begins to become upset rather than acting out.	After the client is able to verbalize feelings, he or she can begin to use expression of feelings to replace acting out.
Teach the client a step-by-step problem-solving process. For example, identify the problem, examine alternatives, weigh the pros and cons of each alternative, select and implement an approach, and evaluate the results.	The client may not know the steps of a logical, orderly process to solve problems. The ability to use the problem-solving process in real-life situations is a useful skill and provides opportunities for the client to have successful experiences.

(continued on page 70)

IMPLEMENTATION (continued)

Nursing Interventions *denotes collaborative interventions	Rationale
*Assist the client to approach someone and ask a question or make a request for assistance. Use real-life situations, such as seeking assistance in a clinic, refilling a prescription, or making an appointment with a health care professional.	If the client lacks these skills, it is more likely that he or she will not access appropriate care when needed. Using real situations makes the exercise more meaningful for the client.
*Assist the client in identifying the resources he or she will access in the community, for example, his or her case manager, pharmacy, support groups, physician, and so forth. Assist the client to make a list with contact information for each resource identified.	Having resource and contact information readily available will facilitate the client's ability to access needed care and support.

Nursing Diagnosis

Ineffective Self-Health Management

Pattern of regulating and integrating into daily living a therapeutic regimen for the treatment of illness and its sequelae that is unsatisfactory for meeting specific health goals.

ASSESSMENT DATA

- Noncompliance with prescribed medications
- Psychogenic polydipsia (excessive intake of water or other fluids)
- Increase or worsening of psychiatric symptoms
- Lack of knowledge or understanding of therapeutic regimen

EXPECTED OUTCOMES

Immediate   The client will

- Ingest all medications as given throughout hospitalization
- Establish fluid intake–output balance within 2 to 3 days

Stabilization   The client will

- Verbalize intent to comply or demonstrate ingestion of prescribed medication
- Demonstrate ability to monitor own fluid intake without staff intervention

Community   The client will

- Take medications as prescribed or seek needed changes from health care providers
- Consume fluids within safe, established guidelines

IMPLEMENTATION

Nursing Interventions *denotes collaborative interventions	Rationale
Observe the client closely to ensure ingestion of medications.	The client must ingest medications as prescribed before their effectiveness can be determined.
Explore the client's reasons for noncompliance with medications: Is the client resistant to taking medications? Can the client afford the medication? Does the client forget to take it?	Identifying the reason for noncompliance will determine your interventions to gain the client's compliance.
*If the client cannot afford to purchase the medication, refer him or her to social services for help to obtain financial assistance.	The client may need financial assistance if that is a significant barrier to compliance.

IMPLEMENTATION (continued)

Nursing Interventions *denotes collaborative interventions	Rationale
If the client cannot remember to take medications, set up a system with him or her to check off the medication times or use a pill box with separate compartments for each dose.	A concrete system for taking medications minimizes problems the client has with trying to remember without being reminded.
*If the client is resistant to taking daily medications, discuss with the physician about the use of long-acting intramuscular medications or attempting to manage without medications.	Noncompliance due to resistance is the most difficult to change. The client does have the right to refuse medications. It is preferable to know that the client is not taking medication rather than to assume compliance.
*Teach the client and his or her family or significant others, if any, about polydipsia or DWB.	The client and his or her significant others may lack knowledge about the severe medical consequences of DWB or may fail to understand how drinking water (or other "harmless" fluids) could be a problem.
If the client is severely water "intoxicated," medical treatment may be required. The client may require seclusion and be allowed only supervised access to water.	Severe water intoxication causes confusion, increased psychosis, hyponatremia, lethargy, and seizures. The client must be "dried out" to a normal baseline of fluid balance before he or she can benefit from any teaching to learn self-control of water intake.
If the client is able to monitor his or her own weight, a target weight protocol can be used in the management of DWB. The client is taught to regulate fluid intake to keep his or her weight under a preset "target" of no more than a 7% weight increase on a day-to-day basis.	Clients with the internal control to regulate water consumption based on the frequent monitoring of body weight have been reported to have success in preventing further episodes of water intoxication (Goldman, 2009).
Setting a designated amount of fluid to be consumed every 30 to 60 minutes throughout the day can be effective in managing DWB. Assist the client to use a checklist to monitor fluid intake.	This structured approach can be useful with clients experiencing difficulty delaying gratification related to drinking fluids, or making decisions about whether or not to drink fluids, how much to drink, and so forth.
If the client experiences anxiety in concert with the desire for increased fluids, teach the client a relaxation technique, such as progressive muscle relaxation.	Relieving the client's anxiety will enhance the ability to resist drinking increased amounts of fluid.
Offer the client calorie-free gum or hard candy if he or she complains of excessive thirst.	Calorie-free gum or hard candy can help the client limit fluid intake.
*Assess the client's use of alcohol or other chemicals. If chemical use is a major problem for the client, consider a referral to a treatment program.	Alcohol and other mood-altering drugs can interfere with the effectiveness of the client's prescribed medication, fluid and electrolyte balance, and general health status.

Nursing Diagnosis

Ineffective Health Maintenance
Inability to identify, manage, and/or seek help to maintain health.

ASSESSMENT DATA

- Lack of independent living skills
- Lack of social skills
- Difficulty handling unstructured time
- Poor nutritional intake
- Lack of or ineffective interpersonal relationships

EXPECTED OUTCOMES

Immediate	The client will
	• Participate in performance of personal hygiene within 24 hours • Eat appropriate, nutritious foods with nursing guidance within 2 to 3 days • Participate in activities or hobbies within 2 to 3 days
Stabilization	The client will
	• Demonstrate adequate personal hygiene skills • Verbalize plans for use of unstructured time, such as walking or going to a community center • Demonstrate basic independent living skills, such as using public transportation
Community	The client will
	• Participate in planned programs, such as vocational or sheltered workshops, recreational or outpatient groups, or community support services • Perform needed activities consistently to maintain community living

IMPLEMENTATION

Nursing Interventions *denotes collaborative interventions	Rationale
Indicate your expectation at the beginning of the hospitalization that the client will return to the community setting.	Your positive approach may help decrease the client's dependence on an institution.
Do not allow the client to become too settled in the hospitalization. Always focus on the client's achievement of expected outcomes and eventual discharge. The client who returns frequently to the hospital should not be greeted as a friend but as a person who is hospitalized on a short-term basis for specific reasons.	The client's hospitalization must be focused on therapeutic work toward expected outcomes and discharge. If the client views hospitalization as a comfortable rest from the challenges of life, he or she is more likely to become dependent on the institution and the staff and less likely to participate in treatment and work toward discharge as a goal.
Encourage the client to develop routines for personal hygiene and grooming activities. Establishing a written schedule for some activities (e.g., bathing, washing hair) may be helpful.	The client is more likely to follow through if he or she is following a routine rather than having to decide each time whether or not to bathe, change clothes, wash hair, and so forth.
Give the client honest praise for accomplishments.	Positive feedback for independent skills will increase the frequency of the behavior and enhance the client's self-esteem.
Encourage the client to eat nutritious meals. Assess the client's selection of food at mealtimes.	You will be able to evaluate the client's knowledge about basic foods needed for a nutritious diet.
*Assess the client's situation with regard to food, cooking, shopping, and so forth. Refer the client to services (such as community centers that serve meals, home-delivered meal services) as appropriate.	The client's ability to procure and prepare nutritious food may be impaired.
*Teach the client about basic nutrition and how to choose more healthful foods. Consultation with a dietitian, if available, may be helpful.	The client may lack knowledge about the nutritional value or health implications of foods. Making better food choices will help the client maintain a better level of overall health.
Help the client plan meals in advance, perhaps for 1 week. Consider the client's food preparation skills and income; does he or she receive financial assistance for food?	Making a plan and following through each week will help the client budget enough money for nutritious food and will avoid the necessity for daily decisions about what to eat.
Assess the client's ability to perform essential daily skills, such as using the telephone book, using the transportation system, knowing how to get emergency assistance, and so forth. Have the client demonstrate these skills when possible.	Assessing the client's skill level will determine how well he or she performs certain skills and help you determine the interventions needed. Demonstrations are helpful because the client may be unable to explain what he or she can do, or the client may say "I know that" because he or she is too embarrassed to admit a knowledge deficit.

IMPLEMENTATION (continued)

Nursing Interventions *denotes collaborative interventions	Rationale
For any skill, the client needs to learn and give simple step-by-step directions.	Small parts of a task are easier to learn than tackling the whole task at once.
Perform the skill with the client initially, and gradually progress to the client's independent performance of the skill.	It may be easier for the client to learn the skill by observing how it is done before he or she can progress to independence.
*Involve the client in social interactions with others to practice social skills. The client may need to learn what topics generally are acceptable for social conversation.	You can be a role model for the client in social interchanges. The client may need to learn to avoid certain topics when in social situations, for example, not discussing hospitalizations when he or she first meets someone.
Ask the client to describe what he or she does during a usual day, week, and weekend. Writing down the activities may be helpful.	You can obtain data regarding the amount of unstructured time the client has available.
Assess the client's previous level of interest and participation in leisure or recreational activities.	If you can build on previous interests, it may be easier to obtain the client's involvement.
Explore possible alternatives for "fun" activities. Help the client try new activities. Keep in mind the cost of the activity and whether it requires the participation of other people.	The client may not have had many successful leisure activities. It would be frustrating to the client to begin a new hobby that he or she could not afford or to learn card games or board games if most of the client's leisure time is solitary.
Encourage the client to engage in daily physical activity, such as walking for at least 30 to 45 minutes each day.	Daily physical activity provides many health benefits, as well as a low-cost leisure activity.
Help the client make a specific plan for unstructured time, including activities alone or with others, leisure activities, or whatever the client desires.	Structuring his or her time will decrease the chance of the client ruminating and becoming more isolated.
*Help the client make plans to deal with changes or problems that may occur while he or she is living in the community. Role-playing might be helpful. Work with the client's community case manager if available.	If the client has an idea of what he or she can anticipate and alternative ways to deal with stress or change, he or she is less likely to return to the hospital as soon as he or she encounters any crisis.

CARE PLAN 8

Partial Community Support

Partial hospitalization and home care programs are widely regarded as representing cost-effective alternatives to inpatient hospitalization. As the US health care system continues to search for cost containment, the use of less costly forms of treatment for mental health problems, such as day treatment or brief respite stays in sheltered community settings, will continue to be emphasized, and more clients can be anticipated to need transitional services as a result of shortened inpatient lengths of stay.

Some clients in partial care will need continued support for an extended time, although it may decrease in frequency or intensity over time. Others need partial hospitalization or home care as a transitional step between an inpatient facility and independent living, or as a less costly alternative to inpatient hospitalization.

Partial hospitalization programs are designed to help clients make a gradual transition from the inpatient setting to living more independently. In day treatment programs, clients return home at night; evening programs are just the reverse. Services in partial programs can vary, but usually include groups for building communication and social skills, problem-solving, medication management, and education. These programs may also offer individual counseling, vocational assistance, and occupational or recreation therapy (Videbeck, 2011).

Partial hospitalization includes day hospitalization, day treatment, and day care programs. Day hospitalization and day treatment programs usually offer more intensive treatment (including crisis care) than day care programs, which focus more on educational, supportive, and rehabilitation needs. The intensity of partial hospitalization programs can meet the needs of some clients who might otherwise require inpatient care, and can result in decreased symptoms, fewer hospitalizations, improved community functioning, and greater satisfaction with services. The structure of day treatment or day care programs can be helpful to clients in transition from inpatient treatment, as well as to clients who need continued structure to maintain community living. Partial hospitalization programs may be offered at various hours (e.g., day, evening, weekends, or overnight) to meet clients' needs for treatment and support while encouraging participation in their community, jobs, school, and so on.

Residential treatment settings offer a wide variety of services, depending on the particular setting. Some offer transitional housing and programs with the expectation that residents will progress to more independence. Other programs offer services for as long as they are needed, even years. Board-and-care homes offer housing, laundry facilities, and one common meal a day, but rarely provide programming. Adult foster homes may care for one to three individuals with mental illness in a family-like atmosphere, including meals and social activities with the family. Halfway houses serve as a temporary placement that provides programming and support as the client prepares for independent living. Group homes usually house 6 to 10 residents who take turns cooking meals and share household chores under the supervision of one or two staff members. Independent living programs are often housed in an apartment complex, where clients share an apartment. Staff members are available to provide crisis intervention, transportation, assistance with finances or other tasks of daily living, drug monitoring, and referrals to other programs and medical services.

Psychiatric or psychosocial rehabilitation programs may be connected to housing arrangements. These services go beyond symptom control and medication management to focus on personal growth, client empowerment, reintegration into the community, and improved quality of life. Community support services include drop-in centers, organized social and educational programs, vocational programs, and assistance with the wide variety of skills and activities needed to live successfully in the community. The clubhouse model, pioneered by Fountain House in New York, is based on four guaranteed rights of members: a place to come to, meaningful work, meaningful relationships, and a place to return to, a lifetime membership.

Assertive community treatment (ACT) is one of the most effective community-based approaches for persons with mental illness. An ACT program has a problem-solving orientation; staff members attend to specific life issues, no matter how mundane. Most services are provided directly rather than relying on referrals to other programs or agencies, and they take place in the client's home or community, not in an office. ACT services are more intense than some other types of programs with three or more face-to-face weekly contacts that are tailored to meet the client's needs. The team approach allows all staff to be equally familiar with all clients, so clients do not have to wait for an assigned staff member. ACT programs also make a long-term commitment to clients, providing services for as long as the need persists, with no time restraints.

Psychiatric home care services offer treatment to clients who are homebound for physical or psychiatric reasons. These services vary in frequency and intensity, and the client's "home" environment may be a hotel room, family home, board and care facility, sheltered living situation, or another residential facility.

It is important to remember that the eventual goal is the client's optimal level of functioning and, if possible, independence from care, even community-based care. Planning for discharge from partial support programs is as much an essential focus as it is for inpatient care.

Many clients living in the community have case managers, whose role is to help these clients obtain or continue treatment, with an emphasis on community settings. The client's case manager may be provided by a health plan, a local government agency (e.g., public health department), or another facility. If possible, the nurse should try to work closely with the case manager to coordinate care planning and resources. If the client does not have an identified case manager, the nurse providing community-based care often assumes this role, including coordinating care, facilitating communication among care providers, identifying appropriate services and resources, supervising nonprofessional caregivers (e.g., in the home care setting), acting as a client advocate (e.g., vis-à-vis payers and service organizations), and making referrals. An interdisciplinary approach to care is especially important in the community setting; the nurse works in collaboration with psychiatrists and other health care providers to plan, provide, evaluate, and revise the client's care. It is important for the nurse to work with the client's community case manager, if any, and the interdisciplinary treatment team to identify and remain aware of all of the types of placement, program, and service resources available to clients in their community and those that can be accessed from their community. Medication management and educating the client and significant others are key components of nursing care in the home setting. Home care provides an opportunity to identify factors that may be contributing to the client's illness, reinforcing problems (e.g., secondary gains), or interfering with progress, and to gain a more complete picture of the client's strengths and sources of support. The nurse also can more fully explore cultural factors relevant to the client's care and functioning in the community. It is especially important to be culturally sensitive in the client's home environment and to be aware of your own reactions and behaviors there.

Important therapeutic goals with clients in partial care include promoting the client's safety and ability to function in the community, promoting compliance with the treatment plan and medications, improving the client's social skills, and decreasing feelings of hopelessness and loneliness. Remember that a client who has few social contacts may not necessarily experience loneliness; that is, if the client is not dissatisfied with limited social activity, he or she may not need interventions to diminish loneliness. However, the client does need to have sufficient interpersonal skills to succeed in daily living activities, and needs to develop these as fully as possible to foster optimal independence.

NURSING DIAGNOSES ADDRESSED IN THIS CARE PLAN
Ineffective Health Maintenance
Risk for Loneliness

RELATED NURSING DIAGNOSES ADDRESSED IN THE MANUAL
Ineffective Coping
Ineffective Self-Health Management
Impaired Home Maintenance
Impaired Social Interaction

Nursing Diagnosis

Ineffective Health Maintenance

Inability to identify, manage, and/or seek out help to maintain health.

ASSESSMENT DATA

- Self-care deficits
- Inadequate independent living skills
- Inadequate social skills
- Ineffective personal and family relationships
- Ineffective management of leisure or unstructured time
- Inadequate compliance with medication or therapeutic regimen
- Inadequate social support
- Inadequate financial resources or inability to manage finances
- Need for continued psychiatric treatment and/or follow-up

EXPECTED OUTCOMES

Immediate

The client will

- Actively participate in partial hospitalization or home treatment program within 24 to 48 hours
- Participate in leisure activities within the program setting within 2 to 3 days

Stabilization

The client will

- Demonstrate skill development, medication compliance, and improved interpersonal interactions
- Demonstrate needed community living skills, such as shopping, cooking, and so forth
- Verbalize plans for problem-solving and managing change

Community

The client will

- Demonstrate adequate social skills and use of leisure time
- Manage medications and therapeutic recommendations independently
- Implement problem-solving skills in the community

IMPLEMENTATION

Nursing Interventions *denotes collaborative interventions	Rationale
Monitor the client's physical health status and response to medications.	The client's physical health is a priority and may affect his or her mental health status.
*Assess the client's level of independence in self-care and community living skills. Assist the client or instruct caregiver(s) to help the client do things that he or she is not yet independent in doing. Caution caregivers about doing things for the client that he or she can do. Discuss the concepts of the client working toward maximum functioning and independence, secondary gain, and positive expectations for the client's behavior, progress, and eventual independent functioning, as appropriate. Teach caregivers a stepwise approach to the client, gradually handing over more responsibility for self-care.	The client's highest level of independent living is the goal. Caregivers may not understand the concepts of the client's eventual independence, secondary gain, and so forth, and may need to learn about how to help the client progress toward self-sufficiency.
*Assess the client's situation with regard to food, cooking, shopping, and so forth. Refer the client to services (such as community centers that serve meals, home-delivered meal services), as appropriate.	The client's ability to procure and prepare nutritious food may be impaired.

IMPLEMENTATION (continued)

Nursing Interventions *denotes collaborative interventions	Rationale
*Teach the client about basic nutrition and how to choose more healthful foods. Consultation with a dietitian, if available, may be helpful.	The client may lack knowledge about the nutritional value or health implications of foods. Making better food choices will help the client maintain a better level of overall health.
*Assess the client's home environment regarding safety issues, including repairs that may be needed (e.g., unsafe stairway) and security (e.g., locks on doors and windows).	The client's ability to assess safety needs may be impaired. The client's safety is a priority.
*Assess the client's transportation needs and resources, especially transportation to and from treatment, physician appointments, obtaining necessary items (e.g., medications, food), and leisure activity opportunities. Make referrals to community resources or social services as needed. Teach the client about using public transportation or transportation services, as appropriate.	The client's ability to comply with continued treatment and medications and to develop community living skills will be impaired if he or she cannot obtain needed transportation. The client may have no knowledge of or experience with public transportation, services, and so on.
Teach the client a simple problem-solving process: identify the problem, consider possible solutions, evaluate these alternatives, select and implement a solution, and evaluate the effectiveness of the solution. Teach the client how to adapt this process for decision making as well.	The client may never have learned a logical approach to problem solving or decision making. These skills are needed for successful community living.
*Help the client use these processes in situations that arise in the home, community life, job, and so forth. Coach the client through the steps of the process in actual situations at first, and then have the client practice the process more and more independently.	The client will learn more effectively if he or she can apply learning to actual life situations.
*Help the client identify appropriate people to contact in the event of a crisis or immediate need. Assist the client as necessary to write down these names and telephone numbers, including a number the client can call to contact someone for help 24 hours a day. Identify a place in the client's environment (such as in the client's home or room) to keep this information and care-related items (such as medication box, calendar for appointments, etc.).	The client's anxiety can be diminished if he or she knows how to obtain help. Simple information that is kept in a consistent place can help the client be successful in remembering and using the information appropriately. The client may be able to avoid unnecessary emergency room visits by contacting identified providers when he or she has a problem or need.
Teach the client about basic manners and social skills, such as how to interact with merchants, prospective landlords and employers, how to eat in restaurants, and so on.	These skills are important for successful community living. The client may never have learned these behaviors, or they may be impaired as a function of the client's illness.
*Use role-modeling and practice sessions, first on a one-on-one basis, then in small groups. Encourage the client to practice skills with other clients or family members, then to use them in real situations.	The client can learn in a nonthreatening atmosphere, and then gradually apply skills in more challenging situations.
At the end of each visit or contact with the client, review with the client his or her plans for the time until the client's next treatment episode. For example, ask the client, "What do you need to do to get through the night until you come back tomorrow?" or "What will you do tomorrow before I see you in the afternoon?"	If the client is anxious about being on his or her own between contacts, helping the client anticipate both the interim activities and the fact that contact will be reestablished can help decrease anxiety.
*Teach the client about seeking a job, interviewing skills, and appropriate behavior at work, both paid and volunteer. Refer the client to a vocational counselor if possible. Encourage the client to seek part-time work initially if he or she has not been employed recently.	The client may lack skills with which to find and perform in a job. Part-time or volunteer work can allow a client to become accustomed to the structure and expectations of a work environment more gradually than full-time employment.

(continued on page 78)

IMPLEMENTATION (continued)

Nursing Interventions *denotes collaborative interventions	Rationale
Teach the client about basic money management (e.g., bank accounts, check cashing, paying rent and bills, budgeting), using the telephone, and shopping for food and other items.	These skills are necessary for successful independent living. The client may be vulnerable to others' trying to take advantage of him or her, and will benefit from knowing how to handle these situations.
*Monitor the client's medication regimen. Ask the client if he or she has an adequate supply of medication. In the client's home, ask the client to show you the medications, assist the client in filling the medication box, or check it if the client is able to fill it independently; ask the client about beneficial effects of the medication and any side effects. Enlist the help of the client's caregivers in monitoring and encouraging compliance with the medication regimen, if necessary.	One of the primary causes of hospital readmission is clients' noncompliance with medications. Structure and reinforcement can help the client continue taking medications correctly.
Teach the client the name of the medication(s), its purpose, desired effects, time frame for effects (e.g., some antidepressants may take weeks to achieve the full desired effect), side effects, signs of toxicity, dosage, and times to take the medication.	The client is more likely to be safe and comply with medications if he or she understands these aspects.
*Tell the client when to call the nurse or physician, for example, for specific toxic effects or if the client has unpleasant side effects and wants to discontinue the medication.	The client needs this information to take medications safely. The client may not be aware that, if a medication causes unpleasant side effects, an alternative often can be found that will provide a similar therapeutic effect and enable the client to continue receiving the benefit of medication treatment.
*If the client is experiencing unpleasant side effects, talk with the client's physician about possible alternative regimens (e.g., take sedating medications at night) or medications.	These measures can assist the client in continuing to take the medications. Often an alternative medication may be better tolerated by the client.
Use simple written information to support teaching about medications and other issues.	Written information can support the client's learning if it is at the appropriate literacy level and does not overwhelm the client with too much information or complexity.
Talk with the client about the importance of continuing to take the medication as prescribed, despite feeling better or despite certain side effects.	Many clients with psychiatric illnesses discontinue their medications because they experience unpleasant side effects, or because they "feel better" and do not understand the need for maintenance of medication therapy.
Ask the client to give you his or her understanding of information, and ask whether he or she is having any difficulties with compliance (if it is an established medication) or whether he or she sees any barriers to compliance (if it is a new medication).	Asking for the client's understanding and perspective will help you assess the degree to which the client has learned the information and his or her feelings about it.
Give the client positive feedback when he or she is compliant with medications, treatment, keeping appointments, learning skills, and so forth, even if success is partial or if the client simply attempts to follow the plan.	Positive feedback can help develop desired behaviors and enhance the client's self-esteem.
Caution the client against changing the medication regimen, trading medications with other clients, or taking additional medications (e.g., medications the client has taken in the past or over-the-counter drugs). Explain the possible consequences of not taking medications or of taking nonprescribed medications.	These behaviors are common ways in which a client can disturb the medication regimen.

IMPLEMENTATION (continued)

Nursing Interventions *denotes collaborative interventions	Rationale
Encourage the client to discuss these issues; stress that honest reporting is most helpful to successful treatment. Give the client positive feedback if he or she brings up these issues.	It is not helpful for the nurse to have incomplete or false information regarding a client's self-care.
Use a written contract with client to enhance compliance with a treatment or medication regimen.	Some clients respond well to the structure and commitment implied by a written contract.
Help the client develop a structure for his or her time that incorporates treatment, medication regimen, work, household chores, leisure activities, and so forth. Help the client learn to use lists (e.g., to manage tasks), a calendar (e.g., to provide date orientation and to record appointments), and so forth.	Following a structured routine can diminish feelings of purposelessness and helplessness. The client also can avoid having to make decisions about whether or not to do each activity each day if he or she is accustomed to a daily routine. The client's organizational skills may be impaired; these tools can help the client succeed with multiple tasks.
*Coordinate referrals to other professional, supportive care, and community resources, such as social services, church or clergy, and recreational programs.	The client's ability to identify and gain access to resources is impaired.
*As the client progresses toward discharge from partial services, make a (written) plan with the client regarding how to identify increasing symptoms, what to do if the client becomes physically ill, who to contact for help in the future, and so on.	A written plan can help diminish the client's anxiety and ensure that he or she will seek help before problems become too severe.
*If you will be terminating your relationship with the client, but the client is to receive services from a new provider, introduce the client to the new provider if possible, before you end your relationship with the client.	Remember that the client's ability to form relationships is impaired. Meeting the new provider with your support can help ensure that the client will continue treatment despite a change in relationships.

Nursing Diagnosis

Risk for Loneliness

At risk for experiencing discomfort associated with a desire or need for more contact with others.

RISK FACTORS

- Social isolation
- Inadequate social and relational skills
- Ineffective personal relationships
- Passivity
- Low self-esteem
- Hopelessness
- Powerlessness
- Anxiety or fear
- Inadequate leisure activity skills
- Inadequate resources for transportation or leisure activities
- Chronic illness or disability

EXPECTED OUTCOMES

Immediate	The client will
	• Participate in the therapeutic relationship, for example, talk with staff for 10 to 15 minutes twice a day within 24 to 48 hours • Initiate interactions with others within 2 to 3 days • Identify strategies to prevent or alleviate feelings of loneliness with nursing assistance within 2 to 3 days
Stabilization	The client will
	• Increase contacts with others • Verbalize decreased feelings of loneliness • Demonstrate increased interpersonal contacts, for example, interact with an increased number of people or for longer periods • Demonstrate increased communication, social, and leisure activity skills
Community	The client will
	• Express satisfaction with leisure and social activities • Maintain ongoing interpersonal relationships that are satisfying

IMPLEMENTATION

Nursing Interventions *denotes collaborative interventions	Rationale
Build a trust relationship with the client (see Care Plan 1: Building a Trust Relationship).	The client may be cautious or wary of a new relationship. The client may have had many relationships with health care providers in the past and may have suffered grief and loneliness when those relationships ended.
Teach the client about the therapeutic relationship, including the purposes and boundaries of such relationships.	The client may not have experienced a therapeutic relationship or may have become dependent on one in the past. The client needs to know that this is not a social relationship, that the goals include eventual termination of the relationship, and so on.
*Assess the client's living situation and support system. Make recommendations for changes that would decrease the client's risk for loneliness, and make referrals as appropriate.	Making a change in the client's living situation to increase contact with other people can be effective in helping the client overcome social isolation and loneliness.
*Teach the client, appropriate caregiver(s), and other support people about the client's illness.	The client and his or her support network may have little or no knowledge of the client's illness. This information can help diminish fears and prevent the client's isolation from supportive relationships.
*Teach the client, caregivers, and other support people about loneliness, and help them develop ways in which to interact to help the client. For example, help the client identify ways to communicate that he or she feels lonely, and help the client's significant others identify ways to respond.	The client and his or her support network may have little knowledge of loneliness or how to communicate and respond to help the client. The client may not know how to ask for help or may have felt unheard in the past.
Encourage the client to express feelings regarding loneliness and other emotions that may be difficult for the client. See other care plans as appropriate.	Expressing feelings verbally or nonverbally can help the client work through emotions that are difficult or painful.
Encourage the client to identify strategies to use when feeling lonely, including things that have alleviated these feelings in the past. If the client has difficulty identifying strategies, make suggestions or ask the client about diversional activities; hobbies; physical activities; household activities; listening to music; volunteer work (especially	Activities like these may be effective in alleviating the client's feelings of loneliness. If the client has a number of activities from which to choose, he or she can learn to anticipate and prevent feelings of loneliness.

IMPLEMENTATION (continued)

Nursing Interventions *denotes collaborative interventions	Rationale
if the client is unable to have a job); solitary activities to express feelings, such as writing in a journal or drawing; social activities; and support groups.	
*Use telephone contact between home care visits as appropriate, or encourage the client to make regular telephone contacts with other people.	Using the telephone for daily contact with others can be more feasible than in-person contacts, yet it can effectively create and maintain a sense of connection with other people.
Encourage the client to develop a structure for daily activities and leisure time, including social activities.	Following a structured routine can diminish feelings of purposelessness and helplessness. The client can avoid having to decide whether or not to do each activity each day if he or she is accustomed to a routine and expects to follow it.
*Help the client identify resources in the community that can provide social functions, offer social support, and meet needs for interpersonal activity, for example, support groups, recreational programs, senior or community centers, cultural or church groups, volunteer work, hobby or special interest groups, and community colleges.	Most communities have resources that can help meet these kinds of needs. The structure of these activities can help the client's daily routine and form a framework within which to develop relationships.
*Explore with the client his or her interests and hobbies (present and past). Help the client identify activities related to these interests, such as going to the library or to concerts, movies, or other entertainment. Help the client learn how to identify free or low-cost activities if finances are limited. Refer the client to a recreational therapy program, if available, to build leisure skills.	Clients often complain of loneliness or feeling worse when they are alone and have nothing to do. Planning and participating in activities can help prevent feelings of loneliness and give the client something to look forward to. These activities can also be shared with others.
Encourage the client to engage in daily physical activity, such as walking for at least 30 to 45 minutes each day.	Daily physical activity provides many health benefits as well as a low cost leisure activity.
*Teach the client about basic manners and social skills, including socially appropriate conversation topics, how to engage someone in a conversation, listening skills, steps in building relationships, how to say no to unwanted attention or relationships, handling rejection by others, and so forth. Use role modeling and group sessions (if available) to help the client learn and practice these skills.	The client may have never learned basic manners or skills in interacting or building relationships, or these may have been adversely affected by the client's illness. Social skills can help the client develop (more satisfying) relationships and alleviate loneliness. The client may also be vulnerable to people who would take advantage of him or her, especially if his or her judgment is impaired by illness.
Spend a part of each contact with the client by addressing the client's general well-being and conveying interest in the client as a person. Inquire about the client's feelings, perceptions, and sense of progress toward his or her goals.	The client can benefit from perceiving that you are interested in him or her as a person and in his or her well-being, as well as in his or her compliance and participation in the treatment program.
At the end of each visit or contact with the client, review with the client what his or her plans are for the time, until your next contact.	Reviewing plans helps remind the client how to use time between contacts with the nurse and can diminish anxiety if the client relies heavily on contacts with the nurse for support.
*Encourage the client to form relationships with a variety of people in the community. Help the client understand that relationships change over time and that he or she will continue to need to form new relationships.	Overreliance on just one or two people can result in the client having inadequate support if the support person is not available and can contribute to a support person becoming "burned out" by excessive demands. The client can anticipate and better deal with relationships that change or end.
*In a group situation, encourage clients to give each other feedback and support. Use role-playing and role-modeling techniques.	Clients can learn and practice interactive skills in a safe, supportive environment.

(continued on page 82)

IMPLEMENTATION (continued)

Nursing Interventions *denotes collaborative interventions	Rationale
Give the client positive feedback for accomplishments (even small ones), for participating in activities, for making efforts (even if not entirely successful), for improving social skills, and so forth. Be honest in your feedback; do not use false flattery.	Positive feedback can reinforce desired behaviors and help enhance the client's self-esteem. The client may not receive positive feedback from others. Clients with low self-esteem are at increased risk for loneliness. Flattery and insincerity are not helpful and can undermine the trust relationship.
*Help the client identify ways in which he or she can give back something to support people or caregivers. For example, the client may be able to make a small gift, write a thank-you note, or do some household chores that the caregiver would ordinarily do.	Reciprocity in support relationships, even if limited, can help prevent burnout of caregivers or support people and enhance the quality of relationships. The client may have limited skills in mutual support and expressing thanks.
Encourage the client to get a pet, if he or she is able to handle the responsibility (or has a significant other or long-term caregiver that is willing to) and is not at risk for harming an animal.	Relationships with pets can be therapeutic, yet not require the level of social skills needed for interpersonal relationships. For example, having a pet can help meet some of the client's needs for affection and physical contact.
*Refer the client to other resources in the community that can address needs for transportation, financial assistance, and so forth.	Clients who lack transportation and financial resources are at increased risk for loneliness. The nurse often is the primary link between the client and other needed services.

SECTION 2 REVIEW QUESTIONS

1. A client with schizophrenia tells the nurse that he usually spends all his time in his apartment since he has no place to go and doesn't know anyone in the apartment complex. Which of the following interventions would be most beneficial for this client?

   a. Arranging for the client to attend day treatment

   b. Encouraging the client to call his family more often

   c. Making an appointment for the client to see the nurse every day for the next week

   d. Telling the client that rehospitalization may be necessary

2. A client with severe and persistent mental illness living in an apartment in the community tells the nurse that he does nothing all day except eat, sleep, and smoke cigarettes. Which of the following interventions would be most appropriate for this client?

   a. Asking a relative to call the client two or three times a day to decrease sleeping

   b. Arranging for the client to move to a group home with structured activities

   c. Having the client make lists of hobbies to pursue to decrease boredom

   d. Helping the client to set up a daily activity schedule that includes setting a wake-up alarm

3. The nurse is working in a psychosocial rehabilitation program for clients with severe and persistent mental illness. Which of the following strategies would the nurse expect to be least beneficial in this type of program?

   a. Assisting clients with living arrangements

   b. Helping clients with insight-oriented therapy

   c. Linking clients with community resources

   d. Teaching independent living skills

4. A client with severe and persistent mental illness tells the nurse he stopped taking his medications 2 weeks ago, stating, "I am tired of not being able to have a few beers with my friends, and besides, I feel fine without them." Which of the following responses by the nurse would be best?

   a. "I know how difficult it must be to live with changes caused by your illness."

   b. "If your friends really care about you, it won't matter if you can't drink with them."

   c. "It is very important that you begin taking your medications again."

   d. "You will have to talk to the doctor about your medications.

SECTION 2 Recommended Readings

Cabassa, L. J., Ezell, J. M., & Lewis-Fernandez, R. (2010). Lifestyle interventions for adults with serious mental illness: A systematic literature review. *Psychiatric Services, 61*(8), 774–782.

Cummings, S. M., & Kropf, N. P. (2009). Formal and informal support for older adults with severe mental illness. *Aging and Mental Health, 13*(4), 619–627.

Hamilton, I. (2010). Ensuring integrated treatment for people with mental health and substance use problems. *Nursing Times, 106*(11), 12–15.

Lloyd, C., King, R., & Moore, L. (2010). Subjective and objective indicators of recovery in severe mental illness: A cross-sectional study. *International Journal of Social Psychology, 56*(3), 220–229.

Lloyd-Evans, B., Slade, M., Jagielska, D., & Johnson, S. (2009). Residential alternatives to acute psychiatric hospital admission: Systematic review. *British Journal of Psychiatry, 195*(2), 109–117.

SECTION 2 Resources for Additional Information

Visit thePoint (http://thePoint.lww.com/Schultz9e) for a list of these and other helpful Internet resources.

American Public Health Association
Assertive Community Treatment Association
Case Management Society of America
Community Access
Community Support Programs
Family Caregiver Alliance
Fountain House
Homelessness Resource Center
National Alliance to End Homelessness
National Association for Home Care & Hospice
National Association of Case Management
National Family Caregivers Association
SAMHSA—Co-Occurring and Homeless Activities Branch
The Way Back

SECTION THREE

Disorders Diagnosed in Childhood or Adolescence

There is widespread agreement that children in our society must face an increasing number of complex challenges, such as drugs and alcohol, violence in the community, and parental problems and issues. These problems only further complicate the already formidable task of "growing up" and forming an identity. The period of growth and development that spans childhood and adolescence can include turmoil, inconsistency, and unpredictability in the normal course of events. However, for some children and adolescents, these difficult times are further complicated by psychosocial or emotional problems that often require professional intervention. The care plans in this section address mental health concerns that are problematic before a youngster reaches adulthood.

CARE PLAN 9

Attention Deficit/Hyperactivity Disorder

Attention deficit/hyperactivity disorder (ADHD) is a neurobehavioral disorder usually first diagnosed in childhood that is characterized by inattention, distraction, restlessness, hyperactivity, and/or impulsivity (Centers for Disease Control [CDC], 2010a). It is important to distinguish ADHD from other childhood disorders, as well as from behavior in a child who is simply difficult to manage; children from chaotic environments, for example, are often mislabeled as hyperactive when problem behaviors are actually occurring due to other factors (e.g., abuse, head injuries, or learning disabilities).

Manifestations of ADHD occur in all of a child's environments (home, school, social situations), whereas other types of problems often occur only in particular situations. At school, the client frequently experiences poor performance, including incomplete assignments, difficulty with organization, and incorrect and messy work. Verbally, the client disrupts others, fails to heed directions, and interrupts in conversations. At home, the client is accident-prone and is intrusive with family members. With peers, the client is unable to follow the rules of games, fails to take turns, and appears oblivious to the desires or requests of others.

The incidence of ADHD in school-aged children is estimated to be between 3% and 7% (American Academy of Child and Adolescent Psychiatry [AACAP] & American Psychiatric Association [APA], 2010a), and the disorder is more common in boys than in girls (APA, 2000). Usually, ADHD is identified when a child enters the educational system. Hyperactivity is often a major component of the disorder in younger children, although this is less common in adolescents. ADHD may occur without hyperactivity, but less frequently. By adolescence, hyperactive behavior usually is reduced to fidgeting and an inability to sit for sustained periods.

Many individuals experience problems with ADHD beyond childhood, especially if no effective treatment was received earlier. About 60% of children with ADHD continue to have problems in adolescence (AACAP, 2007). These problems may include adjustment reactions, depression, anxiety, and conduct problems such as lying, stealing, truancy, and acting out. About 40% of children with ADHD have symptoms that persist into adulthood, including unsuccessful experiences in social, vocational, and academic settings that result from inattention, disinhibition, and lack of persistent effort, motivation, and concentration (AACAP, 2007).

Stimulant medications such as methylphenidate hydrochloride (e.g., Ritalin) or amphetamine sulfate (e.g., Adderall, Concerta), and an antidepressant, atomoxetine (Strattera), frequently are used to decrease hyperactive behavior. Nursing objectives for clients with ADHD include managing symptoms, developing social skills, and providing the client and the significant others with education and resources for continued support. It is important to work with the interdisciplinary treatment team to coordinate follow-up care and communication with school personnel, whose participation is a crucial element in the successful treatment of both adolescents and children.

NURSING DIAGNOSES ADDRESSED IN THIS CARE PLAN
Risk for Injury
Ineffective Role Performance

RELATED NURSING DIAGNOSES ADDRESSED IN THE MANUAL
Ineffective Therapeutic Regimen Management
Chronic Low Self-Esteem
Impaired Social Interaction
Interrupted Family Processes

Nursing Diagnosis

Risk for Injury

At risk for injury as a result of environmental conditions interacting with the individual's adaptive and defensive resources.

RISK FACTORS

• Motor-perceptual dysfunction, for example, poor hand–eye coordination
• Inability to perceive potentially harmful situations
• Intrusive behavior with others
• Impulsivity

EXPECTED OUTCOMES

Immediate   The client will

• Be free of injury or unnecessary risks throughout treatment
• Respond to limits regarding intrusion on others within 2 to 3 days

Stabilization   The client will

• Engage in activities without taking unnecessary risks, for example, walking rather than running down the stairs
• Demonstrate decreased intrusive behavior (e.g., interrupting others)

Community   The client will

• Recognize potentially harmful situations independently
• Use internal controls to manage impulsivity

IMPLEMENTATION

Nursing Interventions *denotes collaborative interventions	Rationale
Do not assume that the client knows proper or expected behavior. State expectations for behavior in clear terms.	Developmentally, the client may be unable to process social cues to guide reasonable behavior choices.
Assess the frequency and severity of accidents.	It is necessary to establish a baseline before planning interventions.
Provide supervision for potentially dangerous situations. Limit the client's participation in activities when safety cannot be ensured.	The client's ability to perceive harmful consequences of a behavior is impaired.
Talk with the client about safe and unsafe behavior. Explain that accidents will result in increased supervision and that purposeful unsafe behavior will have consequences.	This provides the client with clear expectations.
Attempt to distinguish between accidents and behaviors that are deliberate.	Physical safety is a priority. Accidents will require increased supervision, but deliberate actions can be altered with behavioral techniques.
If the situation is determined to be accidental, institute safeguards or limitations as appropriate.	Different interventions are instituted for accidents than for deliberate actions.
If the situation is determined to be deliberate, institute consequences in a nonpunitive manner.	Logical consequences for an undesirable behavior can diminish the occurrence of the behavior.
Make corrective feedback as specific as possible, for example, "Do not jump down the stairs. Walk down one step at a time."	Specific information will help the client understand expectations.

(continued on page 88)

IMPLEMENTATION (continued)

Nursing Interventions *denotes collaborative interventions	Rationale
Provide consequences that are directly related to the undesirable behavior. Institute consequences as soon as possible after the occurrence of the behavior.	The client will be better able to draw the correlation between undesirable behavior and consequences if the two are related to each other.
*Teach the client's parents or caregivers about ADHD and the client's treatment plan and medication, if any.	The client's parents or caregivers may lack knowledge about ADHD and treatment.
*Assist the client's parents or caregivers to make the distinction between accidental and purposeful incidents.	This will enable them to deal with behaviors at home more effectively.

Nursing Diagnosis

Ineffective Role Performance

Patterns of behavior and self-expression that do not match the environmental context, norms, and expectations.

ASSESSMENT DATA

- Short attention span
- High level of distractibility
- Labile moods
- Low frustration tolerance
- Inability to complete tasks
- Inability to sit still or fidgeting
- Excessive talking
- Inability to follow directions

EXPECTED OUTCOMES

Immediate   The client will

- Successfully complete tasks or assignments with assistance within 24 to 36 hours
- Demonstrate acceptable social skills while interacting with staff or family members, for example, listening while others talk rather than interrupting within 2 to 3 days

Stabilization   The client will

- Participate successfully in the educational setting
- Demonstrate the ability to complete tasks with reminders
- Demonstrate successful interactions with family members

Community   The client will

- Verbalize positive statements about himself or herself
- Demonstrate successful interactions with nonfamily members
- Complete tasks independently

IMPLEMENTATION

Nursing Interventions *denotes collaborative interventions	Rationale
Identify the factors that aggravate the client's behavior and those that help the client's performance.	The external stimuli that exacerbate the client's problems can be identified and minimized. Likewise, factors that positively influence the client can be effectively used.
Provide an environment as free from distractions as possible. Institute interventions on a one-to-one basis. Gradually increase the amount of environmental stimuli.	The client's ability to deal with external stimulation is impaired.

IMPLEMENTATION (continued)

Nursing Interventions *denotes collaborative interventions	Rationale
Engage the client's attention before giving instructions (i.e., call the client's name and establish eye contact).	The client must hear the instructions as a first step toward compliance. He or she may not comprehend instructions if his or her attention is distracted by something else.
Give instructions slowly, using simple language and concrete directions.	The client's ability to comprehend instructions (especially if they are complex or abstract) is impaired.
Ask the client to repeat instructions before beginning tasks.	Repetition demonstrates that the client has accurately received the information.
Separate complex tasks into small steps.	The likelihood of success is enhanced with less complicated components of a task.
Provide positive feedback for completion of each step.	The client's opportunity for successful experiences is increased by treating each step as an opportunity for success.
Allow breaks, during which the client can move around.	The client's restless energy can be given an acceptable outlet, so he or she can attend to future tasks more effectively.
State expectations for task completion clearly.	The client must understand the request before he or she can attempt task completion.
Initially, assist the client to complete tasks.	If the client is unable to complete a task independently, having assistance will allow success and will demonstrate how to complete the task.
Progress to prompting or reminding the client to perform tasks or assignments.	The amount of intervention gradually is decreased to increase client independence as the client's abilities increase.
Give the client positive feedback for performing behaviors that come close to task achievement.	This approach, called *shaping*, is a behavioral procedure in which successive approximations of a desired behavior are positively reinforced. It allows rewards to occur as the client gradually masters the actual expectation.
Gradually decrease reminders.	Client independence is promoted as staff participation is decreased.
Assist the client to verbalize by asking sequencing questions to keep on the topic ("Then what happens?" and "What happens next?").	Sequencing questions provide a structure for discussions to increase logical thought and decrease tangentiality.
*Teach the client's family or caregivers to use the same procedures for the client's tasks and interactions at home.	Successful interventions can be instituted by the client's family or caregivers by using this process. This will promote consistency and enhance the client's chances for success.
*Explain and demonstrate "positive parenting" techniques to family or caregivers such as *time-in* for good behavior, or being vigilant in identifying and responding positively to the child's first bid for attention; *special time*, or guaranteed time spent daily with the child with no interruptions and no discussion of problem-related topics; *ignoring minor transgressions* by immediate withdrawal of eye contact or physical contact and cessation of discussion with the child to avoid secondary gains.	It is important for parents or caregivers to engage in techniques that will maintain their loving relationship with the child while promoting, or at least not interfering with, therapeutic goals. Children need to have a sense of being lovable to their significant others that is not crucial to the nurse–client therapeutic relationship.

CARE PLAN 10

Conduct Disorders

Clients with *conduct disorders* exhibit a persistent pattern of behavior in which the "basic rights of others or major age-appropriate societal norms or rules are violated" (APA, 2000, p. 93). The client's difficulties usually exist in all major life areas: at home, at school, with peers, and in the community. Problematic behaviors include aggression that is harmful or threatening to animals or other people, property damage or vandalism, stealing or lying, or breaking rules. However, isolated acts of these types of behaviors do not warrant a diagnosis of conduct disorder.

Conduct disorders are more prevalent in boys than in girls, especially when the disorder presents earlier in childhood. General prevalence is estimated at up to 10% and has apparently increased in recent decades (APA, 2000). The onset of a conduct disorder usually occurs between mid-childhood and mid-adolescence, although it can occur in preschool-aged children; it rarely begins after the age of 16 years. Earlier onset is associated with a poorer prognosis and an increased likelihood that the individual will have antisocial personality disorder as an adult (APA, 2000).

Behavioral symptoms may begin with relatively minor problems such as lying and progress to more severe behaviors such as mugging or rape as the individual moves into later adolescence. As the adolescent grows older, complications often develop, including school suspension, legal difficulties, substance use, sexually transmitted diseases (STDs), pregnancy, injury from accidents and fights, and suicidal behavior. Persistent illegal activity and diagnoses of adult antisocial behavior, antisocial personality disorder, and chemical dependence are common for these individuals as adults.

Treatment should be appropriate to the child's age and developmental stage. It is important to provide education about the disorder and to work with the child's family and school personnel to coordinate care. In cases with mild impairment, improvement is demonstrated as the adolescent matures and may require only special education classes and supportive therapy for the family. Treatment of adolescent clients may include social skills development and anger management, in addition to individual and family therapy. Nurses should work with the interdisciplinary treatment team to identify appropriate follow-up and social services for legal problems, substance abuse, and concurrent, additional mental health disorders.

Referral to supportive community resources and organizations is also important. For example, *TOUGHLOVE* is a national parent support group that assists parents in setting basic rules the adolescent must follow—if the rules are ignored, the adolescent must leave home. These limits are established in an atmosphere of love and caring, hence the name of the organization.

In severe cases, problems related to conduct disorders tend to be chronic and often require placing the client in an institutional setting.

NURSING DIAGNOSES ADDRESSED IN THIS CARE PLAN
Noncompliance
Risk for Other-Directed Violence
Ineffective Coping

RELATED NURSING DIAGNOSES ADDRESSED IN THE MANUAL
Impaired Social Interaction
Chronic Low Self-Esteem
Interrupted Family Processes

Nursing Diagnosis

Noncompliance

Behavior of a person and/or caregiver that fails to coincide with a health-promoting or thera-peutic plan agreed upon by the person (and/or family and/or community) and health care professional. In the presence of an agreed upon, health-promoting or therapeutic plan, the person's or caregiver's behavior is fully or partially nonadherent and may lead to clinically ineffective or partially ineffective outcomes.

ASSESSMENT DATA

- Egocentrism
- Disobedience
- Feelings of frustration
- Lack of remorse for unacceptable behavior
- Manipulative behavior
- Cheating (schoolwork, games, sports)

EXPECTED OUTCOMES

Immediate

The client will

- Participate in treatment program within 2 to 4 days
- Adhere to rules within 2 to 4 days

Stabilization

The client will

- Attend school
- Be truthful
- Demonstrate compliance with negotiated rules and expectations with parents

Community

The client will

- Adhere to expectations independently
- Demonstrate socially acceptable behavior in the community

IMPLEMENTATION

Nursing Interventions *denotes collaborative interventions	Rationale
Inform the client of expectations and limits in a matter-of-fact manner.	This allows the client to be aware of expectations without being "challenged" by them.
Do not make exceptions to stated expectations or rules.	Consistency will discourage manipulative behavior.
Avoid making promises; instead, say, "If possible, I will."	The client may try to use an unfulfilled promise as an example of your not adhering to expectations or commitments.
Contract with the client (ahead of time) for requests or privileges. It may be beneficial to write and sign the agreement.	Using a contract with the client allows him or her to be rewarded for setting a goal and attaining it. A written agreement leaves no room for "forgetting" and minimizes the opportunity for manipulation.
Validate the client's feelings of frustration, but remain firm in denying requests for exceptions to limits.	Validating feelings conveys empathy yet allows consistency in setting and maintaining limits.
Avoid power struggles with the client. Do not engage in lengthy explanations or debating once expectations have been stated.	Debating promotes opportunity for manipulation. If engaged in a power struggle, the adolescent may escalate his or her behavior to "save face" or "win" the struggle.
Demonstrate consistency in your responses to the client, and ensure consistency among all staff members.	Consistent staff response is a primary way to avoid manipulation.

(continued on page 92)

IMPLEMENTATION (continued)

Nursing Interventions *denotes collaborative interventions	Rationale
Designate one staff member each shift to be the primary contact person for the client. Other staff should refer requests to the designated staff person. See "Key Considerations in Mental Health Nursing: Limit Setting."	Designation of one staff person for decisions regarding client behavior decreases the opportunity for lying and manipulating.
Protect other clients from being drawn into the client's influence, especially those who might be nonassertive or vulnerable.	Clients with conduct disorders have established patterns of using others for their own gain.
Institute a daily schedule for getting up, going to bed, studying, activities of daily living, enjoying free time, and so forth.	Increased structure will increase chances for compliance with expectations.
Give positive feedback for completion of each component of the schedule.	Positive reinforcement of a desired behavior increases the frequency of its occurrence.

Nursing Diagnosis

Risk for Other-Directed Violence

At risk for behaviors in which an individual demonstrates that he or she can be physically, emotionally, and/or sexually harmful to others.

RISK FACTORS

- Temper outbursts
- Reckless, thrill-seeking behavior
- Inability to express feelings in a socially acceptable, safe manner
- Lack of remorse for destructive behavior
- Destruction of property
- Cruelty to animals
- Physical aggression
- Running away from home
- Use of tobacco, alcohol, and drugs
- Involvement in violent situations or crimes

EXPECTED OUTCOMES

Immediate

The client will

- Be free of injury throughout hospitalization
- Refrain from harming others or destroying property throughout hospitalization
- Eliminate physically aggressive behavior within 24 to 36 hours

Stabilization

The client will

- Verbalize feelings in a socially acceptable, safe manner, for example, speaking in a calm voice
- Reside in the least restrictive environment necessary for safety of self and others
- Participate in substance dependence treatment, if indicated

Community

The client will

- Demonstrate safe behavior independently
- Engage in age-appropriate activities

IMPLEMENTATION

Nursing Interventions *denotes collaborative interventions	Rationale
Investigate any threats or talk of suicide seriously, and institute interventions as indicated (see Care Plan 26: Suicidal Behavior).	Client safety is a priority.
If the client is losing behavioral control, ask him or her to leave the situation or ask others to leave.	The reinforcement for acting out is diminished when there is no audience.
Institute *time-out* procedure (retreat to a neutral environment to provide the opportunity to regain internal control). Teach the client that time-out is a positive opportunity for "cooling off," not a punishment. Remain matter-of-fact when instituting this procedure.	The purpose of time-out periods is to allow the client to regain control in a neutral setting.
Encourage the client to work toward instituting time-out for himself or herself when unable to handle a situation in any other way.	Self-imposed time-out is a skill the client can use in other situations. This promotes development of the client's internal self-control.
Following the time-out period, when the client is more calm, discuss the situation with him or her.	Any discussion will be more productive when feelings and behavior are not excessive or out of control. Remember that time-out is not a punishment or a "solution," rather a means to facilitate more effective methods of coping.
Encourage the client to keep a diary of his or her feelings, the situation in which the feelings were experienced, what he or she did to handle the situation or feelings, and so forth.	Adolescents often have difficulty identifying and discussing feelings. A written journal provides more concrete information about the connection between the client's feelings and behavior.
Assist the client in examining alternatives to acting-out behavior. Anger management classes or counseling may be appropriate referrals; community or online support groups may be beneficial to the client and his or her family.	This allows the client to develop a repertoire of choices for future situations. The client's behavior impacts his or her family, and the family may benefit from support groups or continued family therapy.

Nursing Diagnosis

Ineffective Coping

Inability to form a valid appraisal of the stressors, inadequate choices of practiced responses, and/or inability to use available resources.

ASSESSMENT DATA

- Few or no meaningful peer relationships
- Inability to empathize with others
- Inability to give and receive affection
- Low self-esteem, masked by "tough" act

EXPECTED OUTCOMES

Immediate   The client will

- Engage in social interaction with staff and other clients, initially with staff assistance for 5 to 10 minutes at least twice a day, gradually increase over time
- Verbalize feelings within 2 to 3 days
- Learn problem-solving process within 2 to 3 days

Stabilization   The client will

- Demonstrate effective problem-solving and coping skills
- Assess own strengths and weaknesses realistically, for example, make a list of strengths and weaknesses and review with the nurse

Community   The client will

• Demonstrate development of relationships with peers
• Verbalize real feelings of self-worth that are age appropriate
• Perform at a satisfactory academic level

IMPLEMENTATION

Nursing Interventions *denotes collaborative interventions	Rationale
Encourage the client to discuss his or her thoughts and feelings.	Verbalizing feelings is an initial step toward dealing with them in an appropriate manner.
Give positive feedback for appropriate discussions.	Positive feedback increases the likelihood of continued performance.
Tell the client that he or she is accepted as a person, although a particular behavior may not be acceptable.	Clients with conduct disorders frequently experience rejection. The client needs support to increase self-esteem, while understanding that behavioral changes are necessary.
Give the client positive attention when behavior is not problematic.	The client may have been receiving the majority of attention from others when he or she was engaged in problematic behavior, a pattern that needs to change.
Teach the client about limit setting and the need for limits. Include time for discussion.	This allows the client to hear about the relationship between aberrant behavior and consequences during a time that the client's behavior is not problematic. The client may have no knowledge of the concept of limits and how limits, including self-imposed limits, can be beneficial.
Teach the client the problem-solving process as an alternative to acting out (identify the problem, consider alternatives, select and implement an alternative, evaluate the effectiveness of the solution).	The client may not know how to solve problems constructively or may not have seen this behavior modeled in the home.
Help the client practice the problem-solving process with situations on the unit, and then with situations the client may face at home, school, and so forth.	The client's ability and skill will increase with practice. He or she will experience success with practice.
Role-model appropriate conversation and social skills for the client.	This allows the client to see what is expected in a non-threatening situation.
Specify and describe the skills you are demonstrating.	Clarification of expectations decreases the chance for misinterpretation.
Practice social skills with the client on a one-to-one basis.	As the client gains comfort with the skills through practice, he or she will increase their use.
Gradually introduce other clients into the interactions and discussions.	Success with others is more likely to occur once the client has been successful with the staff.
Assist the client to focus on age- and situation-appropriate topics.	Peer relationships are enhanced when the client is able to interact as other adolescents do.
Encourage the client to give and receive feedback with others in his or her age group.	Peer feedback can be influential in shaping the behavior of an adolescent.
Facilitate expression of feelings among clients in supervised group situations.	Adolescents are reluctant to be vulnerable to peers and may need encouragement to share feelings.
Teach the client about transmission of human immunodeficiency virus (HIV) infection and other STDs.	Because these clients may act out sexually or use intravenous drugs, it is especially important that they be educated about preventing transmission of HIV and STDs.
*Assess the client's use of alcohol or other substances, and provide referrals as indicated.	Often adolescents with conduct disorders also have substance abuse issues.

CARE PLAN 11

Adjustment Disorders of Adolescence

An *adjustment disorder* involves an excessive reaction to an identified psychosocial stressor, in that the individual experiences more distress than would be expected from the specific stressor or that the individual's functioning is impaired to a greater degree than would be expected. Stressors for adolescents may be easily identifiable, such as separation or divorce of parents, moving to a new community or school, pubertal changes, and so forth. Less-evident stressors, such as emerging sexual feelings, desire for increased autonomy, and the growing significance of peers, can be a primary source of conflict or add stress to other difficulties.

Adjustment disorders are diagnosed in male and female adolescents in approximately equal numbers, and prevalence rates are estimated at between 2% and 8% (APA, 2000). Adjustment disorders occur within 3 months after the onset of the stressor but do not persist longer than 6 months after the stressor is no longer present. Adolescents with adjustment disorders can be at risk for juvenile delinquency, maladaptive sexual behavior, substance use, teen pregnancy, and STDs, including HIV infection. The ultimate problem area for adolescents is suicidal behavior, which is among the three leading causes of death for youth 15 to 24 years of age, according to the U. S. Substance Abuse and Mental Health Services Administration.

Nursing care for the adolescent experiencing an adjustment disorder centers on providing a protective environment in which the client can have corrective emotional experiences. These experiences include limits for behavior, interpersonal relationships, peer-group support and feedback, development of coping skills, and achievement of developmental tasks. The promotion of coping abilities in teens is a major objective in the prevention of teen suicide (Logan, 2009).

NURSING DIAGNOSES ADDRESSED IN THIS CARE PLAN
Ineffective Coping
Interrupted Family Processes
Situational Low Self-Esteem

RELATED NURSING DIAGNOSES ADDRESSED IN THE MANUAL
Risk for Other-Directed Violence
Risk for Suicide
Impaired Social Interaction
Anxiety

Nursing Diagnosis

Ineffective Coping
Inability to form a valid appraisal of the stressors, inadequate choices of practiced responses, and/or inability to use available resources.

ASSESSMENT DATA

- Impulsive behavior
- Acting-out behavior
- Suicidal behavior
- Discomfort with sexual feelings
- Poor social skills
- Anxiety
- Difficulty expressing feelings
- Unmet needs for affection, closeness, and peer-group acceptance
- Ineffective relationships
- Lack of leisure skills

EXPECTED OUTCOMES

Immediate

The client will

- Refrain from harming self or others throughout hospitalization
- Abstain from using alcohol and drugs throughout hospitalization
- Comply with structured daily routine within 24 to 48 hours
- Identify consequences of maladaptive behavior patterns, for example, verbalize limits that have been set and the consequences that have been identified for exceeding limits, within 2 to 3 days

Stabilization

The client will

- Eliminate maladaptive coping patterns (alcohol and drug use, acting out, suicidal behavior)
- Complete daily expectations independently
- Verbalize accurate information regarding substance use, sexual activity, and prevention of HIV and STD transmission

Community

The client will

- Express satisfaction with peer and family relationships
- Demonstrate use of the problem-solving process in decision making

IMPLEMENTATION

Nursing Interventions *denotes collaborative interventions	Rationale
Provide a safe environment for the client. See Care Plan 26: Suicidal Behavior.	The client's safety is a priority.
State rules, expectations, and responsibilities clearly to the client, including consequences for exceeding limits.	The client needs clear expectations regarding behavior and what to expect if he or she exceeds limits.
Use *time-out* (removal to a neutral area) when the client begins to lose behavioral control.	Time-out is not a punishment but an opportunity for the client to regain control. Instituting time-out as soon as the client's behavior begins to escalate may prevent acting out and give the client a successful experience in self-control.
Encourage the client to verbalize feelings.	Identifying and verbalizing feelings is difficult for an adolescent but is a necessary step in resolving difficulties.
Allow the client to express all feelings in an appropriate, nondestructive manner.	The client may have many negative feelings that he or she has not been allowed or encouraged to verbalize.
Use a matter-of-fact approach when discussing these emotionally charged issues with the client.	A matter-of-fact approach will decrease the client's anxiety and demonstrate that these issues are a part of daily life, not topics about which one needs to be ashamed.
Avoid looking shocked or disapproving if the client makes crude or outrageous statements.	Testing behavior, to see your reaction, is common in adolescents.
Ask the client to clarify feelings if he or she is vague or is using jargon ("Can you explain that to me?").	Clarification avoids any misunderstanding of what the client means and helps the client develop skill in verbally expressing himself or herself.

IMPLEMENTATION (continued)

Nursing Interventions *denotes collaborative interventions	Rationale
Encourage a physical activity if the client is better able to discuss difficult issues while doing something physical (e.g., take a walk with the client while talking).	Physical activity such as walking provides an outlet for anxious energy. Eye contact may be difficult if the client feels uncomfortable and is diminished while walking with someone.
Provide factual information about sexual issues, substance use, consequences of high-risk behavior, and preventing transmission of HIV and STD infections.	Adolescents frequently have inadequate or incorrect information. Any client who may be sexually active or who may use intravenous drugs is at increased risk for HIV and other infections.
Written information, such as pamphlets, often is helpful.	Written information allows the client to learn privately, which may be less embarrassing for him or her.
Assess the client's understanding through a return explanation by the client in his or her own words. Do not rely on asking "Did you understand?" or "Do you have any questions?"	Clients may deny questions or say they understand when they do not to decrease discomfort, avoid admitting they do not understand, or avoid further discussion.
Teach the client a simple problem-solving process: describe the problem, list alternatives, evaluate choices, and select and implement an alternative.	The adolescent client has probably not thought about using a systematic approach to solving problems and may not know where to begin.
Have the client list actual concerns or problems he or she has been having.	Listing concerns helps the client to examine the problems that he or she would like to resolve.
Assist the client in applying the problem-solving process to situations in his or her life.	Personal experience in using the problem-solving process is more useful to the client than using hypothetical examples.
Discuss the pros and cons of choices the client has made.	Guiding the client through the process while discussing actual concerns shows him or her how to use the process.
Avoid offering personal opinions. Ask the client, "Knowing what you know now, what might you do next time that happens?"	The client's ability to make more effective decisions is a priority. Your opinions diminish the client's opportunity to develop skills in this area.

Nursing Diagnosis

Interrupted Family Processes
Change in family relationships and/or functioning.

ASSESSMENT DATA

- Inadequate parent–child interactions
- Ineffective communication about family roles, rules, and expectations
- Rigid family roles
- Inability to express feelings openly and honestly
- Situational, developmental, or maturational transition or crisis

EXPECTED OUTCOMES

Immediate

The client will

- Listen to feelings of family members within 24 to 48 hours
- Express feelings within the family group within 3 to 4 days

Stabilization   The client will

• Participate in family problem solving
• Negotiate behavioral rules and expectations with parents

Community   The client will

• Demonstrate compliance with negotiated rules independently
• Report satisfaction with family communication and relationships

IMPLEMENTATION

Nursing Interventions *denotes collaborative interventions	Rationale
Help the client clarify issues he or she would like to discuss with his or her parents. A written list may be helpful.	Anticipatory discussion may decrease the client's discomfort and help the client be specific and avoid generalizations. Writing the ideas ensures that important issues will not be forgotten due to anxiety and provides a focus to keep the client on task.
Encourage the client to use "I" statements to describe what he or she thinks or feels, such as "I think . . .," "I feel . . .," "I need . . .," and so forth, rather than general statements.	Statements using "I" assume responsibility for the statement of feelings, are less likely to be blaming in nature, and can help the client learn how to share his or her thoughts and feelings.
*Encourage the client's parents to communicate with the client in the same way (see above).	Parents also can benefit from assistance in making "I" statements and focus on feelings rather than blaming.
*Facilitate family sessions for sharing feelings, concerns, and ideas. Establish limits for these meetings that encourage mutual support, self-responsibility, and emotional safety.	Such meetings can be a semiformalized method for initiating family interaction. Adolescents and their parents may find this difficult to do without assistance.
*Help the client and parents take turns talking and listening. Do not get drawn into giving opinions or advice.	Your role is to facilitate communication, not to get involved in family dynamics. You must not give the perception of taking sides.
*Help clarify statements made by others. Provide a summary for the family group, for example, saying "Sounds like . . ."	Your communication skills can be helpful in clarifying ideas. A summary statement can reiterate important discussion points and provide closure.
Help the client and family members learn to seek clarification and confirm understanding.	The client and family members can build these skills with your assistance, and then use them in their continuing relationships and discussions.
*Guide the client and parents toward negotiating expectations and responsibilities to be followed at home. A written contract may be helpful.	Negotiating may be unfamiliar to the adolescent and his or her parents, but it is a skill that can help adolescents separate from parents, which is an important developmental task. Writing the agreement increases clarity for all parties and decreases future manipulation or misunderstanding.

Nursing Diagnosis

Situational Low Self-Esteem

Development of a negative perception of self-worth in response to a current situation.

ASSESSMENT DATA

• Negative self-image
• Low self-esteem
• Feelings of doubt
• Minimizing strengths
• Underachievement

- Emotional distancing of significant others
- Absence of satisfactory peer relationships
- Ineffective communication skills

EXPECTED OUTCOMES

Immediate   The client will

- Identify feelings of doubt and uncertainty within 24 to 48 hours
- Give and receive honest feedback with peer group within 2 to 3 days

Stabilization   The client will

- Make realistic, positive self-statements
- Identify own strengths and weaknesses realistically
- Express feelings in an acceptable manner, such as talking or writing in a journal

Community   The client will

- Verbalize increased feelings of self-worth
- Report increased satisfaction with peer relationships

IMPLEMENTATION

Nursing Interventions *denotes collaborative interventions	Rationale
Provide direct, honest feedback on the client's communication skills.	The client may not have had feedback about his or her communication skills. Feedback helps the client understand his or her behavior from others' points of view.
Be specific with feedback (e.g., "You look at the floor when someone is talking to you."). Do not assume the client will know what you mean by general or abstract comments.	General statements are less helpful to the client than specific feedback.
Role-model specific communication skills (i.e., listening, validating meaning, clarifying, etc.).	Modeling desired behaviors and skills gives the client a clear picture of what is expected. Practicing skills in a non-threatening environment enhances comfort with their use.
Encourage clients to practice skills and discuss feelings with each other. Suggest to the client that he or she may have concerns similar to others and that perhaps they could share them with each other.	The stage can be set for honest sharing if the client feels he or she is not too different from peers. Learning that others have similar feelings can help the client accept and express his or her own feelings.
Give positive feedback for honest sharing of feelings and concerns (e.g., "You were able to share your feelings even though it was difficult").	Positive feedback increases the frequency of desired behavior.
Do not allow the client to dwell on past problems, "reliving" mistakes, or self-blame. Help the client separate behavior from the sense of personal worth.	The client may believe that past unacceptable behavior makes him or her a "bad" person.
Help the client change from a focus on the past to a focus on the present. For example, asking "What might you do differently now?" or "What can be learned from . . .?" can help the client with that transition.	Once you have heard the client express feelings about past behavior, it is not useful to allow the client to ruminate—the past cannot be changed.

SECTION 3 REVIEW QUESTIONS

1. An effective nursing intervention for the impulsive and aggressive behaviors that accompany conduct disorders is

   a. Assertiveness training

   b. Consistent limit setting

   c. Negotiation of rules

   d. Open expression of feelings

2. The nurse would expect to see all the following behaviors in a child with ADHD except

   a. Easily distracted and forgetful

   b. Excessive running, climbing, and fidgeting

   c. Moody, sullen, and pouting behavior

   d. Interrupts others and can't take turns

3. A 9-year-old client with ADHD tells the nurse, "No one in my class likes me because they think I'm stupid. And they're right, I am stupid!" Which of the following nursing diagnoses would the nurse identify for this client?

   a. Anxiety

   b. Impaired socialization

   c. Ineffective coping

   d. Low self-esteem

4. Which of the following children is most at risk for an adjustment disorder?

   a. A 10-year-old boy who has never liked school and has a few friends

   b. A 16-year-old boy who has been struggling in school, getting only Cs and Ds

   c. A 13-year-old girl who is upset about not being selected for the cheerleading squad

   d. A 16-year-old girl who recently moved to a new school after her parents' divorce

SECTION 3 Recommended Readings

Bartlett, R., Rowe, T. S., & Shattell, M. M. (2010). Perspectives of college students on their childhood ADHD. *American Journal of Maternal Child Nursing, 35*(4), 226–231.

Bornovalova, M. A., Hicks, B. M., Iacono, W. G., & McGue, M. (2010). Familial transmission and heritability of childhood disruptive disorders. *American Journal of Psychiatry, 167*(9), 1066–1074.

Golder, T. (2010). Tourette syndrome: Information for school nurses. *Journal of School Nursing, 26*(1), 11–17.

Salmeron, P. A. (2009). Childhood and adolescent attention-deficit hyperactivity disorder: Diagnosis, clinical practice guidelines, and social implications. *Journal of the American Academy of Nurse Practitioners, 21*(9), 488–497.

SECTION 3 Resources for Additional Information

Visit thePoint (http://thePoint.lww.com/Schultz9e) for a list of these and other helpful Internet resources.

American Academy of Child and Adolescent Psychiatry
Association of Child and Adolescent Psychiatric Nurses
Attention Deficit Disorder Association
Bipolar Children
Bipolar Disorder Resource Center
Child and Adolescent Bipolar Foundation
Children and Adults with ADHD
Conduct Disorder Resource Center
Inspire USA Foundation
Learning Disabilities Association of America
Learning Disabilities Online
National Center for Learning Disabilities, Inc.
National Center for Mental Health and Juvenile Justice
National Federation of Families
National Institute of Mental Health Information
National Resource Center on AD/HD
Oppositional Defiant Resource Center
Parents Med Guide—American Academy of Child and Adolescent Psychiatry, American Psychiatric Association
Tough Love International

Delirium, Dementia, and Head Injury

Clients with delirium, dementia, or head injury may experience significant cognitive impairment. Delirium is often due to an underlying medical condition, such as alcohol withdrawal, sepsis, head trauma, or metabolic imbalances. The client usually returns to his or her previous level of functioning when the underlying cause is successfully treated.

Dementia usually is a chronic, progressively deteriorating disease, beginning with memory loss and other cognitive difficulties. Nursing interventions are designed to help the client maintain functioning as long as possible and provide support to both the client and his or her family or significant others (see Care Plan 5: Supporting the Caregiver).

Clients who have had a head injury may experience emotional, functional, cognitive, and personality changes that affect both the client and his or her significant others. Care Plan 14 addresses issues specific to clients with head injury and their caregivers.

CARE PLAN 12

Delirium

A *delirium* is defined as "a disturbance of consciousness and a change in cognition that develop over a short period of time" (APA, 2000, p. 135), which is not related to a preexisting or developing dementia. The client has reduced awareness, impaired attention, and changes in cognition or perceptual disturbances. These disturbances may include *misinterpretations* (the client may hear a door slam and believe it is a gunshot), *illusions* (the client may mistake an electric cord on the floor for a snake), or *hallucinations* (the client may "see" someone lurking menacingly in the corner of the room when no one is there). The client may also demonstrate increased or decreased psychomotor activity, fear, irritability, euphoria, labile moods, or other emotional symptoms.

The underlying causes of delirium include medical conditions (e.g., metabolic disturbances, infection), untoward responses to medications, sleep/wake cycle disturbances, sensory deprivation, alcohol or substance intoxication or withdrawal, or a combination of these conditions. Delirium is most common in persons older than 65 years who are hospitalized for a medical condition; prevalence is greater in elderly men than in women. In the general population, delirium occurs in 10% to 30% of hospitalized medically ill patients and as many as 60% of nursing home residents at or over age 75 (APA, 2000). Children on certain medications, such as anticholinergics, and those with febrile illnesses often experience delirium as well.

Delirium usually has an acute onset, from hours to days, and fluctuates throughout the day, with periods of lucidity and awareness alternating with episodes of acute confusion, disorientation, and perceptual disturbances. Clients with delirium may make a full recovery, especially if the underlying etiologic factors are promptly treated and corrected or are self-limited (duration of symptoms ranges from hours to months). However, some clients may have continued cognitive deficits or may develop seizures, coma, or death, especially if the cause of the delirium is not treated (APA, 2000). Medical treatment for clients with delirium is focused on identifying and resolving the underlying cause(s). Nursing care for these clients involves providing safety, preventing injury, providing reality orientation, and supporting physiologic functioning.

NURSING DIAGNOSES ADDRESSED IN THIS CARE PLAN
Acute Confusion
Impaired Social Interaction

RELATED NURSING DIAGNOSES ADDRESSED IN THE MANUAL
Risk for Injury
Ineffective Role Performance
Noncompliance
Interrupted Family Processes
Deficient Diversional Activity
Impaired Home Maintenance
Situational Low Self-Esteem

Nursing Diagnosis

Acute Confusion

Abrupt onset of reversible disturbances of consciousness, attention, cognition, and perception that develop over a short period of time.

ASSESSMENT DATA

- Poor judgment
- Cognitive impairment
- Impaired memory
- Lack of or limited insight
- Loss of personal control
- Inability to perceive harm
- Illusions
- Hallucinations
- Mood swings

EXPECTED OUTCOMES

Immediate

The client will

- Be free of injury throughout hospitalization
- Engage in a trust relationship with staff and caregiver within 24 hours
- Increase reality contact within 24 to 48 hours
- Cooperate with treatment within 8 to 24 hours

Stabilization

The client will

- Establish or follow a routine for activities of daily living
- Demonstrate decreased confusion, illusions, or hallucinations
- Experience minimal distress related to confusion
- Validate perceptions with staff or caregiver before taking action

Community

The client will

- Return to optimal level of functioning
- Manage health conditions, if any, effectively
- Seek medical treatment as needed

IMPLEMENTATION

Nursing Interventions *denotes collaborative interventions	Rationale
Do not allow the client to assume responsibility for decisions or actions if he or she is unsafe.	The client's safety is a priority. He or she may be unable to determine harmful actions or situations.
If limits on the client's actions are necessary, explain limits and reasons clearly, within the client's ability to understand.	The client has the right to be informed of any restrictions and the reasons limits are needed.
Involve the client in making plans or decisions as much as he or she is able to participate.	Compliance with treatment is enhanced if the client is emotionally invested in it.
Assess the client daily or more often if needed for his or her level of functioning.	Clients with organically based problems tend to fluctuate frequently in terms of their capabilities.
Allow the client to make decisions as much as he or she is able.	Decision-making increases the client's participation, independence, and self-esteem.
Assist the client to establish a daily routine, including hygiene, activities, and so forth.	Routine or habitual activities do not require decisions about whether or not to perform a particular task.

(continued on page 104)

IMPLEMENTATION (continued)

Nursing Interventions *denotes collaborative interventions	Rationale
In a matter-of-fact manner, give the client factual feedback on misperceptions, delusions, or hallucinations (e.g., "That is a chair") and convey that others do not share his or her interpretations (e.g., "I don't see anyone else in the room").	When given feedback in a nonjudgmental way, the client can feel validated for his or her feelings, while recognizing that his or her perceptions are not shared by others.
*Teach the client and his or her family or significant others about underlying cause(s) of confusion and delirium.	Knowledge about the cause(s) of confusion can help the client seek assistance when indicated.

Nursing Diagnosis

Impaired Social Interaction
Insufficient or excessive quantity or ineffective quality of social exchange.

ASSESSMENT DATA

- Apathy
- Emotional blandness
- Irritability
- Lack of initiative
- Feelings of hopelessness or powerlessness
- Recognition of functional impairment

EXPECTED OUTCOMES

Immediate

The client will

- Respond to interpersonal contacts in the structured environment, for example, interact with staff for a 5 minutes within 24 hours
- Verbalize feelings of hopelessness or powerlessness with nursing assistance within 24 hours
- Verbalize or express losses with nursing assistance within 24 to 48 hours

Stabilization

The client will

- Demonstrate appropriate social interactions
- Participate in leisure activities with others
- Verbalize or demonstrate increased feelings of self-worth if long-term deficits are present, if possible

Community

The client will

- Progress through stages of grieving within his or her limitations if long-term deficits are present
- Participate in follow-up care as needed

IMPLEMENTATION

Nursing Interventions *denotes collaborative interventions	Rationale
Encourage the client to verbalize feelings, especially feelings of frustration, powerlessness, and so forth.	Expressing feelings is an initial step toward dealing with them constructively.
Give the client positive feedback when he or she is able to identify areas that are difficult for him or her.	Positive reinforcement of a desired behavior helps to increase the frequency of that behavior.

IMPLEMENTATION (continued)

Nursing Interventions *denotes collaborative interventions	Rationale
Ask the client to clarify any feelings that he or she expresses vaguely. Encourage the client to be specific.	Asking for clarification can prevent misunderstanding and help the client more clearly identify and work through feelings.
If the client becomes agitated or seems unable to express himself or herself, redirect the client to a more neutral topic, or engage the client in a calming or pleasurable activity.	The client may be overwhelmed by feelings or unable to express himself or herself in a way that is therapeutic or productive, especially as the organic changes progress.
Encourage the client to interact with staff or other clients on topics of interest.	The client may be reluctant to initiate interaction and may need encouragement to converse with others.
Give the client positive feedback for engaging in social interactions and leisure activities.	Positive feedback increases the likelihood that the client will continue to interact and participate in activities.
*Assist the client to develop plans for follow-up care as needed. Provide referrals to social services and community agencies when indicated.	If recovery from delirium is incomplete, the client may need support or assistance when returning to the community.

CARE PLAN 13

Dementia

The primary feature of *dementia* is impaired memory, with at least one of the following cognitive deficits: *aphasia* (impaired language), *apraxia* (impaired motor function), *agnosia* (impaired object recognition), and impaired *executive functioning* (abstract thinking and the ability to plan and execute complex behaviors). Symptoms of dementia can also include disorientation, poor judgment, lack of insight, socially inappropriate behavior, anxiety, mood disturbances, sleep disturbances, delusions, and hallucinations. Dementia results from the direct effects of one or more medical conditions or the persistent effects of substance use (APA, 2000).

The major disorders that result in dementia include the following:

- *Vascular dementia* results from a decreased blood supply to and hypoxia of the cerebral cortex. Initial symptoms are forgetfulness and a short attention and concentration span. It usually occurs between the ages of 60 and 70, is progressive, and may result in psychosis.
- *Alzheimer's disease* has organic pathology that includes atrophy of cerebral neurons, plaque deposits, and enlargement of the third and fourth ventricles of the brain. It usually begins in people older than 50 years (and incidence increases with increasing age), may last 5 years or more, and includes progressive loss of speech and motor function, profound personality and behavioral changes (such as paranoia, delusions, and hallucinations), and inattention to hygiene.
- *Pick's disease* involves frontal and temporal lobe atrophy and results in a clinical picture similar to Alzheimer's disease. Death usually occurs in 2 to 5 years.
- *Creutzfeldt-Jakob disease* is a central nervous system disorder, an encephalopathy caused by a "slow virus" or prion (APA, 2000). It can occur at any age in adults but most commonly develops between ages 40 and 60. This disease involves altered vision, loss of coordination or abnormal movements, and dementia that usually progresses quite rapidly (over the course of a few months).
- *AIDS dementia complex (ADC)* results from direct invasion of nervous tissue by human immunodeficiency virus as well as from other illnesses that can be present in AIDS, such as toxoplasmosis and cytomegalovirus. ADC can result in a wide variety of symptoms, ranging from mild sensory impairment to gross memory and cognitive deficits.
- *Parkinson's disease* is a progressive disease involving loss of neurons of the basal ganglia that produces tremor, muscle rigidity, and loss of postural reflexes. Psychiatric manifestations include depression, dementia, and delirium, which have become more prevalent as successful medical treatment has extended life expectancy.

The prevalence of severe dementia has been reported to be 3% in adults, with increasing prevalence in older age groups, to as high as 25% in people older than 85 years (APA, 2000). Some minor forgetfulness usually occurs in elderly clients, but this differs drastically from the changes seen in dementia. The prevalence of chronic illnesses, including dementia, increases as average life expectancy increases. However, dementia is not necessarily a component of the aging process, and it is erroneous to assume that because a client is elderly he or she will be confused, forgetful, or demented.

Although dementia is generally considered to be progressive, symptoms can also stabilize for a period or resolve, as sometimes seen in vascular dementia. In progressive dementia, symptoms may begin as mild memory impairment with slight cognitive disturbance and progress to profoundly impaired memory and cognitive functioning. The specific course of dementia varies according to the underlying disorder.

Clients with dementia have an impaired ability to learn new material and eventually forget previously learned material. Deterioration of memory and language function, including loss of the ability to correctly identify familiar people or objects or remember their relationships or function, and the loss of ability to comprehend written or spoken language, as well as speech pattern disturbances (e.g., echolalia, perseveration) present tremendous challenges for both the client and caregiver(s). Wandering, confusion, disorientation, and the inability to correctly use items such as eating utensils produce significant safety issues and profound functional impairment.

Nursing care of a client with dementia is focused on ensuring the client's safety and meeting needs for adequate nutrition, hydration, rest, and activity. Nursing objectives also include helping the client attain and maintain his or her optimal level of functioning, providing support and education to the client and significant others, and working with the rest of the health care team to ensure appropriate follow-up care and continued support in the community.

NURSING DIAGNOSES ADDRESSED IN THIS CARE PLAN
Bathing Self-Care Deficit
Dressing Self-Care Deficit
Feeding Self-Care Deficit
Toileting Self-Care Deficit
Impaired Memory
Impaired Environmental Interpretation Syndrome
Impaired Social Interaction

RELATED NURSING DIAGNOSES ADDRESSED IN THE MANUAL
Risk for Other-Directed Violence
Risk for Injury
Insomnia
Interrupted Family Processes
Ineffective Role Performance

Nursing Diagnosis

Bathing Self-Care Deficit
Impaired ability to perform or complete bathing activities for self.

Dressing Self-Care Deficit
Impaired ability to perform or complete dressing activities for self.

Feeding Self-Care Deficit
Impaired ability to perform or complete self-feeding activities.

Toileting Self-Care Deficit
Impaired ability to perform or complete toileting activities for self.

ASSESSMENT DATA

- Attention deficits
- Apathy
- Impaired performance of daily living activities

EXPECTED OUTCOMES

Immediate	The client will

• Establish adequate nutrition, hydration, and elimination, with nursing assistance, within 24 to 48 hours (e.g., eat at least 30% of meals)
• Establish an adequate balance of rest, sleep, and activity within 48 to 72 hours (e.g., sleep at least 3 hours per night within 48 hours)
• Tolerate personal care activities within 8 to 24 hours

Stabilization   The client will

• Participate in daily activities as independently as possible
• Experience minimal distress over lost abilities

Community   The client will

• Maintain balanced physiologic functions
• Attain his or her optimal level of functioning

IMPLEMENTATION

Nursing Interventions *denotes collaborative interventions	Rationale
Offer the client small amounts of food frequently, including juices, malts, and fortified liquids.	Use of fortified liquids will provide the maximum amount of nutrition without fatiguing the client.
Provide a quiet environment with decreased stimulation for meal times. Assist the client with eating (e.g., feed the client) as necessary.	The client may be easily distracted by external stimuli.
Monitor the client's bowel movements; do not allow impaction to occur.	The client's inactivity, decreased food and fluid intake, lack of awareness of personal needs, and use of major tranquilizers can cause constipation and can lead to impaction if not monitored.
Provide activity and stimulation during the day. Do not allow the client to sleep all day.	The client will be wakeful at night, when confusion is worse, if he or she sleeps excessively during the day.
Provide a regular routine and a quiet environment at bedtime.	These measures facilitate readiness for sleep.
Use bedtime medication for sleep if necessary. Closely observe the client for beneficial effects or potential side effects. Dosages may need to be decreased for the elderly.	Sedatives or hypnotics may be helpful to facilitate sleep but can cause restlessness and confusion. Slow metabolism or decreased liver or kidney function can result in toxicity in elderly clients.
Assess the client's ability to ambulate independently; assist the client until you are sure of physical safety.	Independence is important for the client, but physical safety is a priority.
Explain any task in short, simple steps. Use clear, direct sentences; instruct the client to do one part of the task at a time.	A complex task is easier for the client if it is broken down into a series of steps. The client may not be able to remember all the steps at once.
Tell the client your expectations directly. Do not ask the client to choose unnecessarily (e.g., tell the client it is time to eat rather than asking if he or she wants to eat).	The client may not be able to make choices or may make poor choices.
Do not confuse the client with reasons as to why things are to be done. Abstract ideas will not be comprehended.	Abstract ideas will not be comprehended.
Allow the client an ample amount of time to perform any given task.	It may take the client longer to do even simple tasks because of a short attention or concentration span.
Remain with the client throughout the task; do not attempt to hurry the client.	Trying to rush the client will frustrate him or her and make completing the task impossible.
Assist the client as needed to maintain daily functions and adequate personal hygiene.	The client's sense of dignity and well-being is enhanced if he or she is clean, smells good, looks nice, and so forth.

Nursing Diagnosis

Impaired Memory

Inability to remember or recall bits of information or behavioral skills.

ASSESSMENT DATA

- Inability to recall factual information or events
- Inability to learn new material or recall previously learned material
- Inability to determine if a behavior was performed
- Agitation or anxiety regarding memory loss

EXPECTED OUTCOMES

Immediate   The client will

- Respond positively to memory cues if possible within 48 to 72 hours
- Demonstrate decreased agitation or anxiety within 24 to 48 hours

Stabilization   The client will

- Attain an optimal level of functioning with routine tasks
- Use long-term memory effectively as long as it remains intact
- Verbalize or demonstrate decreased frustration with memory loss

Community   The client will

- Maintain an optimal level of functioning
- Feel respected and supported

IMPLEMENTATION

Nursing Interventions *denotes collaborative interventions	Rationale
Provide opportunities for reminiscence or recall of past events, on a one-to-one basis or in a small group.	Long-term memory may persist after loss of recent memory. Reminiscence is usually an enjoyable activity for the client.
Encourage the client to use written cues such as a calendar, lists, or a notebook.	Written cues decrease the client's need to recall appointments, activities, and so on from memory.
Minimize environmental changes. Determine practical locations for the client's possessions, and return items to this location after use. Establish a usual routine and alter the routine only when necessary.	There is less demand on memory function when structure is incorporated in the client's environment and daily routine.
Provide single-step instructions for the client when instructions are needed.	Clients with memory impairment cannot remember multistep instructions.
Provide verbal connections about using implements. For example, "Here is a washcloth to wash your face," "Here is a spoon you can use to eat your dessert."	The client may not remember what an implement is for; stating its related function is an approach that compensates for memory loss.
Integrate reminders of previous events into current interactions, such as "Earlier you put some clothes in the washing machine; now it's time to put them in the dryer."	Providing links with previous behaviors helps the client make connections that he or she may not be able to make independently.
Assist with tasks as needed, but do not "rush" to do things for the client that he or she can still do independently.	It is important to maximize independent function, yet assist the client when memory has deteriorated further.
Use a matter-of-fact approach when assuming tasks the client can no longer perform. Do not allow the client to work unsuccessfully at a task for an extended time.	It is important to preserve the client's dignity and minimize his or her frustration with progressive memory loss.

Nursing Diagnosis

Impaired Environmental Interpretation Syndrome

Consistent lack of orientation to person, place, time, or circumstances over more than 3 to 6 months necessitating a protective environment.

ASSESSMENT DATA

- Disorientation in known and unknown environments
- Inability to reason
- Inability to concentrate
- Poor judgment
- Misperceptions
- Confusion

EXPECTED OUTCOMES

Immediate   The client will

- Be free of injury throughout hospitalization
- Refrain from injuring others or destroying property throughout hospitalization
- Demonstrate decreased agitation or restlessness within 24 to 48 hours
- Increase reality contact within his or her limitations within 48 to 72 hours

Stabilization   The client will

- Feel comfortable and supported in his or her environment
- Demonstrate accurate awareness of surroundings when possible

Community   The client will

- Attain his or her optimal level of functioning
- Live in the least restrictive environment possible

IMPLEMENTATION

Nursing Interventions *denotes collaborative interventions	Rationale
Observe the client to ascertain his or her whereabouts at all times.	The client may wander off and endanger himself or herself unknowingly.
Check the client frequently at night.	Confusion or disorientation may increase at night.
Provide adequate light in the environment, even at night (e.g., a night-light).	Adequate light decreases the client's misperceptions of shadows, and so forth.
Do not isolate the client. It may be helpful to place the client in a room near the nursing station to facilitate interaction.	Contact with others is reality. Hallucinations usually increase when the client is alone.
Assess the client's disorientation or confusion regularly.	The client's level of orientation may vary.
Provide adequate restraints (Posey, vest, etc.) if necessary for protection. *Note:* Side rails alone may prove dangerous if the client tries to climb over them. Be aware of and follow restraint policies and procedures.	Restraints can increase the client's agitation and fear but may be needed for his or her safety. The client may not understand or remember the purpose of side rails or restraints.
Refer to the date, time of day, and recent activities during your interactions with the client.	Reminders help to orient the client without the client having to ask.
Correct errors in the client's perceptions of reality in a matter-of-fact manner. Do not laugh at the client's misperceptions, and do not allow other clients to ridicule the client.	Failing to correct the client's errors in reality contact or laughing at the client undermines his or her sense of personal worth and dignity.

IMPLEMENTATION (continued)

Nursing Interventions *denotes collaborative interventions	Rationale
*Encourage visits from the client's friends and family, and assess their effect on the client's confusion and memory. You may need to limit the visits if the client tolerates them poorly.	Family and friends usually enhance the client's reality contact. Increased agitation or confusion following visits may signal the need to limit frequency or duration of visits.
Allow the client to have familiar possessions such as pictures and personal clothing in his or her room. Assign the same staff members to work with the client whenever possible.	These measures may help to decrease the client's confusion.

Nursing Diagnosis

Impaired Social Interaction
Insufficient or excessive quantity or ineffective quality of social exchange.

ASSESSMENT DATA

- Confusion with or without periods of awareness and lucidity
- Feelings of frustration
- Feelings of hopelessness
- Impaired memory, particularly concerning recent events
- Disinterest in surroundings
- Socially inappropriate behavior
- Decreased social interaction

EXPECTED OUTCOMES

Immediate   The client will

- Interact with others in the immediate environment within 24 hours
- Express feelings of frustration or hopelessness if possible within 24 to 48 hours
- Demonstrate decreased socially inappropriate behavior within his or her limitations within 48 to 72 hours
- Verbalize fewer negative comments about self within 3 to 5 days

Stabilization   The client will

- Engage in satisfactory interpersonal relationships within his or her limitations
- Verbalize increased feelings of self-worth within his or her limitations

Community   The client will

- Remain involved in his or her surroundings
- Continue to maintain interpersonal relationships within his or her limitations

IMPLEMENTATION

Nursing Interventions *denotes collaborative interventions	Rationale
Intervene as soon as you observe inappropriate behavior (e.g., undressing, advances toward others, urinating somewhere other than the bathroom).	You must protect the client's privacy and dignity when he or she is unable to do so.
Take a matter-of-fact approach; do not chastise or ridicule the client.	Scolding the client (as you might a child) is not helpful, because the client is not willfully misbehaving, and this is something the client cannot understand.

(continued on page 112)

IMPLEMENTATION (continued)

Nursing Interventions *denotes collaborative interventions	Rationale
Offer acceptable alternatives, and redirect the client's activities ("Mr. X, it is not appropriate to undress here, I'll help you to your room to undress").	Providing alternatives guides the client to appropriate behavior, of which he or she may be unaware.
Praise the client for appropriate behavior.	Positive feedback can be supportive for the client, increases the frequency of desired behavior and lets the client know what is acceptable.
*Determine what the client's interests, hobbies, and favorite activities were before hospitalization. (It may be necessary to obtain this information from the client's family or friends.)	It is easier to continue or resume previous interests and hobbies than to develop new ones. Activities that were familiar and enjoyed in the past may bring pleasure to the client.
Assess the client's current capacity for engaging in former hobbies or activities. Make these activities available as much as possible.	Some activities may not be feasible, depending on the client's physical and mental capabilities; however, the client may be able to assume a spectator role for these activities.
Introduce activities during a time of the day when the client seems most able to concentrate and participate.	This will maximize the client's ability to participate successfully.
Approach the client with a calm, positive attitude. Convey the idea that you believe he or she can succeed.	A positive approach enhances the client's confidence.
Begin with small, short-term activities with one staff member, and gradually progress to small groups.	Successful completion is more likely with simple, short activities that involve fewer people.
Increase the length or complexity of the activity or task gradually if the client tolerates increased stimulation.	Gradually increasing complexity challenges the client to his or her maximum potential.
Evaluate the activities and approaches; identify and continue those that are most successful.	Consistency decreases the client's frustration and builds on success.
Encourage small group activities or discussions with clients who share similar interests.	The client's social skills may be enhanced when discussing common interests with others.
*Involve the client with people from the community, such as volunteers, for social interactions. Identify groups outside the hospital in which the client can participate in the future.	The client has an opportunity to become familiar with people in the community with whom he or she may continue to socialize after hospitalization.
Allow the client to ventilate feelings of despair or hopelessness. Do not merely try to cheer up the client or belittle his or her feelings by using pat phrases or platitudes.	It is important to remember that the client is an adult, and disability can be quite frustrating to him or her. Giving false hope of recovery is not helpful to the client.

CARE PLAN 14

Head Injury

A traumatic head injury can result in a multitude of mental health problems for a client, including amnesia; depression; anxiety; irritability; decreased attention, concentration, and cognition; dementia; and mood and personality changes (APA, 2000). Head injuries are usually caused by trauma sustained during falls, diving, vehicular accidents, physical stunts, assault, physical abuse, or contact sports. Traumatic head injury is a leading cause of neurologic disability among adolescents and adults under the age of 35. It is most common in young men and is often associated with substance abuse (APA, 2000).

As medical technology and trauma services have improved, many people now survive an initial injury and must cope with significant alterations in health, lifestyle, employment, and numerous other areas. After physical rehabilitation is completed, residual problems include memory, cognitive and sensory deficits, impulsivity, and profound personality changes.

Most clients with head injuries have some awareness of their previous functioning and the current level of impairment. However, both the client and significant others may need help in identifying and accepting changes, especially if the client looks the same as before the injury, and some symptoms may be subtle.

Following physical recovery, few resources are available for long-term rehabilitation for these clients. Families must cope with drastic changes in the client's ability to earn a living, participate in social activities, or function in previous roles. Others are forced to assume new roles as the family system attempts to reestablish equilibrium.

The nurse must facilitate grief work with the client and significant others for actual, tangible losses, as well as the less tangible losses of potential achievements or aspirations. It is also important for the nurse to teach the client and significant others about head injury and its sequelae, the grief process, and caregiving.

NURSING DIAGNOSES ADDRESSED IN THIS CARE PLAN
Risk for Injury
Risk-Prone Health Behavior

RELATED NURSING DIAGNOSES ADDRESSED IN THE MANUAL
Ineffective Coping
Interrupted Family Processes
Chronic Low Self-Esteem
Deficient Diversional Activity
Noncompliance
Impaired Social Interaction
Risk for Other-Directed Violence
Impaired Memory

Nursing Diagnosis

Risk for Injury
At risk of injury as a result of environmental conditions interacting with the individual's adaptive and defensive resources.

RISK FACTORS

- Lack of awareness of physical or cognitive impairment
- Sensory or memory deficits
- Impulsive behavior
- Impaired cognition
- Inability to distinguish potentially harmful situations
- Inappropriate or unacceptable social behavior

EXPECTED OUTCOMES

Immediate   The client will

- Be safe and free from injury throughout hospitalization
- Respond to limits regarding safety within 24 to 48 hours
- Respond to cues from others regarding acceptable social behaviors within 3 to 4 days

Stabilization   The client will

- Refrain from unnecessary risks
- Perform daily routines safely, including self-care activities, responsibilities, and recreation
- Demonstrate socially appropriate behavior

Community   The client will

- Use community resources to ensure safety
- Collaborate with case manager or significant other in decision making

IMPLEMENTATION

Nursing Interventions *denotes collaborative interventions	Rationale
Provide a safe environment.	The client's safety is a priority. The client's behavior may be unsafe due to impaired judgment or impulsivity.
Protect the client from harming himself or herself by removing the items that could be used in self-destructive behavior or by restraining the client (see Care Plan 47: Aggressive Behavior).	The client's physical safety is a priority.
Remove the client to a quiet area if the client acts out or is exhibiting increased agitation.	The client's ability to deal with stimuli may be impaired.
Intervene if the client is exhibiting behavior that is unsafe. Use a calm, matter-of-fact approach. Do not scold or chastise the client or become angry with him or her.	The client may lack the ability to determine the safety of his or her behavior; he or she is not misbehaving willfully. The client may respond to verbal corrections but have a negative response if you are scolding or angry. Being calm and matter-of-fact decreases embarrassment and avoids a power struggle.
Set and reinforce limits regarding safe behavior.	The client's ability to recognize unsafe actions is impaired.
Teach the client about basic social skills and appropriate social interaction.	The client's injury may have impaired his or her sense of appropriate behavior and social skills. The client may be unaware of his or her deficits.
Give positive feedback for appropriate behavior.	Positive feedback can increase the desired behavior.
Provide the client with safe opportunities to release tension (e.g., exercising in the gym).	Physical activity provides the client with a way to relieve tension in a healthy, safe manner.

Nursing Diagnosis

Risk-Prone Health Behavior
Impaired ability to modify lifestyle/behaviors in a manner that improves health status.

ASSESSMENT DATA

- Irritability
- Mood swings
- Negativism
- Apathy
- Low self-esteem
- Poor judgment
- Impaired cognition
- Resistance to or noncompliance with therapy
- Lack of insight or comprehension

EXPECTED OUTCOMES

Immediate   The client will

- Comply with therapeutic regimen, for example, take medications as given within 24 hours
- Participate in planning treatment within 24 to 48 hours
- Respond to cues from others regarding acceptable social behaviors within 2 to 4 days
- Verbalize feelings openly and honestly within 2 to 4 days
- Demonstrate a daily routine, including self-care activities, responsibilities, and recreation within 3 to 5 days

Stabilization   The client will

- Verbalize increased feelings of self-worth, for example, verbally identify capabilities and strengths
- Demonstrate socially appropriate behavior, for example, listening to others
- Verbalize knowledge of condition and abilities, treatment, or safe use of medication, if any

Community   The client will

- Demonstrate progress in the grief process
- Perform functional role within his or her limitations

IMPLEMENTATION

Nursing Interventions *denotes collaborative interventions	Rationale
Encourage the client to verbalize feelings openly.	Expressing feelings is an essential step toward dealing with those feelings.
Encourage appropriate expression of anger or resentment.	The client may benefit from permission to express negative feelings safely.
Do not attempt to cheer the client with statements such as "At least you're alive; that's something to be thankful for."	The client may not agree with your opinion or could feel that his or her feelings are belittled.
Assist the client to specify his or her losses in concrete terms.	It is easier to deal with a loss stated in specific terms, rather than overwhelming, vague terms.
Give positive feedback for expression of honest feelings. Avoid reinforcing only hopeful or cheerful client statements.	The client must feel free to express actual feelings, not just those that are happy or optimistic.
Assist the client to rediscover past interests or identify new ones that are within his or her abilities.	The client may have forgotten past interests or may lack motivation to pursue interests.

(continued on page 116)

IMPLEMENTATION (continued)

Nursing Interventions *denotes collaborative interventions	Rationale
Ask open-ended questions, rather than questions that can be answered "yes" or "no." For example, ask "What shall we try today?" rather than "Do you want to …?"	Negative responses are common when you ask, "Do you want …?" questions. Open-ended questions put responsibility on the client to respond more fully.
Make needed adaptations to accommodate the client's physical limitations when possible.	Previous interests or hobbies may still be possible with adaptation or assistive devices.
Give the client a list of potential activities from which he or she must make a selection for the day.	Allowing the client a choice among recommended activities gives him or her a sense of control.
Help the client to identify choices.	The client's cognitive impairment may prevent him or her from seeing alternatives.
Respond to negativism with validation for the client's feelings, but maintain positive expectations. For example, if the client says, "I don't know if I'll like …," respond with "I don't know either. I guess you'll have to give it a try."	It often is unsuccessful to convince the client that he or she will like something new. It is more useful to validate his or her feelings, yet encourage the client to try something new.
Teach the client social skills, such as approaching another person for an interaction, appropriate conversation topics, and active listening. Encourage him or her to practice these skills with staff members and other clients, and give the client feedback regarding interactions.	Social awareness and skills frequently are lost or impaired in clients with head injuries.
Introduce the client to other clients in the milieu and facilitate their interactions on a one client to one client basis. Gradually facilitate social interactions between the client and small groups, then larger groups.	Gradually increasing the scope of the client's social interactions will help the client build confidence in social skills.
Intervene if the client is exhibiting behavior that is socially inappropriate.	The client may lack the ability to determine the appropriateness of his or her behavior.
Redirect the client to more socially appropriate behavior.	Redirection provides a socially appropriate alternative for the client.
Role-play real-life situations with which the client has demonstrated difficulty.	Role-playing assists the client to relearn lost skills.
Coach the client toward the development of acceptable behaviors.	Coaching allows shaping of the client's behavior toward successful completion of the behavior.
Provide reinforcement for successful use of social skills.	Reinforcement enhances the likelihood of recurring behavior.
Include the client in planning aspects of daily care (e.g., preference of time for therapy) in which he or she can have input.	The client is more likely to comply if he or she has had input in decision-making.
With the client, make a schedule of daily events or activities. It may be helpful to use a calendar.	Routines require fewer decision points. Written materials provide a concrete visual reminder.
Encourage the client to mark off items that are completed.	A sense of accomplishment can be gained by a concrete activity like crossing off tasks.
Offer verbal reminders, if necessary, referring to the written schedule.	Reminders keep the client focused on the task; referring to the written schedule helps the client remember to use it.
Refer to the day, date, and upcoming events (e.g., "Today is Wednesday; that means occupational therapy will be this afternoon.").	Orientation and memory are enhanced with references to date, place, time, and situation.
*Teach the client, significant others, and caregivers about the client's injury and deficits, giving specific information.	It usually is easier to deal with known facts, even if they are difficult, than to fear the unknown.

IMPLEMENTATION (continued)

Nursing Interventions *denotes collaborative interventions	Rationale
*Reassure the client and significant others that behavior and personality changes are part of the head injury, not willful uncooperativeness.	Changes that occur with head injuries often are baffling to the client and significant others. It may help them to know that these changes are part of the pathology.
Inform the client about what to expect from medications. Decrease reliance on medications to solve problems.	Medications may help to stabilize the client's mood but may not eliminate fluctuations. Clients with head injuries often attempt self-medication to obtain relief.
Instruct the client not to drink alcohol, use drugs, or deviate from the prescribed medication regimen.	Alcohol, drugs, and undesired drug interactions can further impair the client's judgment and cognition.
Encourage the client to continue to express feelings about lost capabilities as new situations arise that make deficits apparent.	Dealing with ongoing effects of a head injury is a continuing process.
Encourage the client to anticipate mood swings, and help him or her to identify ways to manage them.	Mood swings are common in head injuries. Knowing what to expect and having a plan to manage moods increases the client's ability to cope with them.
Assist the client to keep a journal with words or artwork (if he or she is able to write, draw, or use a computer) to document moods, feelings, and so forth.	It is sometimes easier for clients to use nonverbal methods of expression, particularly if aphasic difficulties interfere with verbal abilities.
Respond to the client's statements with validating and reflecting communication techniques. For example, if the client says, "I'll never be able to do…," you might say, "That's probably true. It must be very difficult and frustrating…"	Validating statements acknowledge the reality of the client's situation, which may not improve. Reflection channels the discussion to feelings, with which the client can work.
*Refer the client or family or significant others to a head injury support group in the community or through the Internet.	It often is helpful for clients and significant others to talk with others who have shared similar losses and problems, particularly with chronic conditions such as head injury.

SECTION 4 REVIEW QUESTIONS

1. Which of the following interventions is most appropriate in helping a client with early dementia complete activities of daily living (ADLs)?

   a. Allow enough time for the client to complete ADLs as independently as possible

   b. Provide the client with a written list of all the steps needed to complete ADLs

   c. Plan to provide step-by-step prompting to complete ADLs

   d. Tell the client to finish ADLs before breakfast or the nursing assistant will do them

2. A client with delirium is attempting to remove the intravenous tubing from his arm, saying to the nurse, "Get off me! Go away!" The client is experiencing which of the following?

   a. Delusions

   b. Hallucinations

   c. Illusions

   d. Disorientation

3. The client with dementia says to the nurse, "I know you. You're Judy, the little girl who lives in my apartment building." Which of the following responses would be most therapeutic?

   a. "I'm Maggie, a nurse here at the hospital."

   b. "I've told you before, I'm Maggie and I don't live in your apartment building."

   c. "You can see that I'm a nurse and not a little girl."

   d. "You know who I am, don't you?"

4. Which of the following would be the priority when caring for a client with delirium?

   a. Correcting the underlying causative condition

   b. Controlling behavioral symptoms with low-dose antipsychotic medication

   c. Decreasing fluids to prevent complications

   d. Manipulating the environment to increase stimulation

5. Which of the following would the nurse identify as an immediate goal to be accomplished in 24 to 48 hours for a client with delirium?

   a. Become oriented to person, place, and time

   b. Establish normal bowel and bladder function

   c. Reestablish a normal sleep/wake cycle

   d. Verbalize feelings about the experience of delirium

6. When communicating with clients with dementia, which of the following would the nurse employ to deal with decreased attention and increased confusion?

   a. Ask the client to go for a walk while talking

   b. Eliminate distracting stimuli in the immediate environment

   c. Rephrase questions the client doesn't immediately understand

   d. Use touch to convey empathy and caring

SECTION 4 Recommended Readings

Dewing, J. (2010). Responding agitation in people with dementia. *Nursing Older People, 22*(6), 18–25.

Park, H. (2010). Effect of music on pain for home-dwelling persons with dementia. *Pain Management Nursing, 11*(3), 141–147.

Schreier, A. M. (2010). Nursing care, delirium, and pain management for the hospitalized older adult. *Pain Management Nursing, 11*(3), 177–185.

Snell, F. I., & Halter, M. J. (2010). A signature wound of war: Mild traumatic brain injury. *Journal of Psychosocial Nursing and Mental Health Services, 48*(2), 22–28.

SECTION 4 Resources for Additional Information

Visit thePoint (http://thePoint.lww.com/Schultz9e) for a list of these and other helpful Internet resources.

Alzheimer Society of Canada
Alzheimer's Association
Alzheimer's Disease Education and Referral (ADEAR) Center
Alzheimer's Disease Research Center
American Society on Aging
Brain Injury Association of America
Brainline.org
Centers for Disease Control and Prevention
Family Caregiver Alliance
Gerontological Society of America
Head Injury Association
Institute on Aging and Environment
International Brain Injury Association
National Family Caregivers Association
National Institute on Aging
National Institute of Neurological Disorders and Stroke

Substance-Related Disorders

Abuse of substances may be chronic or acute and may include the use or abuse of alcohol, licit (prescription or over-the-counter) drugs, and illicit drugs. The first two care plans in this section are concerned with acute or short-term treatment plans for the client who is withdrawing from alcohol or another substance. Care Plan 17: Substance Dependence Treatment Program addresses longer-term treatment for clients with substance dependence. Clients who have a dual diagnosis or comorbid (or co-occurring) disorder—a major psychiatric illness and substance use or abuse—have special needs that are not necessarily met by traditional treatment for one or the other major problems. Considerations and care related to these clients are addressed in Care Plan 18: Dual Diagnosis. Considerations related to adult children of alcoholics are found in Care Plan 19: Adult Children of Alcoholics.

CARE PLAN 15

Alcohol Withdrawal

Alcohol is a drug that causes CNS depression. With chronic use and abuse of alcohol, the CNS is chronically depressed. An abrupt cessation of drinking causes a rebound hyperactivity of the CNS, which produces a variety of withdrawal phenomena. The particular phenomena are peculiar to each client, the client's pattern of use, and the chronicity of excessive alcohol intake.

Withdrawal from heavy or prolonged alcohol ingestion can result in a syndrome with a number of characteristic symptoms, including hyperactivity of the autonomic nervous system, hand tremor, sleep disturbance, psychomotor agitation, anxiety, nausea, vomiting, seizures, hallucinations, or illusions (APA, 2000). Clients in alcohol withdrawal can experience symptoms that range from mild to life-threatening, which necessitates careful assessment and monitoring.

In the United States, more than 7% of people 18 years and older—about 13.8 million—have problems with drinking. Of those, 8.1 million have alcoholism (Alcoholism-Statistics. com, 2010). Alcohol dependence is three times higher in men than in women, but the ratio varies in different age groups and among ethnic and cultural groups. Alcohol dependence has been associated with familial, genetic, social, and cultural factors (Alcoholism Information, 2010). Alcohol withdrawal symptoms usually begin within 4 to 12 hours after the last drink or marked reduction in drinking and are usually most severe the day after the last drink and much improved after several days. However, some clients may experience less severe symptoms for up to 6 months, including increased anxiety, sleep disturbance, and autonomic nervous system disturbance (APA, 2000). The most common withdrawal phenomena include the following:

- Physical *symptoms* including rapid pulse, elevated blood pressure, diaphoresis, sleep disturbances, irritability, and coarse tremors, which vary from shaky hands to involvement of the entire body.
- *Alcoholic hallucinosis* or sensory experiences characterized by misperception and misinterpretation of real stimuli in the environment (not to be confused with hallucinations), sleep disturbances, or nightmares. The client remains oriented to person, place, and time.
- *Auditory hallucinations*, true hallucinations caused by a cessation of alcohol intake rather than a psychiatric disorder, such as schizophrenia. The client hears voices, which usually are threatening or ridiculing. These "voices" may sound like someone the client knows.
- *Seizures*, categorized as grand mal, or major motor seizures, although they are transitory in nature. Medical treatment is required.
- *Delirium tremens* (DTs), the most serious phase of alcohol withdrawal. DTs begin with tremors, rapid pulse, fever, and elevated blood pressure, and the client's condition worsens over time. The client becomes confused, is delusional, feels pursued and fearful, and has auditory, visual, and tactile hallucinations (frequently of bugs, snakes, or rodents). DTs may last from 2 to 7 days and also may include physical complications, such as pneumonia, cardiac or renal failure, or death.

Careful assessment of the client's physical health status is essential during the withdrawal process. Use of a global rating scale based on consistent parameters provides a sound basis for clinical decision making. Many practical and effective scales are available and usually include blood pressure, pulse, temperature, hand tremors, tongue tremors, nausea or vomiting, orientation, and level of consciousness.

The client's safety and physical health are priorities in providing nursing care for the client in acute alcohol withdrawal. Other nursing objectives include medication management, assisting the client with personal hygiene and activities of daily living, and providing education and referrals for the client and significant others for follow-up treatment of alcohol dependence and related problems (see Care Plan 17: Substance Dependence Treatment Program and Care Plan 19: Adult Children of Alcoholics).

NURSING DIAGNOSES ADDRESSED IN THIS CARE PLAN
Risk for Injury
Ineffective Health Maintenance

RELATED NURSING DIAGNOSES ADDRESSED IN THE MANUAL
Insomnia
Bathing/Hygiene Self-Care Deficit
Dressing/Grooming Self-Care Deficit
Feeding Self-Care Deficit
Toileting Self-Care Deficit
Risk for Other-Directed Violence
Disturbed Sensory Perception (Specify: Visual, Auditory, Kinesthetic, Gustatory, Tactile, Olfactory)

Nursing Diagnosis

Risk for Injury
At risk for injury as a result of environmental conditions interacting with the individual's adaptive and defensive resources.

RISK FACTORS

- Confusion
- Disorientation
- Feelings of fear, dread
- Belligerent, uncooperative behavior
- Seizures
- Hallucinosis
- Delirium tremens
- Suicidal behavior
- Inability to distinguish potential harm
- Threatening or aggressive behavior
- Environmental misperceptions

EXPECTED OUTCOMES

Immediate   The client will

- Be safe and free from injury throughout hospitalization
- Respond to reality orientation within 12 to 36 hours
- Demonstrate decreased aggressive or threatening behavior within 12 to 36 hours

Stabilization   The client will

- Verbalize knowledge of alcoholism as a disease
- Verbalize risks related to alcohol intake

Community   The client will

- Abstain from alcohol and other drugs
- Accept referral to substance abuse treatment

IMPLEMENTATION

Nursing Interventions *denotes collaborative interventions	Rationale
Place the client in a room near the nurses' station or where the staff can observe the client closely.	The client's safety is a priority.
Institute seizure precautions according to hospital policy (padded side rails up, airway at bedside, etc.).	Seizures can occur during withdrawal. Precautions can minimize chances of injury.
Provide only an electric shaver.	The client may be too shaky to use a razor with blades.
Monitor the client's sleep pattern; he or she may need to be restrained if confused or if he or she attempts to climb out of bed.	The client's physical safety is a priority.
Reorient the client to person, time, place, and situation as needed.	You provide reality orientation by describing situations, stating the date, time, and so forth.
Talk to the client in simple, direct, concrete language. Do not try to discuss the client's feelings, plans for treatment, or changes in lifestyle when the client is intoxicated or in withdrawal.	The client can respond to simple, direct statements from you. The client's ability to deal with complex or abstract ideas is limited by his or her condition.
Reassure the client that the bugs, snakes, and so on are not really there.	You provide reality orientation for the client.
Tell the client that you know these sights appear real to him or her, and acknowledge the client's fears but leave no doubt about hallucinations not being real.	You can demonstrate respect for the client's experience while still providing reality orientation.
Do not moralize or chastise the client for his or her alcoholism. Maintain a nonjudgmental attitude.	Remember that alcoholism is an illness and is out of the client's control at this time. Moralizing belittles the client.

Nursing Diagnosis

Ineffective Health Maintenance
Inability to identify, manage, and/or seek out help to maintain health.

ASSESSMENT DATA

- Physical symptoms (impaired nutrition, fluid and electrolyte imbalance, gastrointestinal disturbances, liver impairment)
- Physical exhaustion
- Sleep disturbances
- Dependence on alcohol

EXPECTED OUTCOMES

Immediate   The client will

- Establish physiologic homeostasis within 24 to 72 hours
- Establish a balance of rest, sleep, and activity within 24 to 72 hours
- Maintain personal hygiene and grooming, for example bathe, wash hair within 24 to 48 hours

Stabilization   The client will

- Maintain physiologic stability
- Establish nutritious eating patterns
- Agree to participate in a treatment program
- Identify needed health resources

Community   The client will

• Follow through with discharge plans regarding physical health, counseling, and legal problems, as indicated
• Abstain from alcohol and other drugs

IMPLEMENTATION

Nursing Interventions *denotes collaborative interventions	Rationale
Complete an initial client assessment; ask what and how much the client usually drinks, as well as the time and amount of the last drink of alcohol. If possible, interview family members or significant others to gain accurate information regarding alcohol intake.	This information can help you anticipate the onset and severity of withdrawal symptoms. The client's memory may be impaired or he or she may not reveal the actual extent of alcohol intake.
*Monitor the client's health status based on standard parameters or rating scale. Administer medications as ordered or as indicated by alcohol withdrawal protocol. Observe the client for behavioral changes. Alert the physician to changes or when assessments exceed parameters.	Blood pressure, pulse, and the presence or absence of tongue tremors are the most reliable data to determine the client's need for medication. Use of predetermined parameters ensures consistent assessments and reliable data on which to evaluate the client's progress.
Monitor the client's fluid and electrolyte balance. Intravenous therapy may be indicated for clients in severe withdrawal.	Clients with alcohol abuse problems are at high risk for fluid and electrolyte imbalances.
Offer fluids frequently, especially juices and protein shakes. Serve only decaffeinated coffee.	Caffeine will increase tremors. Protein shakes and juices offer nutrients and fluids to the client.
Provide food or nourishing fluids as soon as the client can tolerate eating; have something available at night. (Bland food usually is tolerated more easily at first.)	Many clients who use alcohol heavily experience gastritis or anorexia. It is important to reestablish nutritional intake as soon as the client tolerates food.
Administer medication to minimize the progression of withdrawal or complications and to facilitate sleep.	The client will be fatigued and needs rest. Also, he or she should be as comfortable as possible.
Encourage the client to bathe, wash his or her hair, and wear clean clothes.	Personal cleanliness will enhance the client's sense of well-being.
Assist the client as necessary; it may be necessary to provide complete physical care, depending on the severity of the client's withdrawal.	The client's needs should be met with the greatest degree of independence he or she can attain, which is dependent on the severity of withdrawal symptoms.
*After the client's condition has stabilized, teach the client and his or her family or significant others that alcoholism is a disease that requires long-term treatment and follow-up. Refer the client to a substance dependence treatment program.	Detoxification deals only with the client's physical withdrawal from alcohol but does not address the primary disease of alcoholism.
*Refer the client's family or significant others to Al-Anon, Alateen, or Adult Children of Alcoholics, as indicated.	Alcoholism is an illness that affects all family members and significant others.

CARE PLAN 16

Substance Withdrawal

Substance withdrawal, or *drug withdrawal*, is a syndrome that develops when someone stops or greatly reduces use of a drug after heavy and prolonged use. Two characteristics of physiologic addiction to drugs are *tolerance* (the need to increase the dose to achieve the same effect) and *withdrawal* (physiologic and cognitive symptoms occur after drug ingestion ceases). Substance withdrawal can occur in clients of either gender and at any age, as long as a sufficient amount of the substance has been used for a sufficiently long period. Drug abuse is more commonly diagnosed in men, although specific drugs have various ratios of male and female abusers. Adult females and adolescents of both genders often develop drug tolerance and experience complications from drug use more rapidly than adult males.

The timing of onset and duration of withdrawal symptoms after the last dose of the drug vary with the type and dose of substance used and the level of tolerance the client had to the substance. Withdrawal symptoms can occur when drug ingestion is curtailed or eliminated, even when there has been no demonstrable physiologic tolerance.

Clients who abuse prescription drugs have essentially the same problems and difficulties as clients who abuse illicit drugs, although illicit drug abusers have the additional problem of unknowingly taking larger doses than intended, or ingesting additional substances of which they are unaware. Clients with drug use or abuse problems may have poor general health, especially in the area of nutrition, and are at increased risk for infections, gastrointestinal disturbances, and hepatitis.

The symptoms of withdrawal are specific to the drug taken, although in general present effects opposite to the drug taken. Withdrawal signs and symptoms for the major categories of drugs are found in the table below.

Drugs	Withdrawal Symptoms
Sedatives, hypnotics, and anxiolytics (including barbiturates, nonbarbiturate hypnotics, benzodiazepines, Rohypnol, GHB)	Restlessness, anxiety, irritability, autonomic hyperactivity (increased blood pressure, pulse, respiration, temperature), hand tremors, nausea, vomiting, and psychomotor agitation. Delirium, fever, and seizures are rare but occur in severe cases.
Stimulants (including amphetamines, cocaine, methamphetamine). *Note*: Persons using methamphetamine may also experience psychotic symptoms.	Dysphoria, fatigue, vivid and unpleasant dreams, hypersomnia or insomnia, increased appetite, "crashing," possible depressive symptoms with suicidal ideation.
Hallucinogens (including LSD, mescaline, psilocybin, PCP, Ecstasy)	No specific withdrawal symptoms are identified for hallucinogens; however, hyperactivity, hallucinations, delusions, and violent and aggressive behaviors may occur and persist over time.

Treatment of the client with substance withdrawal syndrome focuses on safety, symptom management, and meeting the client's needs for hydration, nutrition, elimination, and rest. After the client has been medically stabilized, it is important for the nurse to work with the interdisciplinary team to fully assess the client's substance abuse–related situation and make appropriate referrals for continued treatment. An additional treatment goal is educating the client and significant others about substance abuse and hepatitis and HIV transmission related to needle sharing and sexual activity.

Note: Do not ask or listen if the client attempts to reveal the names or locations of illicit drug sources to you. You do not need this information to work with the client. If you inadvertently gain knowledge of this nature, it is treated as confidential and not used for legal action.

NURSING DIAGNOSES ADDRESSED IN THIS CARE PLAN
Risk for Injury
Ineffective Health Maintenance

RELATED NURSING DIAGNOSES ADDRESSED IN THE MANUAL
Risk for Other-Directed Violence
Insomnia
Noncompliance
Disturbed Sensory Perception (Specify: Visual, Auditory, Kinesthetic, Gustatory, Tactile, Olfactory)

Nursing Diagnosis

Risk for Injury
At risk for injury as a result of environmental conditions interacting with the individual's adaptive and defensive resources.

RISK FACTORS

- Fearfulness
- Mood alteration, drastic mood swings
- Confusion
- Disorientation
- Seizures
- Hallucinations
- Delusions
- Physical pain or discomfort
- Uncooperative, hostile behavior
- Disturbances of concentration, attention span, or ability to follow directions

EXPECTED OUTCOMES

Immediate

The client will

- Be safe and free from injury throughout hospitalization
- Demonstrate decreased aggressive or hostile behavior within 12 to 36 hours
- Respond to reality orientation within 12 to 36 hours
- Verbally express feelings of fear or anxiety within 12 to 24 hours

Stabilization

The client will

- Verbalize knowledge of substance abuse as a disease
- Verbalize risks related to drug ingestion

Community

The client will

- Abstain from the use of substances
- Accept referral to substance abuse treatment

IMPLEMENTATION

Nursing Interventions *denotes collaborative interventions	Rationale
Place the client in a room near the nurses' station or where the staff can observe the client closely.	The client's safety is a priority.
It may be necessary to assign a staff member to remain with the client at all times.	One-to-one supervision may be required to ensure the client's safety.
Institute seizure precautions as needed, according to hospital policy (padded side rails, airway at bedside).	You should be prepared for the possibility of withdrawal seizures.
Restraints may be necessary to keep the client from harming himself or herself.	If the client cannot be protected from injury in any other manner, restraints may be necessary. Remember, restraints are not to be used punitively.
Decrease environmental stimuli (lights, television, visitors) when the client is agitated. Avoid lengthy interactions; keep your voice soft; speak clearly.	Your presence and use of soft voice tones can be calming to the client. He or she is not able to deal with excessive stimuli.
Do not moralize or chastise the client for substance use. Maintain a nonjudgmental attitude.	Remember that substance use and abuse is an illness and out of the client's control at this time. Moralizing belittles the client.
Talk with the client using simple, concrete language. Do not attempt to discuss the client's feelings, plans for treatment, or changes in lifestyle while the client is influenced by the drug or in acute or severe withdrawal.	The client's ability to process abstractions is impaired during withdrawal. You and the client will be frustrated if you attempt to address interpersonal or complex issues at this point.
Reorient the client to person, time, place, and situation as indicated when the client is confused or disoriented.	Presentation of concrete facts facilitates the client's reality contact.

Nursing Diagnosis

Ineffective Health Maintenance
Inability to identify, manage, and/or seek out help to maintain health.

ASSESSMENT DATA

- Dependence on drugs
- Physical discomfort
- Physical symptoms (impaired nutrition, fluid and electrolyte imbalance)
- Sleep disturbances
- Low self-esteem
- Feelings of apathy
- Ineffective coping strategies

EXPECTED OUTCOMES

Immediate   The client will

- Establish physiologic homeostasis
- Establish a balance of rest, sleep, and activity

Stabilization   The client will

- Establish nutritious eating patterns
- Maintain physiologic stability
- Verbalize knowledge of prevention of HIV transmission
- Agree to participate in a treatment program

Community   The client will

- Follow through with discharge plans regarding employment, legal involvement, family problems, and financial difficulties
- Abstain from alcohol and drugs

IMPLEMENTATION

Nursing Interventions *denotes collaborative interventions	Rationale
*Obtain the client's history, including the kind, amount, route, and time of last drug use. Consult the client's family or significant others to obtain or validate the client's information if necessary.	Baseline data can help you anticipate the onset, type, and severity of physical withdrawal symptoms. The client may report an inaccurate estimate of drug use (either minimized or exaggerated).
Be aware of PRN medication orders to decrease physical symptoms. Do not allow the client to be needlessly uncomfortable, but do not use medications too liberally.	Judicious use of PRN medications can decrease the client's discomfort, but must be used cautiously, as the client is already experiencing drug effects.
You may need to obtain blood or urine specimens for drug screening on admission, per physician order and client consent. Stress that this information is needed to treat the client and is not for legal or prosecution purposes. *Note:* Clients involved in vehicular accidents or charged with criminal activity may be an exception in some states.	Drug screens can positively identify substances the client has ingested. Often other substances are included in illegal drugs, of which the client has no knowledge. The client and family must be reassured that treatment is separate from legal issues. However, depending on state laws, information from laboratory tests may need to be surrendered to authorities.
Remain nonjudgmental in your approach to the client and significant others.	Your nonjudgmental approach can convey acceptance of the client as a person, which is separate from drug-taking behavior.
Monitor the client's intake and output and pertinent laboratory values, such as electrolytes.	The client in withdrawal is at risk for fluid and electrolyte imbalances.
Encourage oral fluids, especially juice, fortified supplements, or milk. If the client is vomiting, intravenous therapy may be necessary.	Milk, juice, and supplements provide a maximum of nutrients in a small volume. Fluids usually are tolerated best by the client initially.
Talk with the client quietly in short, simple terms. Do not chatter or make social conversation. Be comfortable with silence.	Excessive talking on your part may be irritating to the client in withdrawal. The client's ability to deal with stimuli may be impaired.
You may touch or hold the client's hand if these actions comfort or reassure the client.	Your physical presence conveys your acceptance of the client.
Encourage the client to bathe, wash his or her hair, and wear clean clothes.	Personal cleanliness will enhance the client's sense of well-being.
Assist the client as necessary; it may be necessary to provide complete physical care depending on the severity of the withdrawal symptoms.	You should attend to the client's hygiene only to the extent that he or she cannot do so independently.
*Teach the client and his or her family or significant others that substance dependence is an illness and requires long-term treatment and follow-up. Refer the client to a substance dependence treatment program.	Substance withdrawal deals only with the client's physical dependence. Further therapy is needed to address the primary problem of substance dependence.
*Refer the client's family or significant others to Alanon, Alateen, or Adult Children of Alcoholics as indicated.	Family and significant others are affected by the client's substance use and also need help with their own issues.
Teach the client about the prevention of hepatitis and HIV transmission.	Clients who use intravenous drugs are at increased risk for hepatitis and HIV transmission by sharing needles and by sexual activity, especially when judgment is impaired.
*If the client is HIV positive, refer him or her for medical treatment and counseling related to HIV disease.	Clients who are HIV positive face the risk of AIDS as well as related social problems. Clients may be unaware of available medical treatment and supportive resources.

CARE PLAN 17

Substance Dependence Treatment Program

Clients with substance dependence (including alcohol dependence) exhibit symptoms associated with more or less regular use of substances that affect the CNS. This use continues despite negative consequences, such as impaired health, legal or employment difficulties, or family discord. *Substance dependence* or *addiction* is an illness, although some health professionals and others still do not share that view. It is not caused by a lack of willpower, nor is it a moral weakness. Various theories about the etiology of substance dependence include genetic predisposition, body chemistry imbalance, maladaptive response to stress, and personality traits or disorders. Evidence suggests a genetic influence in the etiology, especially in alcohol dependence (APA, 2000).

Clients with substance dependency also often are diagnosed with a personality disorder, but this usually does not preclude success in a treatment program. However, if the client has a major psychiatric disorder, such as bipolar disorder or schizophrenia, there may need to be significant alterations in his or her treatment for substance dependence (see Care Plan 18: Dual Diagnosis).

Young adults are at increased risk for substance use, and onset of dependence is highest between ages 20 and 50. Substance dependence clients are at increased risk for accidents, aggressive behavior, and suicide (APA, 2000).

Clients who have used intravenous drugs are at increased risk for hepatitis C, HIV disease, and AIDS, from sharing needles or unprotected sexual behavior, particularly when judgment is impaired under the influence of alcohol or drugs.

Detoxification must occur before the client can become successfully involved in treatment. The multiple abuse of alcohol and other drugs is common. For recovery to be effective, the client must avoid simply transferring his or her use from one substance to another, that is, if a client quits using alcohol, he or she must not rely on medications to deal with stress. Substance dependence usually has a chronic course that may include periods of exacerbation and remission, although some clients do achieve lasting abstinence (APA, 2000).

Primary nursing interventions are helping the client acknowledge the substance dependence and facilitating development of effective coping skills. In this type of program, the nurse works as an integral part of the treatment team in providing consistent limits, structured support, education, and referrals for continued support in the community. It is important to involve the client's significant others in the treatment (whenever possible) to work toward resolving the problems and feelings surrounding the client's substance use and to facilitate recovery for the client and affected family members (see Care Plan 19: Adult Children of Alcoholics).

NURSING DIAGNOSES ADDRESSED IN THIS CARE PLAN
Ineffective Denial
Ineffective Coping

RELATED NURSING DIAGNOSES ADDRESSED IN THE MANUAL
Ineffective Role Performance
Noncompliance
Impaired Social Interaction

Nursing Diagnosis

Ineffective Denial

Conscious or unconscious attempt to disavow the knowledge or meaning of an event to reduce anxiety and/or fear, leading to the detriment of health.

ASSESSMENT DATA

- Denial or minimization of substance use or dependence
- Blaming others for problems
- Reluctance to discuss self or problems
- Lack of insight
- Failure to accept responsibility for behavior
- Viewing self as different from others
- Rationalization of problems
- Intellectualization

EXPECTED OUTCOMES

Immediate   The client will

- Participate in a treatment program, for example, attend activities and participate in group and therapy sessions within 24 to 36 hours
- Identify negative effects of his or her behavior on others within 24 to 36 hours
- Abstain from drug and alcohol use throughout treatment program
- Verbalize acceptance of responsibility for own behavior, including substance dependence and problems related to substance use (such as losing his or her job) within 24 to 48 hours

Stabilization   The client will

- Express acceptance of substance dependence as an illness
- Maintain abstinence from chemical substances
- Demonstrate acceptance of responsibility for own behavior
- Verbalize knowledge of illness and treatment plan

Community   The client will

- Follow through with discharge plans regarding employment, support groups, and so forth, for example, identify community resources and make initial appointment or schedule time to participate in support group sessions

IMPLEMENTATION

Nursing Interventions *denotes collaborative interventions	Rationale
*Give the client and significant others factual information about substance use in a matter-of-fact manner. Do not argue, but dispel myths such as "I'm not an alcoholic if I only drink on weekends," or "I can learn to just use drugs socially."	Most clients lack factual knowledge about substance use as an illness. If the client can engage you in semantic arguments or debates, the client can keep the focus off himself or herself and personal problems.
Avoid the client's attempts to focus on only external problems (such as marital or employment problems) without relating them to the problem of substance use.	The problem of substance use must be dealt with first because it affects all other areas.
Encourage the client to identify behaviors that have caused problems in his or her life.	The client may deny or lack insight into the relationship between his or her problems and behaviors.
Do not allow the client to rationalize difficulties or to blame others or circumstances beyond the client's control.	Rationalizing and blaming others give the client an excuse to continue his or her behavior.

(continued on page 132)

IMPLEMENTATION (continued)

Nursing Interventions *denotes collaborative interventions	Rationale
Consistently redirect the client's focus to his or her own problems and to what he or she can do about them.	You can facilitate the client's acceptance of responsibility for his or her own behavior.
Positively reinforce the client when he or she identifies and expresses feelings or shows any insight into his or her behaviors and consequences.	You convey acceptance of the client's attempts to express feelings and to accept responsibility for his or her own behavior.
Encourage other clients in the program to provide feedback for each other.	Peer feedback usually is valued by the client because it comes from others with similar problems.

Nursing Diagnosis

Ineffective Coping

Inability to form a valid appraisal of the stressors, inadequate choices of practiced responses, and/or inability to use available resources.

ASSESSMENT DATA

- Isolative behavior
- Low self-esteem
- Lack of impulse control
- Superficial relationships
- Inability to form and maintain intimate personal relationships
- Lack of effective problem-solving skills
- Avoidance of problems or difficult situations
- Ineffective coping skills

EXPECTED OUTCOMES

Immediate   The client will

- Express feelings directly and openly, for example, discuss feelings with staff for at least 30 minutes at least twice a day within 24 to 36 hours
- Engage in realistic self-evaluation, that is, describe strengths and areas needing support or development within 2 to 3 days
- Verbalize process for problem solving within 2 to 3 days

Stabilization   The client will

- Develop a healthful daily routine regarding eating, sleeping, and so forth, for example, sleep for at least 6 hours per night without using sleeping medication
- Practice nonchemical alternatives to dealing with stress or difficult situations
- Verbalize increased self-esteem, based on accurate information

Community   The client will

- Demonstrate effective communication with others
- Demonstrate nonchemical methods of dealing with feelings, problems, and situations, for example, demonstrate and describe the use of the problem-solving process related to an actual life situation
- Participate in follow-up or aftercare programs and support groups

IMPLEMENTATION

Nursing Interventions *denotes collaborative interventions	Rationale
Encourage the client to identify personal strengths as well as areas that need improvement.	The client may lack insight into his or her strengths and weaknesses. Identifying strengths can help the client realize that he or she can successfully cope with life's stressors.
Encourage the client to explore alternative ways of dealing with stress and difficult situations.	The client may have little experience dealing with life stress without chemicals and may be learning for the first time how to cope, solve problems, and so forth.
Talk with the client about coping strategies he or she has used in the past. Explore which strategies have been successful and which may have led to negative consequences.	The client may have had success using coping strategies in the past but may have lost confidence in himself or herself or in his or her ability to cope with stressors and feelings. The client needs to replace negative coping strategies (e.g., self-medication with drugs or alcohol) with activities that are not self-destructive.
Teach the client about positive coping strategies and stress management skills, such as increasing physical exercise, expressing feelings verbally or in a journal, or meditation techniques. Encourage the client to practice these techniques while in treatment.	The client may have limited or no knowledge of stress management techniques or may not have used positive techniques in the past. If the client tries to build skills in the treatment setting, he or she can experience success and receive positive feedback for his or her efforts.
Help the client develop skills in defining problems, planning problem-solving approaches, implementing solutions, and evaluating the process.	The client may not have used a structured problem-solving process. You can provide knowledge and practice of the process in a nonthreatening environment.
Help the client express feelings in acceptable ways, and give positive reinforcement for doing so.	You are a sounding board for the client. Your feedback encourages the client to continue to express feelings.
Involve the client in a group of his or her peers to provide confrontation, positive feedback, and sharing feelings.	Groups of peers are a primary mode of treatment in substance abuse treatment and provide honesty, support, confrontation, and validation, based on common experiences.
Focus attention on the "here-and-now": What can the client do now to redirect his or her behavior and life?	The client cannot change the past. Once he or she acknowledges responsibility for past behavior, it is not helpful or healthy to ruminate or feel guilty about the past.
Avoid discussing unanswerable questions, such as why the client uses substances.	Asking why is frustrating as well as fruitless; there is no answer.
Guide the client to the conclusion that sobriety is a choice he or she can make.	Sobriety, including abstinence from all substances, is associated with greater success in recovery.
Help the client view life and the quest for sobriety in feasible terms, such as "What can I do today to stay sober?"	The client may be overwhelmed by thoughts such as "How can I avoid using substances for the rest of my life?" and can deal more easily with shorter periods. The client needs to talk in terms of today, which is more manageable. The client needs to believe he or she can succeed to do so.
*Refer the client to a chaplain or spiritual advisor of his or her choice, if indicated.	The client may be overwhelmed with guilt or despair. Spiritual resources may help the client maintain sobriety and find social support.
*Teach the client and significant others about prevention of hepatitis and HIV transmission, and refer them for testing and counseling if appropriate.	Clients who use substances are at increased risk for hepatitis and HIV transmission by sharing needles and by sexual activity, especially when judgment is impaired by substance use.
*Refer the client to vocational rehabilitation, social services, or other resources as indicated.	The client may need a variety of services to reestablish successful functioning.

(continued on page 134)

IMPLEMENTATION (continued)

Nursing Interventions *denotes collaborative interventions	Rationale
*Refer the client and significant others to Alcoholics Anonymous, Al-Anon, Alateen, Adult Children of Alcoholics, or other support groups in the community or via the Internet as indicated.	Many clients and significant others benefit from continued support for sobriety after discharge. *Note:* There are many different groups modeled on the basic 12-step program, including gay, lesbian, and non-Christian groups.
*Refer the client for treatment for other problems as indicated.	Substance dependence often is associated with posttraumatic behavior, abusive relationships, and so forth.

CARE PLAN 18

Dual Diagnosis

The term *dual diagnosis or comorbid* (or *co-occurring*) *disorder* is used to describe a client with both substance abuse and another psychiatric illness. (*Note*: Some literature defines dual diagnosis as mental illness and mental retardation. These clients are not included in this discussion.) Clients with mental illness may use substances in an attempt to *self-medicate* (alleviate symptoms of illness), fit in with peers, and reduce social anxiety, or substance dependence may exist as a primary illness. It is common for clients with bipolar disorder or schizophrenia to describe efforts to use drugs or alcohol to self-medicate, attempting to level high and low mood swings. These clients' substance use, however, results in an exacerbation (not relief) of symptoms.

Substance dependence is a complicating factor with many clients who are chronically mentally ill, and substance abuse can occur with many types of mental disorders, including bipolar disorder, schizoaffective disorder, schizophrenia, conduct disorders, and personality disorders. It is estimated that 50% of persons with a substance abuse disorder also have a mental health diagnosis (Horsfall, Cleary, Hunt, & Walter, 2009).

The course of a client's dually diagnosed disorder depends on the psychiatric illness(es), the type of substance abuse, and other factors, including social support and treatment. Literature on the topic of dual diagnosis suggests that these clients are a difficult challenge and that this area needs further research to produce more effective methods of treatment. Traditional methods of treatment for major psychiatric illness or primary chemical dependence treatment programs are reported to have little lasting success in treating clients who have a dual diagnosis (Horsfall et al., 2009). An approach that considers both substance abuse and the specific psychiatric disorder simultaneously, as opposed to either type of treatment alone, may be successful for the client with a dual diagnosis. It is also necessary to tailor the treatment goals to the individual client. For example, the goal for a client to experience the social reward of achieving one or more years of sobriety is not realistic for a client with schizophrenia. For clients with schizophrenia, cognitive impairment and decreased ability to process abstract concepts are barriers to successful participation in substance dependency treatment programs. Likewise, treatment designed to manage psychotic symptoms is less successful when the client uses substances, which may exacerbate symptoms. Some clients with bipolar disorder have difficulty in substance dependence treatment programs with reconciling the concept of being drug free with instructions to remain compliant with lithium or other chemotherapy regimens. In addition, the impulsiveness associated with bipolar disorder interferes with the ability to remain alcohol or drug free. *Note*: The care plan is based on community treatment because, although clients may be readily stabilized in the hospital setting, their treatment presents a greater challenge after discharge.

NURSING DIAGNOSES ADDRESSED IN THIS CARE PLAN
Noncompliance
Ineffective Coping

RELATED NURSING DIAGNOSES ADDRESSED IN THE MANUAL
Ineffective Health Maintenance
Disturbed Thought Processes
Disturbed Sensory Perception (Specify: Visual, Auditory, Kinesthetic, Gustatory, Tactile, Olfactory)
Deficient Diversional Activity
Chronic Low Self-Esteem
Impaired Social Interaction

Nursing Diagnosis

Noncompliance

Behavior of person and/or caregiver that fails to coincide with a health-promoting or therapeutic plan agreed on by the person (and/or family and/or community) and healthcare professional. In the presence of an agreed upon, health-promoting, or therapeutic plan, the person's or caregiver's behavior is fully or partially nonadherent and may lead to clinically ineffective or partially ineffective outcomes.

ASSESSMENT DATA

- Frequent ingestion of alcohol or drugs
- Neuroleptic blood levels outside therapeutic range
- Exacerbation of symptoms
- Failure to keep appointments or follow through on referrals
- Poor impulse control
- Incongruence between therapeutic regimen and personal values or desires
- Knowledge or skill deficit

EXPECTED OUTCOMES

Immediate

The client will

- Verbalize the need for medication compliance throughout the treatment program
- Take medications as directed throughout treatment
- Identify difficulties associated with alcohol or substance use within 24 to 48 hours
- Refrain from alcohol or nonprescribed drug use throughout treatment

Stabilization

The client will

- Report instances of alcohol or drug use accurately
- Report medication compliance accurately
- Experience diminished or absent psychiatric symptoms

Community

The client will

- Participate in community support programs
- Continue compliance with prescribed medications

IMPLEMENTATION

Nursing Interventions *denotes collaborative interventions	Rationale
Complete a nursing assessment; discuss patterns of drug and alcohol use in a nonjudgmental manner.	A nonjudgmental manner increases the chance of obtaining accurate information, builds trust, and lessens the possibility of resistance from the client.
Indicate that your need to know is based on the need for accurate data to assess the client, not for criticism.	This conveys genuine concern for the client, which enhances trust.
Assist the client to draw correlations between increased chemical use and increased psychiatric symptoms.	The effect of increased symptoms caused by alcohol or drug use may not be apparent to the client.
*Inform the client of drug interactions between medications and other substances. It may be helpful to consult with a pharmacist.	Factual information is a sound basis for future problem solving. The client may have used several types of drugs in addition to several medications, creating complex drug interactions.
Encourage the client to ask questions if he or she is uncertain about taking medications when drinking and so forth.	Safety is a priority. The client who uses drugs or alcohol is at a greater risk for an overdose.

IMPLEMENTATION (continued)

Nursing Interventions *denotes collaborative interventions	Rationale
*If the client is having symptoms such as not sleeping, encourage him or her to ask a health professional for assistance before using drugs or alcohol to alleviate the symptoms.	A change in medication or dosage may resolve the client's difficulties without placing him or her at risk. The client may also have sleep apnea or another condition that can be treated successfully without drugs or alcohol.
Give positive feedback for honest reporting.	If the client perceives a greater reward for honesty than for strict adherence, he or she is more likely to report honestly.
*Encourage the client to participate in peer and support groups in the community or on the Internet.	Support from others with dual diagnoses can help the client remain adherent over the long term.

Nursing Diagnosis

Ineffective Coping

Inability to form a valid appraisal of the stressors, inadequate choices of practiced responses, and/or inability to use available resources.

ASSESSMENT DATA

- Poor impulse control
- Low self-esteem
- Lack of social skills
- Dissatisfaction with life circumstances
- Lack of purposeful daily activity

EXPECTED OUTCOMES

Immediate   The client will

- Take only prescribed medication throughout treatment
- Interact appropriately with staff and other clients within 24 to 72 hours
- Express feelings openly within 24 to 48 hours
- Develop plans to manage unstructured time, for example, walking, doing errands, within 2 to 3 days

Stabilization   The client will

- Demonstrate appropriate or adequate social skills, for example, initiate interactions with others
- Identify social activities in drug- and alcohol-free environments
- Assess own strengths and weaknesses realistically

Community   The client will

- Maintain contact or relationship with a professional in the community
- Verbalize plans to join a community support group that meets the needs of clients with a dual diagnosis in the community or on the Internet
- Participate in drug- and alcohol-free programs and activities

IMPLEMENTATION

Nursing Interventions *denotes collaborative interventions	Rationale
Encourage open expression of feelings.	Verbalizing feelings is an initial step toward dealing constructively with those feelings.
Validate the client's frustration or anger in dealing with dual problems (e.g., "I know this must be very difficult").	Expressing feelings outwardly, especially negative ones, may relieve some of the client's stress and anxiety.
Consider alcohol or substance use as a factor that influences the client's ability to live in the community, similar to such factors as taking medications, keeping appointments, and so forth.	Substance use is not necessarily the major problem the client with a dual diagnosis experiences, only one of several problems. Overemphasis on any single factor does not guarantee success.
Maintain frequent contact with the client, even if it is only through brief telephone calls.	Frequent contact decreases the length of time the client feels "stranded" or left alone to deal with problems.
Give positive feedback for abstinence on a daily basis.	Positive feedback reinforces abstinent behavior.
If drinking or substance use occurs, discuss the events that led to the incident with the client in a nonjudgmental manner.	The client may be able to see the relatedness of the events or a pattern of behavior while discussing the situation.
Discuss ways to avoid similar circumstances in the future.	Anticipatory planning may prepare the client to avoid similar circumstances in the future.
Teach the client about positive coping strategies and stress management skills, such as increasing physical exercise, expressing feelings verbally or in a journal, or meditation techniques. Encourage the client to practice this type of technique while in treatment.	The client may have limited or no knowledge of stress management techniques or may not have used positive techniques in the past. If the client tries to build skills in the treatment setting, he or she can experience success and receive positive feedback for his or her efforts.
Assess the amount of unstructured time with which the client must cope.	The client is more likely to experience frustration or dissatisfaction, which can lead to substance use, when he or she has excessive amounts of unstructured time.
Assist the client to plan daily or weekly schedules of purposeful activities: errands, appointments, taking walks, and so forth.	Scheduled events provide the client with something to anticipate or look forward to doing.
Writing the schedule on a calendar may be beneficial.	Visualization of the schedule provides a concrete reference for the client.
Encourage the client to record activities, feelings, and thoughts in a journal.	A journal can provide a focus for the client and yield information that is useful in future planning but may otherwise be forgotten or overlooked.
Teach the client social skills. Describe and demonstrate specific skills, such as eye contact, attentive listening, nodding, and so forth. Discuss the kind of topics that are appropriate for social conversation, such as the weather, news, local events, and so forth.	The client may have little or no knowledge of social interaction skills. Modeling the skills provides a concrete example of the desired skills.
Give positive support to the client for appropriate use of social skills.	Positive feedback will encourage the client to continue socialization attempts and enhance self-esteem.
*Teach the client and his or her significant others about his or her dual diagnosis, conditions, treatment, and medications.	The client's significant others can help provide support and structure. The client and his or her significant others may lack knowledge about his or her conditions, treatment, and medications.
*Refer the client to volunteer, educational, or vocational services if indicated.	Purposeful activity makes better use of the client's unstructured time and can enhance the client's feelings of worth and self-esteem.
*Refer the client to support services in the community or on the Internet that address mental health and substance dependence-related needs.	Clients with dual diagnosis have complicated and long-term problems that require ongoing, extended assistance.

CARE PLAN 19

Adult Children of Alcoholics

The term *adult child of an alcoholic* (ACA) refers to a person who was raised in a family where one or both parents were addicted to alcohol and who was subjected to dysfunctional parenting associated with alcoholism. The National Association for Children of Alcoholics (NACoA) was founded in 1983 to support children of alcoholics and for those in a position to help them—therapists, physicians, nurses, social workers, and so forth. The significance of being an "adult child" has gained attention in only the last several decades, even though alcoholism as a family illness has been recognized for much longer.

Self-help support groups, therapy groups, and a wide variety of popular books were developed in the 1980s to deal with the problems of adult children. In the 1990s, the concept broadened to *codependence*, which included many of the problems previously identified in adult children, but is not as tightly coupled with alcoholism. Although clients are unlikely to be hospitalized for being codependent or an adult child per se, many clients hospitalized or in other treatment settings for other problems may have these issues as complicating factors.

It is estimated that 6.6 million American children younger than 18 years live with at least one alcoholic parent, increasing their own risk for alcoholism fourfold. Forty-three percent of American adults have a child, parent, sibling, or spouse who was or is an alcoholic (Alcoholism Information, 2010). Children of alcoholics are at the highest risk of developing alcoholism and are prone to learning disabilities, eating disorders, stress-related medical problems, and compulsive achieving. Children of alcoholics also often develop an inability to trust, an extreme need to control, an excessive sense of responsibility, and denial of feelings; these problems persist through adulthood. ACAs are more likely to marry individuals who develop alcoholism.

Treatment goals focus on facilitating the client's insight, self-esteem, and coping and problem-solving skills. Other nursing interventions include teaching the client and significant others about substance dependence and working with the treatment team to identify appropriate referrals for continuing support.

NURSING DIAGNOSES ADDRESSED IN THIS CARE PLAN
Ineffective Coping
Chronic Low Self-Esteem

RELATED NURSING DIAGNOSES ADDRESSED IN THE MANUAL
Powerlessness
Post-Trauma Syndrome
Ineffective Role Performance

Nursing Diagnosis

Ineffective Coping

Inability to form a valid appraisal of the stressors, inadequate choices of practiced responses, and/or inability to use available resources.

ASSESSMENT DATA

- Inability to trust
- Excessive need or desire for control, either overtly or covertly expressed
- Very responsible or very irresponsible behavior
- Difficulty with authority
- Impulsive behavior
- Lack of effective assertiveness skills
- Intolerance of changes
- Difficulty setting and keeping limits
- Conflict avoidance behaviors
- Addictive behavior (e.g., to excitement or chaos in daily life or relationships)

EXPECTED OUTCOMES

Immediate   The client will

- Discuss situations involving conflict, identifying the conflict and related feelings within 2 to 3 days or treatment visits
- Demonstrate choices based on self-approval rather than seeking the approval of others within 2 to 3 days or treatment visits

Stabilization   The client will

- Demonstrate appropriate use of assertiveness skills
- Follow through with commitments, for example, keep appointments or make and complete plans with others

Community   The client will

- Demonstrate use of effective problem-solving skills
- Participate in substance dependence treatment, if indicated, or support groups after discharge

IMPLEMENTATION

Nursing Interventions *denotes collaborative interventions	Rationale
Talk with the client about coping strategies he or she has used in the past. Explore which strategies have been successful and which may have led to negative consequences.	The client may have had success using coping strategies in the past but may have lost confidence in himself or herself or in his or her ability to cope with stressors and feelings. Some coping strategies can be self-destructive (e.g., self-medication with drugs or alcohol).
Teach the client about positive coping strategies and stress management skills, such as increasing physical exercise, expressing feelings verbally or in a journal, or meditation techniques. Encourage the client to practice these techniques while in treatment.	The client may have limited or no knowledge of stress management techniques or may not have used positive techniques in the past. If the client tries to build skills in the treatment setting, he or she can experience success and receive positive feedback for his or her efforts.
Teach the client the problem-solving process: identifying a problem, exploring alternatives, making a decision, and evaluating its success.	The client may have limited skills or experience in rational problem solving.

IMPLEMENTATION (continued)

Nursing Interventions *denotes collaborative interventions	Rationale
Have the client make a list of situations that are difficult for him or her.	The client's interest in learning problem-solving skills is enhanced by using actual, rather than hypothetical, situations.
With the client, develop a list of approaches to these situations, followed by the client's feelings about each choice.	Learning to identify his or her feelings and to couple feelings with choices can be a new experience for the client.
Assist the client to determine the pros and cons of each choice.	Practicing the problem-solving process will develop proficiency in its use.
Encourage the client to select a choice and make specific plans for implementation.	ACAs typically have difficulty following through. Specific plans increase the likelihood that the client will do so.
Teach the client about assertiveness skills; differentiate among passive, aggressive, and assertive responses.	The client may be unaware of the basis for assertiveness skills.
Teach the client about setting limits, and encourage the use of limit-setting skills and awareness in relationships.	ACAs often have little or no knowledge, experience, or skill in using limit setting.
Encourage the client to practice using "I" statements to express needs or desires.	Using "I" statements encourages the client to focus on and accept responsibility for his or her own feelings and wishes.
Role-play previously identified difficult or unfamiliar situations with the client, incorporating assertiveness skills.	Anticipatory practice helps the client be better prepared for actual implementation.
Encourage the client to implement an approach to an identified problem situation, beginning with the least threatening situation.	The least threatening situation has the greatest chance of being a successful initial experience for the client.
After the client has made an attempt to deal with the situation, provide time to discuss the client's attempt(s), focusing on how he or she felt.	If the client was successful, his or her self-worth may be enhanced. If unsuccessful, the client learns that one can survive having a negative experience.
Give positive feedback for attempts to use new skills, not just for successful resolution of the situation.	The client needs positive feedback for trying, not just for "winning."
If the client was unsuccessful in resolving the problem, help him or her to evaluate alternatives and make another attempt to solve the problem. Do not punish the client or withdraw your attention when the client is unsuccessful.	This will promote the client's ability to follow through and affords another opportunity for success, even following unsuccessful experiences. The client's early experiences of lack of success may have resulted in punishment or withdrawal of attention.

Nursing Diagnosis

Chronic Low Self-Esteem
Longstanding negative self-evaluating/feelings about self or self-capabilities.

ASSESSMENT DATA

- Excessive need to control emotions
- Denial of feelings
- Difficulty expressing feelings
- Fear of emotional abandonment
- Chronic feelings of insecurity
- Reluctance to discuss personal issues
- Guilt feelings
- Harsh judgment of own behavior
- Consistent feelings of failure

- Impaired spontaneity or ability to have fun
- Reluctance to try new things
- Dysfunctional or unsatisfactory relationships (e.g., the client may play the role of the victim or have difficulty with intimacy)
- Views self as "different" from other people
- Extreme loyalty to others, even when undeserved

EXPECTED OUTCOMES

Immediate

The client will

- Verbalize recognition of alcoholism as an illness within 12 to 24 hours
- Demonstrate a focus on self in the present rather than past experiences within 2 to 3 days
- Verbally identify his or her feelings in a nonjudgmental manner within 3 to 4 days

Stabilization

The client will

- Verbalize realistic self-evaluation, for example, make a written list of strengths, abilities, and areas needing support or development and discuss with staff
- Demonstrate the ability to engage in spontaneous activities for the sake of having fun
- Verbalize knowledge about alcoholism and related family problems

Community

The client will

- Make decisions and solve problems independently
- Express feelings to others without guilt

IMPLEMENTATION

Nursing Interventions *denotes collaborative interventions	Rationale
*Provide education to the client and significant others about alcoholism as a family illness.	Accurate information helps the client to recognize that parental alcoholism, not the client, is a source of many family problems.
Encourage the client to remember and discuss experiences of growing up, family interactions, and so forth.	ACAs often have kept "family secrets," especially related to alcoholism, and shared them with no one.
Encourage the client to identify characteristics of himself or herself and family members as individuals.	The client's sense of identity may be enmeshed with the entire family. The client may have difficulty seeing himself or herself as a separate person.
Assist the client to view himself or herself realistically in the present and to allow the past to become history.	Once the client has expressed past feelings and experiences, he or she can put them in the past and "let go" of them, which can provide opportunities for growth.
Encourage the client to verbalize all feelings, especially negative ones, such as anger, resentment, and so forth.	ACAs often have learned to "stuff" or deny feelings and are not skilled at identifying or expressing them.
Give positive feedback for honest expression of feelings.	Positive feedback increases the frequency of desired behavior.
Involve the client in small group discussions with others having similar issues, if possible.	Groups of ACAs allow clients to find that they are not alone in their feelings and experiences.
Suggest appropriate ways of expressing feelings, such as talking and writing in a journal.	The client needs to identify the most comfortable and beneficial ways of appropriately expressing feelings.
Encourage the client to use a journal to focus on present thoughts, feelings, and their relatedness.	Using a journal can help increase awareness of feelings and behavior, promote insight, and help the client focus on self-approval, rather than the approval of others.
With the client, review journal entries as a basis for identifying aspects of personal growth for the client, including efforts made and successes, even if small.	The client is struggling with issues that often are many years old. Progress can be more easily identified if he or she has a means for recognizing steps in growth and positive change.

IMPLEMENTATION (continued)

Nursing Interventions *denotes collaborative interventions	Rationale
See Care Plan 49: Sexual, Emotional, or Physical Abuse.	ACAs often have issues involving abuse.
Encourage the client to make a list of his or her strengths and areas he or she would like to change.	A written list gives the client a concrete focus, so he or she is not so likely to feel overwhelmed. The client may have the most difficulty identifying positive qualities.
Practice giving and receiving compliments with the client.	Receiving compliments may be new to the client and can increase self-esteem. Giving compliments helps the client build communication skills and relationships.
Assist the client to set small achievable daily or weekly goals.	Small goals seem possible to attain and will not discourage or overwhelm the client. Attaining even small goals provides successful experiences for the client.
*Provide the client with a reading list of resources related to ACAs.	The client cannot assimilate all possible information in a short time. A list provides an ongoing resource.
*Encourage the client to continue to seek support after the treatment episode. Refer the client to ACA support group(s) in the community or on the Internet.	The client is dealing with issues that have accumulated over a lifetime. Resolving these issues is a long process, facilitated by the ongoing support of others in similar situations.

SECTION 5 REVIEW QUESTIONS

1. Which of the following would the nurse recognize as signs of alcohol withdrawal?

   a. Coma, disorientation, and hypervigilance

   b. Tremulousness, sweating, and elevated blood pressure

   c. Increased temperature, lethargy, and hypothermia

   d. Talkativeness, hyperactivity, and blackouts

2. A client who is intoxicated is admitted to the hospital for alcohol withdrawal. Which of the following would the nurse do to help the client become sober?

   a. Give the client black coffee to drink

   b. Have the client take a cold shower

   c. Provide the client with a quiet room to sleep in

   d. Walk around the unit with the client

3. Which of the following would be contraindicated for a client who is experiencing severe symptoms of alcohol withdrawal?

   a. Ambulating the client

   b. Lowering environmental stimuli

   c. Monitoring intake and output

   d. Using short, direct statements

4. Which of the following foods would the nurse eliminate from the diet of a client with alcohol withdrawal?

   a. Ice cream

   b. Milk

   c. Orange juice

   d. Regular coffee

5. Which of the following interventions would the nurse include in the plan of care for the client in severe alcohol withdrawal?

   a. Continuous use of restraints for safety

   b. Informing the client about alcohol treatment programs

   c. Remaining with the client when he or she is confused

   d. Touching the client before saying anything

6. When caring for a client who has been using PCP, the nurse would be especially alert for which of the following behaviors?

   a. Auditory hallucinations

   b. Bizarre behavior

   c. Loud screaming

   d. Violent behavior

SECTION 5 Recommended Readings

Finfgeld-Connett, D. (2009). Web-based treatment for rural women with alcohol problems: Preliminary findings. *Computers, Informatics, Nursing, 27*(6), 345–353.

Nordfjaern, T., Rundmo, T., & Hole, R. (2010). Treatment and recovery as perceived by patients with substance addiction. *Journal of Psychiatric and Mental Health Nursing, 17*(1), 46–64.

Jane, L. (2010). How is alcohol withdrawal syndrome best managed in the emergency department? *International Emergency Nursing, 18*(2), 89–98.

Wallace, C. (2010). Integrated assessment of older adults who misuse alcohol. *Nursing Standard, 24*(33), 51–57.

SECTION 5 Resources for Additional Information

Visit thePoint (http://thePoint.lww.com/Schultz9e) for a list of these and other helpful Internet resources.

Addiction Technology Transfer Center Network
Adult Children of Alcoholics World Service Organization
Al-Anon/Alateen
Alcoholics Anonymous World Service Organization
American Society of Addiction Medicine
Association of Nurses in Substance Abuse
Co-Occurring Center for Excellence
Dual Diagnosis Resources
Dual Diagnosis Web Site
International Nurses Society on Addictions
National Association for Children of Alcoholics
National Clearinghouse for Alcohol and Drug Information
National Council on Alcoholism and Drug Dependence, Inc.
National Institute on Alcohol Abuse and Alcoholism
National Institute on Drug Abuse
Substance Abuse and Mental Health Services Administration
SAMSA—Co-Occurring and Homeless Activities Branch

Schizophrenia and Psychotic Disorders/ Symptoms

Schizophrenia is a thought disorder that includes psychotic symptoms such as delusions, hallucinations, and disordered thought processes. Psychotic behavior also can be encountered in clients who are experiencing other problems or disorders, such as bipolar disorder, alcohol withdrawal, or dementia. The care plans in this section address common psychotic symptoms, such as delusions and hallucinations, as well as problems and disorders that may produce psychotic symptoms, such as schizophrenia and certain medical conditions.

CARE PLAN 20

Schizophrenia

Schizophrenia is a disorder that involves characteristic psychotic symptoms (e.g., delusions, hallucinations, and disturbances in mood and thought) and impairment in the individual's level of functioning in major life areas. The characteristic symptoms of schizophrenia (APA, 2000) are listed below. Clients typically experience symptoms in several of these areas.

1. *Thought content.* Delusional thoughts are fragmented, sometimes bizarre, and frequently unpleasant for the client. Many clients believe that their thoughts are "broadcast" to the external world, so others are able to hear them *(thought broadcasting)*, that the thoughts are not their own but are placed there by others *(thought insertion)*, and that thoughts are being removed from their head *(thought withdrawal).* The client believes all this *thought control* occurs against his or her will and feels powerless to stop it.
2. *Perception.* The major perceptual disturbance is hallucinations, most commonly auditory (voices). The voices may be familiar to the client and may command the client to do things that may be harmful to the client or others; there may be more than one voice "speaking" at once. Visual, tactile, gustatory, kinesthetic, and olfactory hallucinations also can occur, but less commonly.
3. *Language and thought process.* The client is unable to communicate meaningful information to others. There may be *loose associations*, or jumping from one topic to an unrelated topic. *Poverty of speech* or *alogia* (little verbalization), *poverty of content* (much verbalization but no substance), *neologisms* (invented words), *perseveration* (repetitive speech), *clanging* (rhyming speech), or *blocking* (inability to verbalize thoughts) may occur. The client may be unaware that others cannot comprehend what he or she is saying.
4. *Psychomotor behavior.* The client may respond excitedly to the environment, demonstrating agitated pacing or other movements, or may be almost unresponsive to the environment and exhibit motor retardation, posturing, or stereotyped movements. These disturbances are usually seen during acute psychotic episodes and in severely chronically ill clients.
5. *Affect.* The client has a restricted mood, may feel numb or lack the intensity of normal feelings, and demonstrates a flat or inappropriate affect. The client with a flat affect has a lack of expression, monotonous tone of voice, and immobile facies. (*Note*: Many psychotropic medications produce effects that resemble a flat affect.) An inappropriate affect occurs when the client's expression is incongruent with the situation; for example, the client may talk of a sad event yet be laughing loudly.
6. *Avolition.* The client's ability to engage in self-initiated, goal-directed activity is disturbed. This can persist into a residual phase, resulting in marked impairment in the client's social, vocational, and personal functioning.

The symptoms of schizophrenia often are categorized as *hard* or *soft signs.* Hard signs include delusions and hallucinations, which are more amenable to the therapeutic effects of medication. Soft signs, such as lack of volition, impaired socialization, and affective disturbances, can persist after major symptoms of psychosis have abated and cause the client continued distress. The major types of schizophrenia and associated characteristics are as follows:

- *Catatonic*: generalized motor inhibition, stupor, mutism, negativism, waxy flexibility, or excessive, sometimes violent motor activity
- *Disorganized*: grossly inappropriate or flat affect, incoherence, loose associations, and extremely disorganized behavior

- *Paranoid*: persecutory or grandiose delusions, hallucinations, sometimes excessive religiosity, or hostile, aggressive behavior
- *Undifferentiated*: mixed schizophrenic symptoms along with disturbances of thought, affect, and behavior
- *Residual*: symptoms are not currently psychotic, but the client has had at least one previous psychotic episode and currently has other symptoms, which may include social withdrawal, flat affect, or looseness of associations

Schizoaffective disorder is no longer categorized as a subtype of schizophrenia (APA, 2000). The symptoms are neither exclusively those of a major mood disorder nor of schizophrenia; rather, they are a combination of both.

Schizophrenia is equally prevalent in men and women; it affects approximately 1.1% of adults in the United States in a given year. The average age of onset is in the late teens or early twenties for men and the twenties or early thirties for women (National Institute of Mental Health, 2010). Schizophrenia is not diagnosed until relevant symptoms have been present for at least six months. Most clients continue to have symptoms that necessitate long-term management; these symptoms may wax and wane, be relatively stable, or progressively worsen over time (APA, 2000). The prognosis for a client with schizophrenia is better when onset is acute; a precipitating event is present; or the client has a history of good social, occupational, and sexual adjustment.

Interventions with clients with schizophrenia focus on safety, meeting the client's basic needs, symptom management, medication management (see Appendix E: Defense Mechanisms), and long-term care planning. It is extremely important for the nurse to work closely with the interdisciplinary treatment team to coordinate acute care, referrals for continued care, and appropriate resources for support in the community.

NURSING DIAGNOSES ADDRESSED IN THIS CARE PLAN
Disturbed Personal Identity
Social Isolation
Bathing Self-Care Deficit
Dressing Self-Care Deficit
Feeding Self-Care Deficit
Toileting Self-Care Deficit

Nursing Diagnosis

Disturbed Personal Identity
Inability to maintain an integrated and complete perception of self.

ASSESSMENT DATA

- Bizarre behavior
- Regressive behavior
- Loss of ego boundaries (inability to differentiate self from the external environment)
- Disorientation
- Disorganized, illogical thinking
- Flat or inappropriate affect
- Feelings of anxiety, fear, or agitation
- Aggressive behavior toward others or property

EXPECTED OUTCOMES

Immediate

The client will

- Be free from injury throughout hospitalization
- Refrain from harming others or destroying property throughout hospitalization
- Establish contact with reality within 48 to 72 hours

- Demonstrate or verbalize decreased psychotic symptoms within 24 to 48 hours
- Demonstrate decreased feelings of anxiety, agitation, and so forth within 3 to 5 days
- Participate in the therapeutic milieu, for example, respond verbally to simple questions, within 48 to 72 hours

Stabilization   The client will

- Take medications as prescribed
- Express feelings in an acceptable manner, for example, talk with staff about feelings for a specific time period or frequency

Community   The client will

- Reach or maintain his or her optimal level of functioning
- Cope effectively with the illness
- Continue compliance with prescribed regimen, such as medications and follow-up appointments

IMPLEMENTATION

Nursing Interventions *denotes collaborative interventions	Rationale
Protect the client from harming himself or herself or others. See Care Plan 26: Suicidal Behavior.	Client safety is a priority. Self-destructive ideas may come from hallucinations or delusions.
Reassure the client that the environment is safe by briefly and simply explaining routines, procedures, and so forth.	The client is less likely to feel threatened if the surroundings are known.
Decrease excessive stimuli in the environment. The client may not respond favorably to competitive activities or large groups if he or she is actively psychotic.	The client is unable to deal with excess stimuli. The environment should not be threatening to the client.
Be aware of as needed (PRN) medications and the client's varying need for them.	Medication can decrease psychotic symptoms and can help the client gain control over his or her own behavior.
Reorient the client to person, place, and time as indicated (call the client by name, tell the client where he or she is, etc.).	Repeated presentation of reality is concrete reinforcement for the client.
Spend time with the client even when he or she is unable to respond coherently. Convey your interest and caring.	Your physical presence is reality. Nonverbal caring can be conveyed even when verbal caring is not understood.
Limit the client's environment to enhance his or her feelings of security.	Unknown boundaries or a perceived lack of limits can foster insecurity in the client.
Help the client establish what is real and unreal. Validate the client's real perceptions, and correct the client's misperceptions in a matter-of-fact manner. Do not argue with the client, but do not give support for misperceptions.	The unreality of psychosis must not be reinforced; reality must be reinforced. Reinforced ideas and behavior will recur more frequently.
Stay with the client when he or she is frightened. Touching the client can sometimes be therapeutic. Evaluate the effectiveness of the use of touch with the client before using it consistently.	Your presence and touch can provide reassurance from the real world. However, touch may not be effective if the client feels that his or her boundaries are being invaded.
Remove the client from the group if his or her behavior becomes too bizarre, disturbing, or dangerous to others.	The benefit of involving the client with the group is outweighed by the group's need for safety and protection.
Help the client's group accept the client's "strange" behavior. Give simple explanations to the client's group as needed (e.g., "[Client] is very sick right now; he [or she] needs our understanding and support").	The client's group benefits from awareness of others' needs and can help the client by demonstrating empathy.
Consider the other clients' needs. Plan for at least one staff member to be available to other clients if several staff members are needed to care for this client.	Remember that other clients have their own needs and problems. Be careful not to give attention only to the "sickest" client.

IMPLEMENTATION (continued)

Nursing Interventions *denotes collaborative interventions	Rationale
Explain to other clients that they have not done anything to warrant the client's verbal or physical threats; rather, the threats are the result of the client's illness.	Other clients may interpret verbal or physical threats as personal or may feel that they are doing something to bring about the threats.
Set limits on the client's behavior when he or she is unable to do so (when the behavior interferes with other clients or becomes destructive). Do not set limits to punish the client.	Limits are established by others when the client is unable to use internal controls effectively. Limits are intended to protect the client and others, not to punish inappropriate behaviors.
Make only promises that you can realistically keep.	Breaking your promise can result in increasing the client's mistrust.
Be simple, direct, and concise when speaking to the client.	The client is unable to process complex ideas effectively.
Talk with the client about simple, concrete things; avoid ideological or theoretical discussions.	The client's ability to deal with abstractions is impaired.
Direct activities toward helping the client accept and remain in contact with reality.	Increased reality contact decreases the client's retreat into unreality.
Initially, assign the same staff members to work with the client.	Consistency can reassure the client.
Begin with one-to-one interactions, and then progress to small groups as tolerated (introduce slowly).	Initially, the client will better tolerate and deal with limited contact.
Establish and maintain a daily routine; explain any variation in this routine to the client.	The client's ability to adapt to change is impaired.
Make the client aware of your expectations for him or her.	The client must know what is expected before he or she can work toward meeting those expectations.
Set realistic goals. Set daily goals and expectations.	Unrealistic goals will frustrate the client. Daily goals are short term and therefore easier for the client to accomplish.
At first, do not offer choices to the client ("Would you like to go to activities?" "What would you like to eat?"). Instead, approach the client in a directive manner ("It is time to eat. Please pick up your fork.").	The client's ability to make decisions is impaired. Asking the client to make decisions at this time may be very frustrating.
Gradually, provide opportunities for the client to accept responsibility and make personal decisions.	The client needs to gain independence as soon as he or she is able. Gradual addition of responsibilities and decisions gives the client a greater opportunity for success.

Nursing Diagnosis

Social Isolation
Aloneness experienced by the individual and perceived as imposed by others and as a negative or threatening state.

ASSESSMENT DATA

- Inappropriate or inadequate emotional responses
- Poor interpersonal relationships
- Feeling threatened in social situations
- Difficulty with verbal communication
- Exaggerated responses to stimuli

EXPECTED OUTCOMES

Immediate	The client will

- Engage in social interaction, for example, verbally interact with other clients for specified periods or specified frequency, for example, for 5 minutes at least twice a day within 2 days
- Identify at least two strengths or assets with nursing assistance within 2 to 3 days
- Verbalize increased feelings of self-worth within 5 to 7 days

Stabilization	The client will

- Demonstrate appropriate emotional responses
- Communicate effectively with others
- Demonstrate basic social skills, for example, talk with others about weather, local events, or activities

Community	The client will

- Demonstrate use of strengths and assets
- Establish interpersonal relationships in the community

IMPLEMENTATION

Nursing Interventions *denotes collaborative interventions	Rationale
Provide attention in a sincere, interested manner.	Flattery can be interpreted as belittling by the client.
Support any successes, responsibilities fulfilled, interactions with others, and so forth.	Sincere and genuine praise that the client has earned can improve self-esteem.
Avoid trying to convince the client verbally of his or her own worth.	The client will respond to genuine recognition of a concrete behavior rather than to unfounded praise or flattery.
Initially, interact with the client on a one-to-one basis. Manage nursing assignments so that the client interacts with a variety of staff members, as the client tolerates.	Your social behavior provides a role model for the client. Interacting with different staff members allows the client to experience success in interactions within the safety of the staff–client relationship.
Introduce the client to other clients in the milieu and facilitate their interactions on a one client to one client basis. Gradually facilitate social interactions between the client and small groups, then larger groups.	Gradually increasing the scope of the client's social interactions will help the client build confidence in social skills.
Teach the client social skills. Describe and demonstrate specific skills, such as approaching another person for interaction, eye contact, attentive listening, and so forth. Discuss the type of topics that are appropriate for casual social conversation, such as the weather, local events, and so forth.	The client may have little or no knowledge of social interaction skills. Modeling provides a concrete example of the desired skills.
Talk with the client about his or her interactions and observations of interpersonal dynamics.	Awareness of interpersonal and group dynamics is an important part of building social skills. Sharing observations provides an opportunity for the client to express his or her feelings and receive feedback about his or her progress.
Help the client improve his or her grooming; assist when necessary in bathing, doing laundry, and so forth.	Good physical grooming can enhance confidence in social situations.
Help the client accept as much responsibility for personal grooming as he or she can (do not do something for the client that he or she can do alone).	The client must be encouraged to be as independent as possible to foster self-esteem and continued self-care practices.

Nursing Diagnosis

Bathing Self-Care Deficit
Impaired ability to perform or complete bathing activities for self.

Dressing Self-Care Deficit
Impaired ability to perform or complete dressing activities for self.

Feeding Self-Care Deficit
Impaired ability to perform or complete self-feeding activities.

Toileting Self-Care Deficit
Impaired ability to perform or complete toileting activities for self.

ASSESSMENT DATA

- Poor personal hygiene
- Lack of awareness of or interest in personal needs
- Disturbance of appetite or regular eating patterns
- Disturbance of self-initiated, goal-directed activity
- Inability to follow through with completion of daily tasks
- Apathy
- Anergy, or inability to use energy productively

EXPECTED OUTCOMES

Immediate	The client will

- Establish an adequate balance of rest, sleep, and activity with nursing assistance within 2 to 4 days.
- Establish nutritional eating patterns with nursing assistance within 2 to 4 days.
- Participate in self-care activities, such as bathing, washing hair, toileting within 48 to 72 hours.

Stabilization	The client will

- Complete daily tasks with minimal assistance
- Initiate daily tasks

Community	The client will

- Maintain adequate routines for physiologic well-being
- Demonstrate independence in self-care activities

IMPLEMENTATION

Nursing Interventions *denotes collaborative interventions	Rationale
Be alert to the client's physical needs.	The client may be unaware of or unresponsive to his or her needs. Physical needs must be met to enhance the client's ability to meet emotional needs.
Monitor the client's food and fluid intake; you may need to record intake, output, and daily weight.	The client may be unaware of or may ignore his or her needs for food and fluids.
Offer the client foods that are easily chewed, fortified liquids such as nutritional supplements, and high-protein malts.	If the client lacks interest in eating, highly nutritious foods that require little effort to eat may help meet nutritional needs.

(continued on page 152)

IMPLEMENTATION (continued)

Nursing Interventions *denotes collaborative interventions	Rationale
Try to find out what foods the client likes, including culturally based foods or foods from family members, and make them available at meals and for snacks.	The client may be more apt to eat foods he or she likes or has been accustomed to eating.
Monitor the client's elimination patterns. You may need to use PRN medication to establish regularity.	Constipation frequently occurs with the use of major tranquilizers, decreased food and fluid intake, and decreased activity levels.
Encourage good fluid intake.	Constipation may result from inadequate fluid intake.
Explain any task in short, simple steps.	A complex task will be easier for the client if it is broken down into a series of steps.
Using clear, direct sentences, instruct the client to do one part of the task at a time.	The client may not be able to remember all the steps at once.
Tell the client your expectations directly. Do not ask the client to choose unnecessarily, that is, tell the client it is time to eat or get dressed rather than asking if he or she wants to eat or dress.	The client may not be able to make choices or may make poor choices.
Do not confuse the client with reasons as to why things are to be done.	Abstract ideas will not be comprehended and will interfere with task completion.
Allow the client ample time to complete any task.	It may take the client longer to complete tasks because of a lack of concentration and short attention span.
Remain with the client throughout the task; do not attempt to hurry the client.	Trying to rush the client will frustrate him or her and make completion of the task impossible.
Assist the client as needed to maintain daily functions and adequate personal hygiene.	The client's sense of dignity and well-being is enhanced if he or she is clean, smells good, looks nice, and so forth.
Gradually withdraw assistance and supervise the client's grooming or other self-care skills. Praise the client for initiating and completing activities of daily living.	It is important for the client to gain independence as soon as possible. Positive reinforcement increases the likelihood of recurrence.

CARE PLAN 21

Delusions

Delusions are false beliefs that are misperceptions or are not based in reality. *Bizarre delusions* "are clearly implausible and are not understandable and do not derive from ordinary life experiences" or represent a belief of "loss of control over mind or body" (APA, 2000, p. 299). *Nonbizarre delusions* are beliefs that are false in the present situation but could possibly happen in other circumstances.

The client may have delusional ideas in more than one area or may have insight into the delusional state but is unable to alter it. Sometimes the delusion is the antithesis of what the client thinks or feels. For example, a client who feels unimportant may believe himself or herself to be Jesus Christ, or a client who is destitute may believe himself or herself to be a wealthy financier.

Delusions can occur as one of several symptoms as in schizophrenia or bipolar disorder, or the primary symptom, as in a delusional disorder. Common categories of delusions are persecutory, grandiose, somatic, religious, poverty or wealth, contamination, and infidelity.

Delusions can also result from sensory deprivation or overload, sleep deprivation, substance withdrawal, and metabolic disorders. The client may be attempting to meet some need through the delusion, such as increased self-esteem, punishment, or freedom from anxiety associated with feelings of guilt or fear.

Some clients (especially those with paranoia) may have *fixed delusions*—delusions that may persist throughout their lives. Most delusions that occur during psychotic episodes are *transient delusions*—delusions that do not persist over time, especially when the client is compliant in taking prescribed medications.

Three phases have been identified in the process of delusional thinking. First, the client is totally involved in the delusions. Second, reality testing and trust in others coexist with the delusions. Third, the client no longer experiences the delusions (or is not bothered by them in the case of fixed delusions).

Treatment may be primarily focused on the underlying disorder, such as schizophrenia or bipolar disorder, and includes providing a safe environment and medication management. It is important to remember that delusions are a protection that can be abandoned only when the client feels more safe in the reality of his or her environment, and that delusions are not within the client's conscious, voluntary control.

NURSING DIAGNOSES ADDRESSED IN THIS CARE PLAN
Disturbed Thought Processes
Ineffective Health Maintenance

RELATED NURSING DIAGNOSES ADDRESSED IN THE MANUAL
Ineffective Therapeutic Regimen Management
Anxiety

Nursing Diagnosis

Disturbed Thought Processes*
Disruption in cognitive operations and activities.

*Note:** This nursing diagnosis was retired in *NANDA-I Nursing Diagnoses: Definitions & Classification 2009–2011*, but the NANDA-I Diagnosis Development Committee encourages work to be done on retired diagnoses toward resubmission for inclusion in the taxonomy.

ASSESSMENT DATA

- Non–reality-based thinking
- Disorientation
- Labile affect
- Short attention span
- Impaired judgment
- Distractibility

EXPECTED OUTCOMES

Immediate

The client will

- Be free from injury throughout hospitalization
- Demonstrate decreased anxiety level within 24 to 48 hours
- Respond to reality-based interactions initiated by others, for example, verbally interact with staff for 5 to 10 minutes within 24 to 48 hours

Stabilization

The client will

- Interact on reality-based topics, such as daily activities or local events
- Sustain attention and concentration to complete tasks or activities

Community

The client will

- Verbalize recognition of delusional thoughts if they persist
- Be free from delusions or demonstrate the ability to function without responding to persistent delusional thoughts

IMPLEMENTATION

Nursing Interventions *denotes collaborative interventions	Rationale
Be sincere and honest when communicating with the client. Avoid vague or evasive remarks.	Clients with delusions are extremely sensitive about others and can recognize insincerity. Evasive comments or hesitation reinforces mistrust or delusions.
Be consistent in setting expectations, enforcing rules, and so forth.	Clear, consistent limits provide a secure structure for the client.
Do not make promises that you cannot keep.	Broken promises reinforce the client's mistrust of others.
Encourage the client to talk with you, but do not pry for information.	Probing increases the client's suspicion and interferes with the therapeutic relationship.
Explain procedures, and try to be sure the client understands the procedures before carrying them out.	When the client has full knowledge of procedures, he or she is less likely to feel tricked by the staff.
Give positive feedback for the client's successes.	Positive feedback for genuine success enhances the client's sense of well-being and helps make nondelusional reality a more positive situation for the client.
Recognize the client's delusions as the client's perception of the environment.	Recognizing the client's perceptions can help you understand the feelings he or she is experiencing.
Initially, do not argue with the client or try to convince the client that the delusions are false or unreal.	Logical argument does not dispel delusional ideas and can interfere with the development of trust.

IMPLEMENTATION (continued)

Nursing Interventions *denotes collaborative interventions	Rationale
Interact with the client on the basis of real things; do not dwell on the delusional material.	Interacting about reality is healthy for the client.
Engage the client in one-to-one activities at first, and then activities in small groups, and gradually activities in larger groups.	A distrustful client can best deal with one person initially. Gradual introduction of others as the client tolerates is less threatening.
Recognize and support the client's accomplishments (projects completed, responsibilities fulfilled, or interactions initiated).	Recognizing the client's accomplishments can lessen anxiety and the need for delusions as a source of self-esteem.
Show empathy regarding the client's feelings; reassure the client of your presence and acceptance of his or her feelings.	The client's delusions can be distressing. Empathy conveys your caring, interest, and acceptance of the client without conveying that the delusions are reality.
Do not be judgmental or belittle or joke about the client's beliefs.	It is not appropriate to be judgmental toward a client or his or her beliefs. The client's delusions and feelings are not funny to him or her. The client may not understand or may feel rejected by attempts at humor.
Never convey to the client that you accept the delusions as reality.	Indicating belief in the delusion reinforces the delusion (and the client's illness).
Directly interject doubt regarding delusions as soon as the client seems ready to accept this (e.g., "I find that hard to believe."). Do not argue, but present a factual account of the situation.	As the client begins to trust you, he or she may become willing to doubt the delusion if you express your doubt.
As the client begins to doubt the delusions or is willing to discuss the possibility that they may not be accurate, talk with the client about his or her perceptions and feelings. Give the client support for expressing feelings and concerns.	As the client begins to relinquish delusional ideas, he or she may have increased anxiety or be embarrassed about the beliefs.
Ask the client if he or she can see that the delusions interfere with or cause problems in his or her life.	Discussion of the problems caused by the delusions is a focus on the present and is reality based.
If the delusions are persistent but the client can acknowledge the consequences of expressing the beliefs, help him or her understand the difference between holding a belief and acting on it or sharing it with others. See Care Plan 23: Delusional Disorder.	Learning to choose to not act on a delusional belief and not discuss it with others outside the therapeutic relationship may help the client avoid hospitalization and other consequences in the future.

Nursing Diagnosis

Ineffective Health Maintenance
Inability to identify, manage, and/or seek out help to maintain health.

ASSESSMENT DATA

- Poor diet
- Insomnia, unrestful sleep
- Inadequate food and fluid intake
- Inability to follow through with activities of daily living

EXPECTED OUTCOMES

Immediate	The client will
	• Establish a balance of rest, sleep, and activity with nursing assistance within 2 to 4 days
	• Ingest adequate amounts of food and fluids within 2 to 4 days
	• Take medications as administered within 24 to 48 hours
Stabilization	The client will
	• Complete necessary daily activities with minimal assistance
	• Take medications as prescribed
Community	The client will
	• Maintain a balance of rest, sleep, and activity
	• Maintain adequate nutrition, hydration, and elimination
	• Seek assistance from health care professionals at the onset of problems

IMPLEMENTATION

Nursing Interventions *denotes collaborative interventions	Rationale
If the client has delusions that prevent adequate rest, sleep, or food or fluid intake, you may need to institute measures to maintain or regain physical health. For example, provide food in containers the client can open (i.e., prepackaged foods), sleep medications, or life-saving medical treatment such as intravenous, enteral, or total parenteral nutrition feedings in severe situations.	The client's safety and physical health are a priority.
If the client thinks that his or her food is poisoned or that he or she is not worthy of food, you may need to alter routines to increase the client's control over issues involving food. As the client's trust develops, gradually reintroduce routine procedures.	Any steps to directly increase the client's nutritional intake must be taken without validating the client's delusions. They must be taken unobtrusively and should be used if the client's nutritional status is severely impaired.
If the client is too suspicious to sleep, try to allow the client to choose a place and time in which he or she will feel most comfortable sleeping. Sedatives as needed may be indicated.	If the client feels he or she can select the most comfortable place to sleep, he or she may feel secure enough to sleep. Again, avoid validating the client's delusions.
If the client is reluctant to take medications, allow him or her to open prepackaged (unit-dose) medications.	The client can see the medications sealed in packages, which may decrease suspicion or alleviate anxiety. The client's sense of control is enhanced.
Design a chart or schedule that indicates the prescribed medications and times of administration. The client can record medications as they are taken.	Taking responsibility for recording medications increases the client's participation in his or her care. The client can continue using a chart after discharge to enhance compliance with prescribed medications.
As the client establishes adequate intake, sleep, and medication compliance, gradually decrease the amount of prompting to accomplish these activities.	Once the client is meeting minimal health needs, it is important to maximize the client's independence in performing these activities.
*Assist the client to compile a checklist to use after discharge that describes when the client should seek assistance from health professionals. The list should be as specific as possible, for example, "Call case manager if there are problems getting prescriptions filled."	When the client is stressed, he or she is less likely to engage in effective problem solving. Having a specific preplanned list enhances the client's chances for effective problem resolution before the problem reaches crisis proportions.

CARE PLAN 22

Hallucinations

Hallucinations are perceptions of an external stimulus without a source in the external world. They may involve any of the senses—hearing, sight, smell, touch, or taste. Clients often act on these inner perceptions, which may be more compelling to them than external reality.

Hallucinations may occur with any of the following conditions:

* Schizophrenia
* Bipolar disorder, severe mania
* Hallucinogenic drugs
* Drug toxicity or adverse effects (e.g., digitalis toxicity)
* Withdrawal from alcohol, barbiturates, and other substances
* Alcoholic hallucinosis
* Sleep or sensory deprivation
* Neurologic diseases
* Endocrine imbalance (e.g., thyrotoxicosis)

Current theories of the etiology of hallucinations include a metabolic response to stress, neurochemical disturbances, brain lesions, an unconscious attempt to defend the ego, and symbolic expressions of dissociated thoughts.

Hallucinations usually diminish and may resolve in response to treatment, which centers on the underlying disorder or problem, such as schizophrenia or alcohol withdrawal. Goals include ensuring the client's safety, managing medications, and meeting the client's needs for nutrition, hydration, and so forth. Because the client may perceive the hallucination as reality and reject the reality of the surrounding environment, it is important for the nurse to interrupt the hallucinations with reality by encouraging contact with real people, activities, and interactions. Occasionally, the client may be aware that he or she is hallucinating, but often does not recognize hallucinations per se until they subside. The client may then feel ashamed when he or she remembers psychotic behavior.

NURSING DIAGNOSES ADDRESSED IN THIS CARE PLAN
Disturbed Sensory Perception (Specify: Visual, Auditory, Kinesthetic, Gustatory, Tactile, Olfactory)
Risk for Other-Directed Violence

RELATED NURSING DIAGNOSES ADDRESSED IN THE MANUAL
Fear
Ineffective Health Maintenance
Disturbed Thought Processes
Risk for Suicide

Nursing Diagnosis

Disturbed Sensory Perception (Specify: Visual, Auditory, Kinesthetic, Gustatory, Tactile, Olfactory)*
Change in the amount or patterning of incoming stimuli accompanied by a diminished, exaggerated, distorted, or impaired response to such stimuli.

> ***Note:** This nursing diagnosis was retired in *NANDA-I Nursing Diagnoses: Definitions & Classification 2012–2014*, but the NANDA-I Diagnosis Development Committee encourages work to be done on retired diagnoses toward resubmission for inclusion in the taxonomy.

ASSESSMENT DATA

- Hallucinations (auditory, visual, tactile, gustatory, kinesthetic, or olfactory)
- Listening intently to no apparent stimuli
- Talking out loud when no one is present
- Rambling, incoherent, or unintelligible speech
- Inability to discriminate between real and unreal perceptions
- Attention deficits
- Inability to make decisions
- Feelings of insecurity
- Confusion

EXPECTED OUTCOMES

Immediate

The client will

- Demonstrate decreased hallucinations within 24 to 48 hours
- Interact with others in the external environment, for example, talk with staff about present reality (e.g., tangible objects in the environment) for a specified time period or specified frequency (e.g., for 5 to 10 minutes within 24 hours)
- Participate in the real environment, for example, sit with other clients and help with a specific activity (e.g., crafts projects) for a specified time period (e.g., 10 minutes) within a specified time period (e.g., 48 to 72 hours)

Stabilization

The client will

- Verbalize plans to deal with hallucinations, if they recur
- Verbalize knowledge of hallucinations or illness and safe use of medications

Community

The client will

- Make sound decisions based in reality
- Participate in community activities or programs

IMPLEMENTATION

Nursing Interventions *denotes collaborative interventions	Rationale
Be aware of all surrounding stimuli, including sounds from other rooms (e.g., television in adjacent areas).	Many seemingly normal stimuli will trigger or intensify hallucinations. The client can be overwhelmed by stimuli.
Try to decrease stimuli or move the client to another area.	Decreased stimuli decreases chances of misperception. The client has a diminished ability to deal with stimuli.
Avoid conveying to the client the belief that hallucinations are real. Do not converse with the "voices" or otherwise reinforce the client's belief in the hallucinations as reality.	You must be honest with the client, letting him or her know the hallucinations are not real.
Explore the content of the client's hallucinations to determine what kind of stimuli the client is receiving, but do not reinforce the hallucinations as real. You might say, "I don't hear any voices—what are you hearing?"	It is important to determine if auditory hallucinations are "command" hallucinations that direct the client to hurt himself or herself or others. Safety is always a priority.
If the client appears to be hallucinating, attempt to engage the client in conversation or a concrete activity.	It is more difficult for the client to respond to hallucinations when he or she is engaged in real activities and interactions.

IMPLEMENTATION (continued)

Nursing Interventions *denotes collaborative interventions	Rationale
Maintain simple topics of conversation to provide a base in reality.	The client is better able to talk about basic things; complexity is more difficult.
Use concrete, specific verbal communication with the client. Avoid gestures, abstract ideas, and innuendos.	The client's ability to deal in abstractions is diminished. The client may misinterpret your gestures or innuendos.
Avoid asking the client to make choices. Don't ask "Would you like to talk or be alone?" Rather, suggest that the client talk with you.	The client's ability to make decisions is impaired, and the client may choose to be alone (and hallucinate) rather than deal with reality (talking to you).
Respond verbally and reinforce the client's conversation when he or she refers to reality.	Positive reinforcement increases the likelihood of desired behaviors.
Encourage the client to tell staff members about hallucinations.	The client has the chance to seek others (in reality) and to cope with problems caused by hallucinations.
Show acceptance of the client's behavior and of the client as a person; do not joke about or judge the client's behavior.	The client may need help to see that hallucinations were a part of the illness, not under the client's control. Joking or being judgmental about the client's behavior is not appropriate and can be damaging to the client.
If the client tolerates it, use touch in a nonthreatening manner and allow the client to touch your hand. Remember, some clients are too threatened by touch; evaluate each client's response carefully.	Your physical touch is reality, and it can help the client to reestablish boundaries between self and nonself.
Provide simple activities that the client can realistically accomplish (such as uncomplicated craft projects).	Long or complicated tasks may be frustrating for the client. He or she may be unable to complete them.
Encourage the client to express any feelings of shame or embarrassment once he or she is aware of psychotic behavior; be supportive.	It may help the client to express such feelings, particularly if you are a supportive, accepting listener.
Note: Not all clients will remember previous psychotic behavior, and they may ask you what they did. Be honest in your answers, but do not dwell on the psychotic behavior.	Honest answers may relieve the client. Many times the client's fears about his or her behavior are worse than the actual behavior.

Nursing Diagnosis

Risk for Other-Directed Violence

At risk for behaviors in which an individual demonstrates that he or she can be physically, emotionally, and/or sexually harmful to others.

RISK FACTORS

- Fear
- Mistrust or suspicion
- Agitation
- Rapid, shallow breathing
- Clenched teeth or fists
- Rigid or taut body
- Hostile or threatening verbalizations
- History of aggression toward property or others
- History of violent family patterns
- Low neuroleptic level

EXPECTED OUTCOMES

Immediate	The client will

- Be free from injury throughout hospitalization
- Refrain from injuring others or destroying property throughout hospitalization
- Verbally express feelings of anger, frustration, or confusion within 24 to 48 hours
- Express decreased feelings of agitation, fear, or anxiety within 48 to 72 hours

Stabilization	The client will

- Take medications as prescribed
- Demonstrate appropriate methods of relieving anxiety, for example, talking about feelings with staff or keeping a journal

Community	The client will

- Demonstrate satisfying relationships with others
- Demonstrate effective coping strategies

IMPLEMENTATION

Nursing Interventions *denotes collaborative interventions	Rationale
Provide protective supervision for the client, but avoid hovering over him or her.	The safety of the client and others is a priority. Allowing the client to have some personal distance may diminish agitation.
Be aware of indications that the client is hallucinating (intent listening or talking to someone when no one is present, muttering to self, inappropriate facial expression).	The client may act on what he or she "hears." Your early response to cues indicating active hallucinations decreases the chance of acting out or aggressive behavior.
Provide a structured environment with scheduled routine activities of daily living. Explain unexpected changes. Make your expectations clear to the client in simple, direct terms.	Lack of structure and unexplained changes may increase agitation and anxiety. Structure enhances the client's security.
Be alert for signs of increasing fear, anxiety, or agitation and intervene as soon as possible.	The earlier you can intervene, the easier it is to calm the client and prevent harm.
Avoid backing the client into a corner either verbally or physically.	If the client feels threatened or trapped, he or she is more likely to be aggressive.
Intervene with one-to-one contact, seclusion, and medication as needed.	The safety of the client and others is a priority.
Do not expect more (or less) of the client than he or she is capable of doing.	Expecting too much will frustrate the client, and he or she may not even try to comply. Expecting too little may undermine the client's self-esteem, confidence, and growth.
As agitation subsides, encourage the client to express his or her feelings, first in one-to-one contacts, and then in small and larger groups as tolerated.	The client will be more at ease with just one person and will gradually tolerate more people when he or she feels less threatened.
Help the client identify and practice ways to relieve anxiety, such as deep breathing or listening to music. See Care Plan 26: Suicidal Behavior and Care Plan 47: Aggressive Behavior.	With decreased anxiety, the client will be more successful in solving problems and establishing relationships.

CARE PLAN 23

Delusional Disorder

The primary feature of a *delusional disorder* is the persistence of a *delusion* or a false belief that is limited to a specific area of thought and is not related to any organic or major psychiatric disorder. The different types of delusional disorders are categorized (APA, 2000) according to the main theme of the delusional belief:

Erotomania. This is an erotic delusion that one is loved by another person, usually a famous person. The client may come into contact with the law as he or she writes letters, makes telephone calls, or attempts to "protect" the object of the delusion.

Grandiose. The client is usually convinced that he or she is uniquely talented, has created a fantastic invention, has a religious calling, or believes himself or herself to be a famous person, claiming the actual person is an imposter.

Jealous. The client believes that a spouse or partner is unfaithful, when that is not true. The client may follow the partner, read mail, and so forth, to find "proof" of the infidelity. The client may become physically violent or demand that the partner never go anywhere alone.

Persecutory. This type of delusion is the most common. The client believes that he or she is being spied on, followed, harassed, drugged, and so forth, and may seek to remedy these perceived injustices through police reports, court action, and sometimes violence.

Somatic. The client believes falsely that he or she emits a foul odor from some body orifice, has infestations of bugs or parasites, or that certain body parts are ugly or deformed. These clients often seek help from medical (nonpsychiatric) sources.

Delusional disorders are uncommon with prevalence under 0.1% (APA, 2000) and are most prevalent in people 40 to 55 years of age, although the age of onset ranges from adolescence to old age.

The client with a delusional disorder has no other psychiatric symptoms and often can function quite well when not discussing or acting on the delusional belief. Occupational and intellectual functioning are rarely affected, but these individuals often are dysfunctional in social situations and close relationships. The course of delusional disorder varies: some clients have a remission without a relapse; some experience relapses after a remission or their symptoms wax and wane over time; and some have chronic persistent delusions.

Because the delusion may persist despite efforts to extinguish it, the goal is not to eliminate the delusion but to contain its effect on the client's life. It is important to identify a safe person with whom the client can discuss the delusional belief and validate perceptions or plans of action in order to prevent the client from acting (irrationally) based on the delusional belief.

NURSING DIAGNOSIS ADDRESSED IN THIS CARE PLAN
Disturbed Thought Processes

RELATED NURSING DIAGNOSES ADDRESSED IN THE MANUAL
Ineffective Role Performance
Impaired Social Interaction
Risk for Other-Directed Violence

Nursing Diagnosis

Disturbed Thought Processes*
Disruption in cognitive operations and activities.

> *Note: This nursing diagnosis was retired in *NANDA-I Nursing Diagnoses: Definitions & Classification 2009–2011*, but the NANDA-I Diagnosis Development Committee encourages work to be done on retired diagnoses toward resubmission for inclusion in the taxonomy.

ASSESSMENT DATA

- Erratic, impulsive behavior
- Poor judgment
- Agitation
- Feelings of distress
- Illogical thinking, irrational ideas leading to faulty conclusions
- Extreme, intense feelings
- Refusal to accept factual information from others
- Described by others as "normal" most of the time
- Socially inappropriate or odd behavior in certain situations

EXPECTED OUTCOMES

Immediate

The client will

- Demonstrate decreased agitation and aggressive behavior within 24 hours
- Verbally recognize that others do not see his or her belief as real within 48 to 72 hours
- Express the delusion and related feelings only to therapeutic staff within 4 to 5 days
- Refrain from acting on the delusional belief within 5 to 7 days

Stabilization

The client will

- Verbalize plans to maintain contact with a therapist to provide an avenue for discussing the delusion as needed
- Verbally validate decisions or conclusions about the delusional area before taking action, for example, talk with a staff member before acting on thoughts related to the delusion

Community

The client will

- Refrain from any public discussion of the delusional belief
- Attain his or her optimal level of functioning

IMPLEMENTATION

Nursing Interventions *denotes collaborative interventions	Rationale
Let the client know that all feelings, ideas, and beliefs are permissible to share with you.	The client can identify the nurse as someone who will not be judgmental of feelings and ideas, even if bizarre or unusual.
Do not validate delusional ideas. Let the client know that his or her feelings are real, but that the delusional ideas are not real even though they seem real.	The client may begin to recognize that not all people share his or her belief, but his or her feelings will still be respected.
Avoid trying to convince the client that the delusions are not real. Rather, convey that the ideas seem real to the client, but others do not share or accept that belief.	The client believes the delusions to be true and cannot intellectually be convinced otherwise. Debating this issue can damage the therapeutic relationship and is futile.

IMPLEMENTATION (continued)

Nursing Interventions *denotes collaborative interventions	Rationale
Give the client feedback that others do not share his or her perceptions and beliefs.	This feedback is reality, and it can assist the client to begin problem solving.
Contract with the client to limit the amount of time he or she will spend thinking about the delusion, such as 5 minutes an hour or 15 minutes a day. Encourage the client to gradually decrease this amount of time as he or she tolerates.	It is not feasible to expect the client to forget about the delusion entirely. By limiting the time focused on the delusion, the client feels less frustrated than if he or she is "forbidden" to think about it, but will spend less time dwelling on the delusion.
Explore with the client ways he or she can redirect some of the energy or anxiety generated by the delusional ideas.	Energy from the client's anxious feelings needs to be expressed in a constructive manner.
Assist the client to identify difficulties in daily life that are caused by or related to the delusional ideas.	The client might be motivated to contain behaviors related to the delusion if he or she feels distress about life areas that are disrupted.
Have the client identify the events that led to his or her current difficulties. Discuss the relationship between these events and the delusional beliefs.	If the client can begin to see the relationship between delusions and life difficulties, he or she might be more willing to consider making some behavioral changes.
Focus interactions and problem-solving on how the client can avoid further difficulties at home, work, or other situations in which problems are experienced.	The client's agreement that he or she would like to avoid further problems can provide a basis for making changes while avoiding the issue of whether or not the delusion is true.
*Help the client identify people with whom it is safe to discuss the delusional beliefs, such as the therapist, nurse, psychiatrist, and so forth.	By talking with nurses, therapists, and designated others, the client has a nonthreatening outlet for expression of feelings and ideas.
*Assist the client to select someone whom he or she trusts and validate perceptions with him or her before taking any action that may precipitate difficulties.	If the client can avoid acting on the delusional beliefs by checking his or her perceptions with someone, many difficulties at home, work, and so forth can be avoided.
*Encourage the client to use his or her contact person as often as needed. It may be helpful to use telephone or e-mail contact rather than always scheduling an appointment.	If the client can quickly call the person he or she trusts and receive immediate feedback, he or she is more likely to be able to contain behavior related to the delusion.

CARE PLAN 24

Psychotic Behavior Related to a Medical Condition

The client's behavior closely resembles that seen in schizophrenia, especially delusions and hallucinations. However, these symptoms are not due to a psychiatric disorder; they are related to a medical condition, such as fluid and electrolyte imbalance, hepatic or renal disease, sleep deprivation, or metabolic, endocrine, neurologic, or drug-induced disorders (APA, 2000).

The major types of psychoses in this category are as follows:

Korsakoff syndrome results from chronic alcoholism and the associated vitamin B_1 (thiamine) deficiency, usually occurring after a minimum of 5 to 10 years of heavy drinking. The brain damage it causes is irreversible, even with no further alcohol intake.

Drug-induced psychosis usually occurs following massive doses or chronic use of amphetamines and usually clears in 1 to 2 weeks when drug intake is discontinued. It also may result from use of hallucinogenic drugs and lasts from 12 hours to 2 days. With repeated hallucinogen use, psychosis may occur briefly without recent drug ingestion.

Endocrine imbalances such as those resulting from doses of steroids resulting in toxic blood levels or the abrupt withdrawal of steroids. Thyroid disturbances (e.g., thyrotoxicosis) can produce psychotic behavior that subsides when thyroxine is brought to a therapeutic level.

Sleep deprivation and lack of rapid eye movement (REM) cycle sleep, such as occur in *critical care unit psychosis*, related to the constant stimuli (lights, sounds), disruptions of diurnal patterns, frequent interruption of sleep, and so on, experienced in critical care units.

Psychotic behavior caused by chemical, toxic, or physical damage or sleep deprivation usually is acute and will subside in a short time with treatment of the underlying cause. Residual damage may remain after the psychotic behavior subsides, in cases of Korsakoff syndrome or heavy metal ingestion such as lead poisoning, and requires long-term treatment.

Although the behaviors seen with these types of psychoses are clinically similar to those seen with schizophrenia, treatment of these psychoses is aimed at correcting the underlying cause. The client may improve quite rapidly as the cause is treated or removed. Nursing care is focused on promoting reality orientation, allaying the client's fears and anxiety, and supporting the client's family and significant others.

NURSING DIAGNOSES ADDRESSED IN THIS CARE PLAN
Disturbed Sensory Perception (Specify: Visual, Auditory, Kinesthetic, Gustatory, Tactile, Olfactory)
Risk for Injury

RELATED NURSING DIAGNOSES ADDRESSED IN THE MANUAL
Ineffective Health Maintenance
Bathing Self-Care Deficit
Dressing Self-Care Deficit
Feeding Self-Care Deficit
Toileting Self-Care Deficit
Acute Confusion
Impaired Environmental Interpretation Syndrome

Nursing Diagnosis

Disturbed Sensory Perception (Specify: Visual, Auditory, Kinesthetic, Gustatory, Tactile, Olfactory)*

Change in the amount of patterning of incoming stimuli accompanied by a diminished, exaggerated, distorted, or impaired response to such stimuli.

*Note: This nursing diagnosis was retired in *NANDA-I Nursing Diagnoses: Definitions & Classification 2012–2014*, but the NANDA-I Diagnosis Development Committee encourages work to be done on retired diagnoses toward resubmission for inclusion in the taxonomy.

ASSESSMENT DATA

- Hallucinations
- Disorientation
- Fear
- Inability to concentrate
- Inattention to personal hygiene or grooming

EXPECTED OUTCOMES

Immediate

The client will

- Be oriented to person, time, place, and situation within 24 to 48 hours
- Establish a balance of rest, sleep, and activity with nursing assistance within 24 to 48 hours
- Establish adequate nutrition, hydration, and elimination with nursing assistance within 24 to 48 hours
- Participate in self-care activities, such as eating, bathing within 48 to 72 hours

Stabilization

The client will

- Maintain adequate, balanced physiologic functioning
- Communicate effectively with others

Community

The client will

- Demonstrate independence in self-care activities
- Manage chronic illnesses, if any, effectively
- Avoid use of alcohol, drugs, or other factors that could precipitate recurrence of symptoms

IMPLEMENTATION

Nursing Interventions *denotes collaborative interventions	Rationale
Be alert to the client's physical needs.	The client's physical needs are crucial. He or she may not be aware of or attend to hunger, fatigue, and so forth.
Monitor the client's food and fluid intake; you may need to record intake, output, and daily weight.	Adequate nutrition is important for the client's well-being.
Offer the client foods that are easily chewed, fortified liquids such as nutritional supplements, and high-protein malts.	If the client lacks interest in eating, highly nutritious foods that require little effort to eat may help meet nutritional needs.
Try to find out what foods the client likes, including culturally based foods or foods from family members, and make them available at meals and for snacks.	The client may be more apt to eat foods he or she likes or has been accustomed to eating.

(continued on page 166)

IMPLEMENTATION (continued)

Nursing Interventions *denotes collaborative interventions	Rationale
Monitor the client's elimination patterns. You may need to use PRN medication to maintain bowel regularity.	Constipation is a frequent side effect of major tranquilizers.
Institute relaxing, quieting activities before bedtime (tepid bath, warm milk, quiet environment).	Calming activities before bedtime facilitate rest and sleep.
Spend time with the client to facilitate reality orientation.	Your physical presence is reality.
Reorient the client to person, place, and time as necessary, by using the client's name often and by telling the client your name, the date, the place and situation, and so forth.	Reminding the client of surroundings, people, and time increases reality contact.
Evaluate the use of touch with the client.	Touch can be reassuring and may provide security for the client.
Be simple, direct, and concise when speaking to the client. Talk with the client about concrete or familiar things; avoid ideologic or theoretical discussions.	The client's ability to process abstractions or complexity is impaired.
*Direct activities toward helping the client accept and remain in contact with reality; use recreational or occupational therapy when appropriate.	The greater the client's reality contact and involvement in activities, the less time he or she will deal in unreality.
*Provide information and explanations to the client's family or significant others.	The family or significant others may have difficulty understanding that psychotic behavior is related to medical illness.

Nursing Diagnosis

Risk for Injury
At risk of injury as a result of environmental conditions interacting with the individual's adaptive and defensive resources.

RISK FACTORS

- Feelings of hostility
- Fear
- Cognitive deficits
- Emotional impairment
- Integrative dysfunction
- Sensory or motor deficits
- History of combative or acting-out behavior
- Inability to perceive harmful stimuli

EXPECTED OUTCOMES

Immediate

The client will

- Be free from injury throughout hospitalization
- Refrain from harming others or destroying property throughout hospitalization
- Be free from toxic substances, such as alcohol or illicit drugs throughout hospitalization

Stabilization

The client will

- Demonstrate adherence to the treatment regimen
- Verbalize plans for further treatment, if indicated

Community	The client will

- Avoid toxic or chemical substances
- Participate in treatment or follow-up care as needed

IMPLEMENTATION

Nursing Interventions *denotes collaborative interventions	**Rationale**
Protect the client from harming himself or herself by removing the items that could be used in self-destructive behavior or by restraining the client. See Care Plan 26: Suicidal Behavior and Care Plan 47: Aggressive Behavior.	The client's physical safety is a priority.
Remove the client to a quiet area or withdraw your attention if the client acts out, provided there is no potential danger to the client or others.	Decreased attention from you and others may help to extinguish unacceptable behavior.
Be alert for signs of increasing fear, anxiety, or agitation and intervene as soon as possible.	The earlier you can intervene, the easier it is to calm the client and prevent harm.
Reassure the client that the environment is safe by briefly and simply explaining procedures, routines, and so forth.	The client may be fearful and act out as a way to protect himself or herself.
Set limits on the client's behavior when he or she is unable to do so if the behavior interferes with other clients or becomes self-destructive. Do not set limits to punish the client.	Limit setting is the positive use of external control to promote safety and security; it should never be used as a punishment.
*Evaluate the client's response to the presence of family and significant others. If their presence helps to calm the client, maximize visit time, but if the client becomes more agitated, limit visits to short periods with one or two people at a time.	The client may not tolerate the additional stimulation of visitors. The client's safety and the safety of others is a priority. If visits are limited, the family or significant others need to know the client's response is not a personal reaction to them, but part of the illness.

SECTION 6 REVIEW QUESTIONS

1. Which of the following nursing diagnoses would the nurse identify for a client who says, "The mafia is following me because I know all their secrets"?

   a. Disturbed Sensory Perceptions

   b. Disturbed Thought Processes

   c. Impaired Verbal Communication

   d. Social Isolation

2. A client who is paranoid tells the nurse, "Move away from the window. They're watching us." The nurse recognizes that moving away from the window is contraindicated for which of the following reasons?

   a. It is essential to show the client that the nurse is not afraid

   b. Moving away from the window would indicate nonverbal agreement with the client's idea

   c. The client will think he is in control of the nurse's behavior

   d. The nurse would be demonstrating a lack of control of the situation

3. The client reports that she hears God's voice telling her that she has sinned and must be punished. Which of the following nursing diagnoses would the nurse identify?

   a. Anxiety

   b. Disturbed Thought Processes

   c. Disturbed Sensory Perceptions

   d. Ineffective Coping

4. A client with schizophrenia tells the nurse, "The aliens are sending messages to everyone that I am stupid and need to be killed." Which of the following responses would be most appropriate initially?

   a. "I know those voices are real to you, but I don't hear them."

   b. "I want you to let staff know when you hear those voices."

   c. "Those voices are hallucinations that are just part of your illness."

   d. "Your medications will help control the voices you are hearing."

5. A client with schizophrenia is admitted to the unit wearing torn and soiled clothing and looking confused. She is suspicious of others, has a flat affect, and talks very little. Which of the following would the nurse identify as the initial priority for this client?

   a. Giving the client information about the hospital program

   b. Helping the client feel safe and secure

   c. Introducing the client to other clients on the unit

   d. Providing the client with clean, comfortable clothes

SECTION 6 Recommended Readings

Buccheri, R. K., Trygstad, L. N., Buffum, M. D., Lyttle, K., & Dowling, G. (2010). Comprehensive evidence-based program teaching self-management of auditory hallucinations on inpatient psychiatric units. *Journal of Psychosocial Nursing and Mental Health Services, 47*(12), 42–48.

Chu., C. I., Liu, C. Y., Sun, C. T., & Lin, J. (2009). The effect of animal assisted activity on inpatients with schizophrenia. *Journal of Psychosocial Nursing and Mental Health Services, 47*(12), 42–48.

Leutwyler, H. C., Chaftez, L., & Wallhagen, M. (2010). Older adults with schizophrenia finding a place to belong. *Issues in Mental Health Nursing, 31*(8), 507–513.

Meerwijk, E. L., van Meijel, B., van den Bout, J., Kerkhof, A., de Vogel, W., & Grypdonck, M. (2010). Development and evaluation of a guideline for nursing care of suicidal patients with schizophrenia. *Perspectives in Psychiatric Care, 46*(1), 65–73.

SECTION 6 Resources for Additional Information

Visit thePoint (http://thePoint.lww.com/Schultz9e) for a list of these and other helpful Internet resources.

Mayo Clinic Schizophrenia resources
Mental Health America schizophrenia resources
Mental Health Today Schizophrenia Resources
NARSAD: The Mental Health Research Association
National Alliance on Mental Illness
National Institute of Mental Health

Mood Disorders and Related Behaviors

Mood can be described as an overall emotional feeling tone. Disturbances in mood can be manifested by a wide range of behaviors, such as suicidal thoughts and behavior, withdrawn behavior, or a profound increase or decrease in the level of psychomotor activity. The care plans in this section address the disorders and behaviors most directly related to mood, but care plans in other sections of the *Manual* may also be appropriate in the planning of a client's care (e.g., Care Plan 45: Withdrawn Behavior).

CARE PLAN 25

Major Depressive Disorder

Depression is an affective state characterized by feelings of sadness, guilt, and low self-esteem. It may be a chronic condition or an acute episode, often related to loss. This loss may or may not be recent and may be observable to others or perceived only by the client, such as disillusionment or loss of a dream. Depression may be seen in *grief*, the process of a normal response to a loss; *premenstrual syndrome* (PMS), a complex of symptoms that begins the week prior to menstrual flow; and *postpartum depression*, which occurs after childbirth and may involve symptoms from mild depressive feelings to acute psychotic behavior.

A *major depressive episode* is characterized by a depressed mood or loss of interest or pleasure in almost all activities for at least 2 weeks, in addition to at least four other depressive symptoms. These include appetite, weight, or sleep changes; a decrease in energy or activity; feelings of guilt or worthlessness; decreased concentration; or suicidal thoughts or activities. A *major depressive disorder* is diagnosed when one or more of these episodes occur without a history of manic (or hypomanic) episodes. When there is a history of manic episodes, the diagnosis is *bipolar disorder* (see Care Plan 27: Bipolar Disorder, Manic Episode). The duration and severity of symptoms and degree of functional impairment of depressive behavior vary widely, and the diagnosis of major depressive disorder is further described as *mild, moderate, severe without psychotic features*, or *severe with psychotic features* (APA, 2000).

Major depressive disorder occurs more frequently in people with chronic or severe medical illnesses (e.g., diabetes, stroke) and in people with a family history of depression. Theories of the etiology of depression focus on genetic, neurochemical, hormonal, and biologic factors, as well as psychodynamic, cognitive, and social/behavioral influences.

Prevalence of major depressive disorder in adults is estimated to be between 2% and 3% in men and between 5% and 9% in women. The lifetime risk of major depressive disorder is estimated at 8% to 12% in men and 20% to 26% in women (Gorman, 2006). Depressive behavior frequently occurs in clients during withdrawal from alcohol or other substances, and in clients with anorexia nervosa, phobias, schizophrenia, a history of abuse, post-traumatic behavior, poor social support, and so forth.

The average age of a person with an initial major depressive episode is in the midtwenties, although it can occur at any age. Approximately 66% of clients experience a full recovery from a depressive episode, but most have recurrent episodes over time. Symptoms of depressive episodes last a year or more in many clients (APA, 2000).

Treatment usually involves antidepressant medications (see Appendix E: Psychopharmacology). It is important for the nurse to be knowledgeable about medication actions, timing of effectiveness (certain drugs may require up to several weeks to achieve the full therapeutic effect), and side effects. Teaching the client and family or significant others about safe and consistent use of medications is essential. Other therapeutic goals include maintaining the client's safety; decreasing psychotic symptoms; assisting the client in meeting physiologic needs and hygiene; promoting self-esteem, expression of feelings, socialization, and leisure skills; and identifying sources of support.

NURSING DIAGNOSES ADDRESSED IN THIS CARE PLAN
Ineffective Coping
Impaired Social Interaction
Bathing Self-Care Deficit
Dressing Self-Care Deficit

Feeding Self-Care Deficit
Toileting Self-Care Deficit
Chronic Low Self-Esteem

RELATED NURSING DIAGNOSES ADDRESSED IN THE MANUAL
Social Isolation
Disturbed Thought Processes
Risk for Other-Directed Violence
Risk for Suicide
Complicated Grieving
Insomnia
Hopelessness

Nursing Diagnosis

Ineffective Coping

Inability to form a valid appraisal of the stressors, inadequate choices of practiced responses, and/or inability to use available resources.

ASSESSMENT DATA

- Suicidal ideas or behavior
- Slowed mental processes
- Disordered thoughts
- Feelings of despair, hopelessness, and worthlessness
- Guilt
- Anhedonia (inability to experience pleasure)
- Disorientation
- Generalized restlessness or agitation
- Sleep disturbances: early awakening, insomnia, or excessive sleeping
- Anger or hostility (may not be overt)
- Rumination
- Delusions, hallucinations, or other psychotic symptoms
- Diminished interest in sexual activity
- Fear of intensity of feelings
- Anxiety

EXPECTED OUTCOMES

Immediate

The client will

- Be free from self-inflicted harm throughout hospitalization
- Engage in reality-based interactions within 24 hours
- Be oriented to person, place, and time within 48 to 72 hours
- Express anger or hostility outwardly in a safe manner, for example, talking with staff members within 5 to 7 days

Stabilization

The client will

- Express feelings directly with congruent verbal and nonverbal messages
- Be free from psychotic symptoms
- Demonstrate functional level of psychomotor activity

Community

The client will

- Demonstrate compliance with and knowledge of medications, if any
- Demonstrate an increased ability to cope with anxiety, stress, or frustration
- Verbalize or demonstrate acceptance of loss or change, if any
- Identify a support system in the community

IMPLEMENTATION

Nursing Interventions *denotes collaborative interventions	Rationale
Provide a safe environment for the client.	Physical safety of the client is a priority. Many common items may be used in a self-destructive manner.
Continually assess the client's potential for suicide. Remain aware of this suicide potential at all times.	Clients with depression may have a potential for suicide that may or may not be expressed and that may change with time.
Observe the client closely, especially under the following circumstances: • After antidepressant medication begins to raise the client's mood. • During unstructured time on the unit or times when the number of staff on the unit is limited. • After any dramatic behavioral change (sudden cheerfulness, relief, or giving away personal belongings). See Care Plan 26: Suicidal Behavior.	You must be aware of the client's activities at all times when there is a potential for suicide or self-injury. Risk of suicide increases as the client's energy level is increased by medication, when the client's time is unstructured, and when observation of the client decreases. These changes may indicate that the client has come to a decision to commit suicide.
Reorient the client to person, place, and time as indicated (call the client by name, tell the client your name, tell the client where he or she is, etc.).	Repeated presentation of reality is concrete reinforcement for the client.
Spend time with the client.	Your physical presence is reality.
If the client is ruminating, tell him or her that you will talk about reality or about the client's feelings, but limit the attention given to repeated expressions of rumination.	Minimizing attention may help decrease rumination. Providing reinforcement for reality orientation and expression of feelings will encourage these behaviors.
Initially, assign the same staff members to work with the client whenever possible.	The client's ability to respond to others may be impaired. Limiting the number of new contacts initially will facilitate familiarity and trust. However, the number of people interacting with the client should increase as soon as possible to minimize dependency and to facilitate the client's abilities to communicate with a variety of people.
When approaching the client, use a moderate, level tone of voice. Avoid being overly cheerful.	Being overly cheerful may indicate to the client that being cheerful is the goal and that other feelings are not acceptable.
Use silence and active listening when interacting with the client. Let the client know that you are concerned and that you consider the client a worthwhile person. See Care Plan 45: Withdrawn Behavior.	The client may not communicate if you are talking too much. Your presence and use of active listening will communicate your interest and concern.
Be comfortable sitting with the client in silence. Let the client know you are available to converse, but do not require the client to talk.	Your silence will convey your expectation that the client will communicate and your acceptance of the client's difficulty with communication.
When first communicating with the client, use simple, direct sentences; avoid complex sentences or directions.	The client's ability to perceive and respond to complex stimuli is impaired.
Avoid asking the client many questions, especially questions that require only brief answers.	Asking questions and requiring only brief answers may discourage the client from expressing feelings.
Do not cut off interactions with cheerful remarks or platitudes (e.g., "No one really wants to die," or "You'll feel better soon."). Do not belittle the client's feelings. Accept the client's verbalizations of feelings as real, and give support for expressions of emotions, especially those that may be difficult for the client (like anger).	You may be uncomfortable with certain feelings the client expresses. If so, it is important for you to recognize this and discuss it with another staff member rather than directly or indirectly communicating your discomfort to the client. Proclaiming the client's feelings to be inappropriate or belittling them is detrimental.

IMPLEMENTATION (continued)

Nursing Interventions *denotes collaborative interventions	Rationale
Encourage the client to ventilate feelings in whatever way is comfortable—verbal and nonverbal. Let the client know you will listen and accept what is being expressed.	Expressing feelings may help relieve despair, hopelessness, and so forth. Feelings are not inherently good or bad. You must remain nonjudgmental about the client's feelings and express this to the client.
Allow (and encourage) the client to cry. Stay with and support the client if he or she desires. Provide privacy if the client desires and it is safe to do so.	Crying is a healthy way of expressing feelings of sadness, hopelessness, and despair. The client may not feel comfortable crying and may need encouragement or privacy.
Interact with the client on topics with which he or she is comfortable. Do not probe for information.	Probing or topics that are uncomfortable for the client may be threatening and discourage communication. After trust has been established, the client may be able to discuss more difficult topics.
Talk with the client about coping strategies he or she has used in the past. Explore which strategies have been successful and which may have led to negative consequences.	The client may have had success using coping strategies in the past but may have lost confidence in himself or herself or in his or her ability to cope with stressors and feelings. Some coping strategies can be self-destructive (e.g., self-medication with drugs or alcohol).
Teach the client about positive coping strategies and stress management skills, such as increasing physical exercise, expressing feelings verbally or in a journal, or meditation techniques. Encourage the client to practice this type of technique while in the hospital.	The client may have limited or no knowledge of stress management techniques or may not have used positive techniques in the past. If the client tries to build skills in the treatment setting, he or she can experience success and receive positive feedback for his or her efforts.
Teach the client about the problem-solving process: explore possible options, examine the consequences of each alternative, select and implement an alternative, and evaluate the results.	The client may be unaware of a systematic method for solving problems. Successful use of the problem-solving process facilitates the client's confidence in the use of coping skills.
Provide positive feedback at each step of the process. If the client is not satisfied with the chosen alternative, assist the client to select another alternative.	Positive feedback at each step will give the client many opportunities for success, encourage him or her to persist in problem-solving, and enhance confidence. The client also can learn to "survive" making a mistake.

Nursing Diagnosis

Impaired Social Interaction
Insufficient or excessive quantity or ineffective quality of social exchange.

ASSESSMENT DATA

- Withdrawn behavior
- Verbalization diminished in quantity, quality, or spontaneity
- Rumination
- Low self-esteem
- Unsatisfactory or inadequate interpersonal relationships
- Verbalizing or exhibiting discomfort around others
- Social isolation
- Inadequate social skills
- Poor personal hygiene

EXPECTED OUTCOMES

Immediate	The client will

• Communicate with others, for example, respond verbally to question(s) asked by staff within 24 to 48 hours
• Participate in activities within 48 to 72 hours

Stabilization	The client will

• Initiate interactions with others, for example, approach a staff member to talk at least once per shift
• Assume responsibility for dealing with feelings

Community	The client will

• Re-establish or maintain relationships and a social life
• Establish a support system in the community, for example, initiate contacts with others by telephone

IMPLEMENTATION

Nursing Interventions *denotes collaborative interventions	**Rationale**
Initially, interact with the client on a one-to-one basis. Manage nursing assignments so that the client interacts with a variety of staff members, as the client tolerates.	Your social behavior provides a role model for the client. Interacting with different staff members allows the client to experience success in interactions within the safety of the staff–client relationship.
Introduce the client to other clients in the milieu and facilitate their interactions on a one client to one client basis. Gradually facilitate social interactions between the client and small groups, then larger groups.	Gradually increasing the scope of the client's social interactions will help the client build confidence in social skills.
Talk with the client about his or her interactions and observations of interpersonal dynamics.	Awareness of interpersonal and group dynamics is an important part of building social skills. Sharing observations provides an opportunity for the client to express his or her feelings and receive feedback about his or her progress.
Teach the client social skills, such as approaching another person for an interaction, appropriate conversation topics, and active listening. Encourage him or her to practice these skills with staff members and other clients, and give the client feedback regarding interactions.	The client may lack social skills and confidence in social interactions; this may contribute to the client's depression and social isolation.
Encourage the client to identify relationships, social, or recreational situations that have been positive in the past.	The client may have been depressed and withdrawn for some time and have lost interest in people or activities that provided pleasure in the past.
*Encourage the client to pursue past relationships, personal interests, hobbies, or recreational activities that were positive in the past or that may appeal to the client. Consultation with a recreational therapist may be indicated.	The client may be reluctant to reach out to someone with whom he or she has had limited contact recently and may benefit from encouragement or facilitation. Recreational activities can serve as a structure for the client to build social interactions as well as provide enjoyment.
*Encourage client to identify supportive people outside the hospital and to develop these relationships.	In addition to re-establishing past relationships or in their absence, increasing the client's support system by establishing new relationships may help decrease future depressive behavior and social isolation.

Nursing Diagnosis

Bathing Self-Care Deficit
Impaired ability to perform or complete bathing activities for self.

Dressing Self-Care Deficit
Impaired ability to perform or complete dressing activities for self.

Feeding Self-Care Deficit
Impaired ability to perform or complete self-feeding activities.

Toileting Self-Care Deficit
Impaired ability to perform or complete toileting activities for self.

ASSESSMENT DATA

- Anergy (overall lack of energy for purposeful activity)
- Decreased motor activity
- Lack of awareness or interest in personal needs
- Self-destructive feelings
- Withdrawn behavior
- Psychological immobility
- Disturbances of appetite or regular eating patterns
- Fatigue

EXPECTED OUTCOMES

Immediate

The client will

- Establish adequate nutrition, hydration, and elimination with nursing assistance within 2 to 4 days
- Establish an adequate balance of rest, sleep, and activity with nursing assistance within 2 to 4 days
- Establish adequate personal hygiene, for example, tolerate bathing and grooming as assisted by staff within 24 to 48 hours

Stabilization

The client will

- Maintain adequately balanced physiologic functioning
- Maintain adequate personal hygiene independently, for example, follow structured routine for bathing and hygiene, initiate self-care activities

Community

The client will

- Maintain a daily routine that meets physiologic and personal needs, including nutrition, hydration, elimination, hygiene, sleep, activity

IMPLEMENTATION

Nursing Interventions *denotes collaborative interventions	Rationale
Closely observe the client's food and fluid intake. Record intake, output, and daily weight if necessary.	The client may not be aware of or interested in meeting physical needs, but these needs must be met.
Offer the client foods that are easily chewed, fortified liquids such as nutritional supplements, and high-protein malts.	If the client lacks interest in eating, highly nutritious foods that require little effort to eat may help meet nutritional needs.

(continued on page 176)

IMPLEMENTATION (continued)

Nursing Interventions *denotes collaborative interventions	Rationale
Try to find out what foods the client likes, including culturally based or foods from family members, and make them available at meals and for snacks.	The client may be more apt to eat foods he or she likes or has been accustomed to eating.
Do not tell the client that he or she will get sick or die from not eating or drinking.	The client may hope to become ill or die from not eating or drinking.
If the client is overeating, limit access to food, schedule meals and snacks, and serve limited portions. Give the client positive feedback for adhering to the prescribed diet.	The client may need limits to maintain a healthful diet.
Observe and record the client's pattern of bowel elimination.	Severe constipation may result from the depression; inadequate exercise, food, or fluid intake; or the effects of some medications.
Encourage good fluid intake.	Constipation may result from inadequate fluid intake.
Be aware of PRN laxative orders and the possible need to offer medication to the client.	The client may be unaware of constipation and may not ask for medication.
Provide the client with his or her own clothing and personal grooming items when possible.	Familiar items will decrease the client's confusion and promote task completion.
Initiate dressing and grooming tasks in the morning.	Clients with depression may have the most energy and feel best in the morning and may have greater success at that time.
Maintain a routine for dressing, grooming, and hygiene.	A routine eliminates needless decision making, such as whether or not to dress or perform personal hygiene.
The client may need physical assistance to get up, dress, and spend time on the unit.	The client's ability to arise, initiate activity, and join in the milieu is impaired.
Be gentle but firm in setting limits regarding time spent in bed. Set specific times when the client must be up in the morning, and when and for how long the client may rest.	Specific limits let the client know what is expected and indicate genuine caring and concern for the client.
Provide a quiet, peaceful time for resting. Decrease environmental stimuli (conversation, lights) in the evening.	Limiting noise and other stimuli will encourage rest and sleep.
Provide a nighttime routine or comfort measures (back rub, tepid bath, warm milk) just before bedtime.	Use of a routine may help the client expect to sleep.
Talk with the client for only brief periods during night hours to help alleviate anxiety and to provide reassurance before the client returns to bed.	Talking with the client for long periods during the night will stimulate the client, give the client attention for not sleeping, and interfere with the client's sleep.
Do not allow the client to sleep for long periods during the day.	Sleeping excessively during the day may decrease the client's need for and ability to sleep at night.
Use PRN medications as indicated to facilitate sleep. *Note:* Some sleep medications may worsen depression or cause agitation.	Medications may be helpful in facilitating sleep.

Nursing Diagnosis

Chronic Low Self-Esteem
Longstanding negative self-evaluating/feelings about self or self-capabilities.

ASSESSMENT DATA

- Feelings of inferiority
- Defeatist thinking
- Self-criticism
- Lack of involvement
- Minimizing of own strengths
- Guilt
- Feelings of despair, worthlessness

EXPECTED OUTCOMES

Immediate

The client will

- Verbalize increased feelings of self-worth within 2 to 5 days
- Express feelings directly and openly with nursing facilitation within 2 to 4 days
- Evaluate own strengths realistically, for example, describe three areas of personal strength, with nursing assistance, within 2 to 4 days

Stabilization

The client will

- Demonstrate behavior consistent with increased self-esteem, for example, make eye contact, initiate conversation or activity with staff or other clients
- Make plans for the future consistent with personal strengths

Community

The client will

- Express satisfaction with self and personal qualities

IMPLEMENTATION

Nursing Interventions *denotes collaborative interventions	Rationale
Encourage the client to become involved with staff and other clients in the milieu through interactions and activities.	When the client can focus on other people or interactions, cyclic, negative thoughts are interrupted.
Give the client positive feedback for completing responsibilities and interacting with others.	Positive feedback increases the likelihood that the client will continue the behavior and begin to internalize positive feelings, such as the satisfaction of completing a task successfully.
If negativism dominates the client's conversations, it may help to structure the content of interactions, for example, by making an agreement to listen to 10 minutes of "negative" interaction, after which the client will interact on a positive topic.	The client will feel you are acknowledging his or her feelings yet will begin practicing the conscious interruption of negativistic thought and feeling patterns.
Explore with the client his or her personal strengths. Making a written list is sometimes helpful.	While you can help the client discover his or her strengths, it will not be useful for you to list the client's strengths. The client needs to identify them but may benefit from your supportive expectation that he or she will do so.
Involve the client in activities that are pleasant or recreational as a break from self-examination.	The client needs to experience pleasurable activities that are not related to self and problems. Such experiences can demonstrate the usefulness of incorporating leisure activities into his or her life.
*At first, provide simple activities that can be accomplished easily and quickly. Begin with a solitary project; progress to group occupational and recreational therapy sessions. Give the client positive feedback for participation.	The client may be limited in his or her ability to deal with complex tasks or stimuli. Any task that the client is able to complete provides an opportunity for positive feedback to the client.

(continued on page 178)

IMPLEMENTATION (continued)

Nursing Interventions *denotes collaborative interventions	Rationale
It may be necessary to stress to the client that he or she should begin doing things to feel better, rather than waiting to feel better before doing things.	The client will have the opportunity to recognize his or her own achievements and will receive positive feedback. Without this stimulus, the client may lack motivation to attempt activities.
Give the client honest praise for accomplishing small responsibilities by acknowledging how difficult it can be for the client to perform these tasks.	Clients with low self-esteem do not benefit from flattery or undue praise. Positive feedback provides reinforcement for the client's growth and can enhance self-esteem.
Gradually increase the number and complexity of activities expected of the client; give positive feedback at each level of accomplishment.	As the client's abilities increase, he or she can accomplish more complex activities and receive more feedback.

CARE PLAN 26

Suicidal Behavior

Suicide is defined as a death that results from an act that the victim commits believing that the act will cause death. Clients who are depressed may certainly be suicidal, but many clients who are suicidal are not depressed. The client may view suicide as an escape from extreme despair or from a (perceived) intolerable life situation, such as a terminal illness. Suicide may be the culmination of self-destructive urges that have resulted from the client's internalizing anger; a desperate act by which to escape a perceived intolerable psychological state or life situation. The client may be asking for help by attempting suicide, or the client may be seeking attention or attempting to manipulate someone with suicidal behavior.

The risk of suicide is increased when:

- A plan is formulated
- The client has the ability to carry out the plan
- There is a history of suicide attempts or a family history of suicide
- Suicide attempts become more painful, more violent, or lethal
- The client is white, male, adolescent, or older than 55 years
- The client is divorced, widowed, separated, or living without family
- The client is terminally ill, addicted, or psychotic
- The client gives away personal possessions, settles accounts, and so forth
- The client is in an early stage of treatment with antidepressant medications, and his or her mood and activity level begin to elevate
- The client's mood or activity level suddenly changes

Suicide is a significant cause of death worldwide; it is the eighth leading cause of death for men in the United States and the third leading cause of death among people aged 15 to 24. Men commit suicide more often than women, and Caucasians commit suicide more often than African Americans. Suicide rates for adults in the United States rise with increasing age, and people over 65 years of age have the highest rate. Clients with certain mental disorders are at increased risk for suicide, including clients with depression, bipolar disorder, schizophrenia, and substance abuse.

Many people who commit suicide have given a verbal warning or clue. It is not true that "anyone who talks about suicide doesn't actually commit suicide." However, not everyone who attempts or commits suicide has given any warning at all. *Remember:* Threatening suicide may be an effort to bring about a fundamental change in the client's life situation or to elicit a response from a significant person, but it may indeed be an indication of real intent to commit suicide.

Suicidal ideation is defined as thoughts of committing suicide or of methods to commit suicide.

Suicidal gesture is a behavior that is self-destructive, as though it was a suicide attempt, but is not lethal (e.g., writing a suicide note and taking 10 aspirin tablets). This often is considered to be manipulative behavior, but the nonlethality of the behavior may be a result of the client's ignorance of the effects of such behavior or methods; the client may indeed wish to die.

Suicide attempt is a self-destructive behavior that is potentially lethal.

Suicide precautions are specific actions taken to protect a client from suicidal gestures and attempts and to ensure close observation of the client.

The paramount therapeutic goal is to prevent death or harm to the client. The specific precautions taken by nursing staff to protect a client from suicidal attempts will vary with each client's needs, but will include being alert to possible signs that might indicate suicidal behavior and maintaining close supervision of the client. Many in-hospital suicides occur during unstructured time and when relatively few staff members are on duty (e.g., nights and weekends). It is especially important to observe the client closely, to document his or her behavior carefully, and to communicate *any* pertinent information to others who are making decisions about the client (especially if the client is to go on activities, on pass, or be discharged). There may be legal ramifications associated with a hospitalized client who is suicidal, especially if the client successfully commits suicide. *Remember:* Every client has the potential for suicide.

Beyond preventing suicide, nursing goals focus on identifying and addressing the factors underlying the client's suicidal behavior, which may include deep religious or cultural conflicts, interpersonal issues, life situation difficulties, problems with self-esteem, substance use, or other psychiatric disorders. Other important interventions are helping the client develop skills with which to deal with these problems and other life stresses and teaching the client and the family or significant others about suicidal behavior. Discharge planning may include arrangements for long-term support, such as referral to support groups, vocational or other training, or continued individual or family therapy.

NURSING DIAGNOSES ADDRESSED IN THIS CARE PLAN
Risk for Suicide
Ineffective Coping
Chronic Low Self-Esteem

RELATED NURSING DIAGNOSES ADDRESSED IN THE MANUAL
Hopelessness
Powerlessness
Impaired Social Interaction

Nursing Diagnosis

Risk for Suicide
At risk for self-inflicted, life-threatening injury.

RISK FACTORS

- Suicidal ideas, feelings, ideation, plans, gestures, or attempts
- Lack of impulse control
- Lack of future orientation
- Self-destructive tendencies
- Feelings of anger or hostility
- Agitation
- Aggressive behavior
- Feelings of worthlessness, hopelessness, or despair
- Guilt
- Anxiety
- Sleep disturbance
- Substance use
- Perceived or observable loss
- Social isolation
- Problems of depression, withdrawn behavior, eating disorders, psychotic behavior, personality disorder, manipulative behavior, post-traumatic stress, or other psychiatric problems

EXPECTED OUTCOMES

Immediate	The client will

- Be safe and free from injury throughout hospitalization
- Refrain from harming others throughout hospitalization
- Identify alternative ways of dealing with stress and emotional problems, for example, talking with staff or significant others, within 48 to 72 hours

Stabilization	The client will

- Demonstrate use of alternative ways of dealing with stress and emotional problems, for example, initiating interaction with staff when feeling stressed
- Verbalize knowledge of self-destructive behavior(s), other psychiatric problems, and safe use of medication, if any

Community	The client will

- Develop a plan of community support to use if crisis situations arise in the future, for example, make a written list of resources or contacts

IMPLEMENTATION

Nursing Interventions *denotes collaborative interventions	Rationale
Determine the appropriate level of suicide precautions for the client. Institute these precautions immediately on admission by nursing or physician order. Some suggested levels of precautions follow:	Physical safety of the client is a priority.
1. A staff member provides one-to-one supervision of the client at all times, even when in the bathroom and sleeping. The client is restricted to the unit and is permitted to use nothing that may cause harm to him or her (e.g., sharp objects, a belt).	1. A client who is at high risk for suicidal behavior needs constant supervision and strict limitation of opportunities to harm himself or herself.
2. A staff member provides one-to-one supervision of the client at all times, but the client may attend activities off the unit (maintaining one-to-one contact).	2. A client at a somewhat lower risk of suicide may join in activities and use potentially harmful objects (such as sharp objects) but still must have close supervision.
3. Special attention—the client must be accompanied by a staff member while off the unit but may be in a staff–client group on the unit, though the client's whereabouts and activities on the unit should be known at all time.	3. A client with a lower level of suicide risk still requires observation, though one-to-one contact may not be necessary at all times when the client is on the unit.
Assess the client's suicidal potential, and evaluate the level of suicide precautions at least daily.	The client's suicidal potential varies; the risk may increase or decrease at any time.
In your initial assessment, note any previous suicide attempts and methods, as well as family history of mental illness or suicide. Obtain this information in a matter-of-fact manner; do not discuss at length or dwell on details.	Information on past suicide attempts, ideation, and family history is important in assessing suicide risk. The client may be using suicidal behavior as a manipulation or to obtain secondary gain. It is important to minimize reinforcement given to these behaviors.
Ask the client if he or she has a plan for suicide. Attempt to ascertain how detailed and feasible the plan is.	Suicide risk increases when the client has a plan, especially one that is feasible or lethal.
Explain suicide precautions to the client.	The client is a participant in his or her care. Suicide precautions demonstrate your caring and concern for the client.
Know the whereabouts of the client at all times. Designate a specific staff person to be responsible for the client at all times. If this person must leave the unit for any reason, information and responsibility regarding supervision of the client must be transferred to another staff person.	The client at high risk for suicidal behavior needs close supervision. Designating responsibility for observation of the client to a specific person minimizes the possibility that the client will have inadequate supervision.

(continued on page 182)

IMPLEMENTATION (continued)

Nursing Interventions *denotes collaborative interventions	Rationale
Be especially alert to sharp objects and other potentially dangerous items (e.g., glass containers, vases, and matches); items like these should not be in the client's possession.	The client's determination to commit suicide may lead him or her to use even common objects in self-destructive ways. Many seemingly innocuous items can be used, some lethally.
The client's room should be near the nurses' station and within view of the staff, not at the end of a hallway or near an exit, elevator, or stairwell.	The client at high risk for suicidal behavior requires close observation.
Make sure that the client cannot open windows. (The maintenance department may have to seal or otherwise secure the windows.)	The client may attempt to open and jump out of a window or throw himself or herself through a window if it is locked.
If the client needs to use a sharp object, sign out the object to the client, and stay with the client during its use.	The client may use a sharp object to harm himself or herself or may conceal it for later use.
Have the client use an electric shaver if possible.	Even disposable razors can be quickly disassembled and the blades used in a self-destructive manner.
If the client is attempting to harm himself or herself, it may be necessary to restrain the client or to place him or her in seclusion with no objects that can be used to self-inflict injury (electric outlets, silverware, and even bed clothing).	Physical safety of the client is a priority.
Stay with the client when he or she is meeting hygienic needs such as bathing, shaving, and cutting nails.	Your presence and supervision may prevent self-destructive activity, or you can immediately intervene to protect the client.
Check the client at frequent, *irregular* intervals during the night to ascertain the client's safety and whereabouts.	Checking at irregular intervals will minimize the client's ability to predict when he or she will (or will not) be observed.
Maintain especially close supervision of the client at any time there is a decrease in the number of staff, the amount of structure, or the level of stimulation (nursing report at the change of shift, mealtime, weekends, nights). Also, be especially aware of the client during any period of distraction and when clients are going to and from activities.	Risk of suicide increases when there is a decrease in the number of staff, the amount of structure, or the level of stimulation. The client may use times of turmoil or distraction to slip away or to engage in self-destructive behavior.
Be alert to the possibility of the client saving up his or her medications or obtaining medications or dangerous objects from other clients or visitors. You may need to check the client's mouth after medication administration or use liquid medications to ensure that they are ingested.	The client may accumulate medication to use in a suicide attempt. The client may manipulate or otherwise use other clients or visitors to obtain medications or other dangerous items.
Observe, record, and report any changes in the client's mood (elation, withdrawal, sudden resignation).	Risk of suicide increases when mood or behavior suddenly changes. *Remember:* As depression decreases, the client may have the energy to carry out a plan for suicide.
Observe the client and note when the client is more animated or withdrawn with regard to the time of day, structured versus unstructured time, interactions with others, activities, and attention span. Use this information to plan nursing care and the client's activities.	Assessment of the client's behavior can help to determine unusual behavior and may help to identify times of increased risk for suicidal behavior.
Be alert to the client's behaviors, especially decreased communication, conversations about death or the futility of life, disorientation, low frustration tolerance, dependency, dissatisfaction with dependence, disinterest in surroundings, and concealing articles that could be used to harm self.	These behaviors may indicate the client's decision to commit suicide.

IMPLEMENTATION (continued)

Nursing Interventions *denotes collaborative interventions	Rationale
Be aware of the relationships the client is forming with other clients and be alert to any manipulative or attention-seeking behavior. Note who may become his or her confidant. See Care Plan 48: Passive–Aggressive Behavior.	The client may warn another client about a suicide attempt or may use other clients to elicit secondary gain.
Note: The client may ask you not to tell anyone something he or she tells you. Avoid promising to keep secrets in this way; make it clear to the client that you must share all information with the other staff members on the treatment team, but assure the client of confidentiality with regard to anyone outside the treatment team.	The client may attempt to manipulate you or may seek attention for having a "secret" that may be a suicide plan. You must not assume responsibility for keeping secret a suicide plan the client may announce to you. If the client hints at but will not reveal a plan, it is important to minimize attention given to this behavior, but suicide precautions may need to be used.
Tell the client that although you are willing to discuss emotions or other topics, you will not discuss details of prior suicide attempts repeatedly; discourage such conversations with other clients also. Encourage the client to talk about his or her feelings, relationships, or life situation.	Reinforcement given to suicidal ideas and rumination must be minimized. However, the client needs to identify and express the feelings that underlie the suicidal behavior.
Convey that you care about the client and that you believe the client is a worthwhile human being.	The client is acceptable as a person regardless of his other behaviors, which may or may not be acceptable.
Do not joke about death, belittle the client's wishes or feelings, or make insensitive remarks, such as "Everybody really wants to live."	The client's ability to understand and use abstractions such as humor is impaired. The client's feelings are real to him or her. The client may indeed not want to live; remarks like this may further alienate the client or contribute to his or her low self-esteem.
Do not belittle the client's prior suicide attempts, which other people may deem "only" attention-seeking gestures.	People who make suicidal gestures are gambling with death and need help.
Convey your interest in the client and approach him or her for interaction at least once per shift. If the client says, "I don't feel like talking," or "Leave me alone," remain with him or her in silence or state that you will be back later and then withdraw. You may tell the client that you will return at a specific time.	Your presence demonstrates interest and caring. The client may be testing your interest or pushing you away to isolate himself or herself. Telling the client you will return conveys your continued caring.
Give the client support for efforts to remain out of his or her room, to interact with other clients, or to attend activities.	The client's ability to interact with others is impaired. Positive feedback gives the client recognition for his or her efforts.
Encourage and support the client's expression of anger. (*Remember:* Do not take the anger personally.) Help the client deal with the fear of expressing anger and related feelings.	Self-destructive behavior can be seen as the result of anger turned inward. Verbal expression of anger can help to externalize these feelings.
Do not make moral judgments about suicide or reinforce the client's feelings of guilt or sin.	Feelings such as guilt may underlie the client's suicidal behavior.
*Referral to the facility chaplain, clergy, or other spiritual resource person may be indicated.	Discussing spiritual issues with an advisor who shares his or her belief system may be more comfortable for the client and may enhance trust and alleviate guilt.
Remain aware of your own feelings about suicide. Talk with other staff members to deal with your feelings if necessary.	Many people have strong feelings about taking one's own life, such as disapproval, fear, seeing suicide as a sin, and so forth. Being aware of and working through your feelings will diminish the possibility that you will inadvertently convey these feelings to the client.
Involve the client as much as possible in planning his or her own treatment.	Participation in planning his or her care can help to increase the client's sense of responsibility and control.

(continued on page 184)

IMPLEMENTATION (continued)

Nursing Interventions *denotes collaborative interventions	Rationale
*Examine with the client his or her home environment and relationships outside the hospital. What changes are indicated to decrease the likelihood of future suicidal behavior? Include the client's family or significant others in teaching, skill development, and therapy, if indicated.	The client's significant others may be reinforcing the client's suicidal behavior, or the suicidal behavior may be a symptom of a problem involving others in the client's life.
*Plan with the client how he or she will recognize and deal with feelings and situations that have precipitated suicidal feelings or behavior. Include whom the client will contact (ideally, someone in the home environment) and what to do in order to alleviate suicidal feelings (identify what has worked in the past).	Concrete plans may be helpful in averting suicidal behavior. Recognizing feelings that lead to suicidal behavior may help the client seek help before reaching a critical point.

NURSING DIAGNOSIS

Ineffective Coping

Inability to form a valid appraisal of the stressors, inadequate choices of practiced responses, and/or inability to use available resources.

ASSESSMENT DATA

- Dysfunctional grieving
- Feelings of worthlessness or hopelessness
- Inability to solve problems
- Feelings of anger or hostility
- Difficulty identifying and expressing emotions
- Guilt
- Self-destructive behavior
- Anxiety
- Lack of trust
- Lack of future orientation
- Depression
- Withdrawn behavior
- Low self-esteem
- Perceived crisis in life, situation, or relationships

EXPECTED OUTCOMES

Immediate

The client will

- Participate in the treatment program within 24 to 48 hours
- Express feelings in a non–self-destructive manner, for example, talk with staff or write about feelings, within 24 to 48 hours
- Identify alternative ways of dealing with stress and emotional problems, within 48 to 72 hours

Stabilization

The client will

- Demonstrate use of the problem-solving process
- Verbalize plans for using alternative ways of dealing with stress and emotional problems when they occur after discharge
- Verbalize plans for continued therapy after discharge if appropriate, for example, identify a therapist, make an initial appointment

Community

The client will

- Maintain satisfying relationships in the community

IMPLEMENTATION

Nursing Interventions *denotes collaborative interventions	Rationale
Encourage the client to express his or her feelings; convey your acceptance of the client's feelings.	Expressing feelings can help the client to identify, accept, and work through feelings, even if these are painful or otherwise uncomfortable. Feelings are not inherently bad or good. You must remain nonjudgmental about the client's feelings and express this attitude to the client.
Help the client identify situations in which he or she would feel more comfortable expressing feelings; use role-playing to practice expressing emotions.	The client may not have experienced a safe environment in which to express emotions and may benefit from practicing with staff members and other clients. Role playing allows the client to try out new behaviors in a supportive environment.
Convey your interest in the client and approach him or her for interaction at least once per shift. If the client says, "I don't feel like talking," or "Leave me alone," remain with him or her in silence or state that you will be back later and then withdraw. You may tell the client that you will return at a specific time.	Your presence demonstrates interest and caring. The client may be testing your interest or pushing you away to isolate himself or herself. Telling the client you will return conveys your continued caring.
Give the client support for efforts to remain out of his or her room, to interact with other clients, or to attend activities.	The client's ability to interact with others is impaired. Positive feedback gives the client recognition for his or her efforts.
Encourage the client to express fears, anxieties, and concerns.	The client's behavior may be related to fear or anxieties that he or she has not expressed or is unaware of, or that seem overpowering. Identifying and expressing these emotions can help the client learn how to deal with them in a non–self-destructive way.
Provide opportunities for the client to express emotions and release tension in non–self-destructive ways such as discussions, activities, and physical exercise.	The client needs to develop skills with which to replace self-destructive behavior.
Involve the client as much as possible in planning his or her own treatment.	Participating in his or her plan of care can help increase the client's sense of responsibility and control.
Teach the client about depression, self-destructive behavior, or other psychiatric problems (see other care plans as appropriate).	The client may have very little knowledge of or insight into his or her behavior and emotions.
Teach the client about the problem-solving process: identify a problem, identify and evaluate alternative solutions, choose and implement a solution, and evaluate its success.	The client may never have learned a logical, step-by-step approach to problem resolution.
Teach the client social skills, such as approaching another person for an interaction, appropriate conversation topics, and active listening. Encourage him or her to practice with staff members and other clients. Give the client feedback regarding social interactions.	The client may lack skills and confidence in social interactions; this may contribute to the client's anxiety, depression, or social isolation.
*Encourage the client to pursue personal interests, hobbies, and recreational activities. Consultation with a recreational therapist may be indicated.	Recreational activities can help increase the client's social interaction and provide enjoyment.
Discuss the future with the client; consider hypothetical situations, emotional concerns, significant relationships, and future plans. Use role-playing and ask the client about plans for time outside the hospital, on a trial basis and for discharge.	Anticipatory guidance can help the client prepare for future stress, crises, and so forth. *Remember:* Although the client may not be suicidal, he or she may not yet be ready for discharge. The client may have increased anxiety when outside of the therapeutic milieu or may be planning self-destructive behavior when no longer being supervised.
*Encourage the client to identify and develop relationships with supportive people outside the hospital environment. See Care Plan 2: Discharge Planning.	Increasing the client's support system may help decrease future suicidal behavior. The risk of suicide is increased when the client is socially isolated.

Nursing Diagnosis

Chronic Low Self-Esteem

Longstanding negative self-evaluating/feelings about self or self-capabilities.

ASSESSMENT DATA

- Verbalization of low self-esteem, negative self-characteristics, or low opinion of self
- Verbalization of guilt or shame
- Feelings of worthlessness, hopelessness, or rejection

EXPECTED OUTCOMES

Immediate

The client will

- Express feelings related to self-esteem and self-worth issues within 2 to 5 days
- Identify personal strengths with nursing assistance within 2 to 4 days

Stabilization

The client will

- Demonstrate behavior congruent with increased self-esteem, for example, approach staff or other clients for interactions, maintain eye contact, verbalize personal strengths
- Assess own strengths and weaknesses realistically
- Verbalize plans to continue therapy regarding self-esteem issues, if needed

Community

The client will

- Participate in follow-up care or community support groups
- Express satisfaction with self and personal qualities

IMPLEMENTATION

Nursing Interventions *denotes collaborative interventions	Rationale
Convey that you care about the client and that you believe the client is a worthwhile human being.	The client is acceptable as a person regardless of his or her behaviors, which may or may not be acceptable.
Encourage the client to express his or her feelings; convey your acceptance of the client's feelings.	The client's self-evaluation may be related to feelings that he or she finds unacceptable. The client's expression and your acceptance of these feelings can help him or her separate the feelings from his or her self-image and learn that feelings are not inherently bad (or good).
Initially, provide opportunities for the client to succeed at activities that are easily accomplished and give positive feedback. *Note:* The client's self-esteem may be so low that he or she may feel able to make things only for others at first, not for his or her own use.	Positive feedback provides reinforcement for the client's growth and can enhance self-esteem. The client's ability to concentrate, complete tasks, and interact with others may be impaired.
Encourage the client to take on progressively more challenging activities. Give the client positive support for participating in activities or interacting with others.	As the client's abilities increase, he or she may be able to feel increasing self-esteem related to his or her accomplishments. Your verbal feedback can help the client recognize his or her role in accomplishments and take credit for them.
Acknowledge and support the client for efforts to interact with others, participate in the treatment program, and express emotions.	Regardless of the level of "success" of a given activity, the client can benefit from acknowledgement of his or her efforts.
Help the client identify positive aspects about himself or herself. You may point out these aspects, behaviors, or activities as observations, without arguing with the client about his or her feelings.	The client may see only his or her negative self-evaluation and not recognize positive aspects. While the client's feelings are real to him or her, your positive observations present a different viewpoint that the client can examine and begin to integrate.

IMPLEMENTATION (continued)

Nursing Interventions *denotes collaborative interventions	Rationale
Do not flatter the client or be otherwise dishonest. Give honest, genuine, positive feedback to the client whenever possible.	The client will not benefit from insincerity; dishonesty undermines trust and the therapeutic relationship.
*Encourage the client to pursue personal interests, hobbies, and recreational activities. Consultation with a recreational therapist may be indicated.	Recreational activities can help increase the client's social interaction and provide enjoyment.
*Referral to a clergy member or spiritual advisor of the client's own faith may be indicated.	The client may have feelings of shame or guilt related to his or her religious beliefs.
*Encourage the client to pursue long-term therapy for self-esteem issues, if indicated.	Self-esteem problems can be deeply rooted and require long-term therapy.

Bipolar Disorder, Manic Episode

Bipolar disorder is usually characterized by manic and depressive episodes with periods of relatively normal functioning in between. Manic behavior is characterized by an "abnormally and persistently elevated, expansive, or irritable mood" (APA, 2000, p. 357). Clients who exhibit manic behavior may:

- be agitated
- have no regard for eating, drinking, hygiene, grooming, resting, or sleeping
- have extremely poor judgment
- exhibit seductive or aggressive behavior
- have psychotic symptoms such as hallucinations or delusions
- be at increased risk for injury

Clients with bipolar disorder also are at high risk for suicide: 10% to 15% of these clients successfully commit suicide (APA, 2000).

Bipolar disorder occurs at about the same rate in men and women and affects between 0.4% and 1.6% of the population (APA, 2000). Research indicates a genetic component to bipolar disorder and an increased incidence of major depressive disorder (APA, 2000). Clients often manifest or have a family history of alcoholism or other substance abuse. Substance abuse may be an attempt to self-medicate, or the client may have a *dual diagnosis* (bipolar disorder and substance abuse); each disorder requires treatment (see Care Plan 18: Dual Diagnosis). Bipolar disorder is also associated with eating disorders, attention deficit/hyperactivity disorder, and anxiety disorders (APA, 2000).

Pediatric bipolar disorder is estimated to affect 1% of children and adolescents (Stanford School of Medicine, 2010). It differs from the adult form of the disorder: longer episodes; rapid cycling; and irritability. AD/HD and anxiety disorders are often seen co-morbidly with) pediatric bipolar disorder (Carbray & McGuinness, 2009).

The average age of the first manic episode in bipolar disorder is 20 years old. Manic and depressive episodes are recurrent in most clients; periods between episodes are characterized by significantly reduced symptoms, but some symptoms can cause chronic problems in the client's life (APA, 2000).

Initial nursing goals include preventing injury and meeting the client's basic physiologic needs. It is important to remember that clients with manic behavior may have very low self-esteem, often in contradiction to their euphoric or grandiose behavior. After the client's agitation has subsided, teaching the client and family or significant others about the client's illness and medication regimen is an important goal, because successful long-term treatment often depends on medication compliance.

NURSING DIAGNOSES ADDRESSED IN THIS CARE PLAN
Risk for Other-Directed Violence
Defensive Coping
Disturbed Thought Processes
Bathing Self-Care Deficit
Dressing Self-Care Deficit
Feeding Self-Care Deficit
Toileting Self-Care Deficit
Deficient Knowledge (Specify)

RELATED NURSING DIAGNOSES ADDRESSED IN THE MANUAL
Risk for Injury
Disturbed Sensory Perception (Specify: Visual, Auditory, Kinesthetic, Gustatory,
   Tactile, Olfactory)
Chronic Low Self-Esteem
Ineffective Therapeutic Regimen Management
Impaired Social Interaction
Imbalanced Nutrition: Less Than Body Requirements
Insomnia

Nursing Diagnosis

Risk for Other-Directed Violence
At risk for behaviors in which an individual demonstrates that he or she can be physically,
emotionally, and/or sexually harmful to others.

RISK FACTORS

- Restlessness
- Hyperactivity
- Agitation
- Hostile behavior
- Threatened or actual aggression toward self or others
- Low self-esteem

Immediate

EXPECTED OUTCOMES
The client will

- Be safe and free from injury throughout hospitalization
- Demonstrate decreased restlessness, hyperactivity, and agitation within 24 to 48 hours
- Demonstrate decreased hostility within 2 to 4 days
- Refrain from harming others throughout hospitalization

Stabilization

The client will

- Be free of restlessness, hyperactivity, and agitation
- Be free of threatened or actual aggression toward self or others

Community

The client will

- Demonstrate level moods
- Express feelings of anger or frustration verbally in a safe manner

IMPLEMENTATION

Nursing Interventions *denotes collaborative interventions	Rationale
Provide a safe environment. See Care Plan 26: Suicidal Behavior, Care Plan 46: Hostile Behavior, and Care Plan 47: Aggressive Behavior.	Physical safety of the client and others is a priority. The client may use many common items and environmental situations in a destructive manner.
Administer PRN medications judiciously, preferably before the client's behavior becomes destructive.	Medications can help the client regain self-control but should not be used to control the client's behavior for the staff's convenience or as a substitute for working with the client's problems.

(continued on page 190)

IMPLEMENTATION (continued)

Nursing Interventions *denotes collaborative interventions	Rationale
Set and maintain limits on behavior that is destructive or adversely affects others.	Limits must be established by others when the client is unable to use internal controls effectively. The physical safety and emotional needs of other clients are important.
Decrease environmental stimuli whenever possible. Respond to cues of agitation by removing stimuli and perhaps isolating the client; a private room may be beneficial.	The client's ability to deal with stimuli is impaired.
Provide a consistent, structured environment. Let the client know what is expected of him or her. Set goals with the client as soon as possible.	Consistency and structure can reassure the client. The client must know what is expected before he or she can work toward meeting those expectations.
Give simple direct explanations (e.g., for procedures, tests, etc.). Do not argue with the client.	The client is limited in the ability to deal with complex stimuli. Stating a limit tells the client what is expected. Arguing interjects doubt and undermines limits.
Encourage the client to verbalize feelings such as anxiety and anger. Explore ways to relieve tension with the client as soon as possible.	Ventilation of feelings may help relieve anxiety, anger, and so forth.
Encourage supervised physical activity.	Physical activity can diminish tension and hyperactivity in a healthy, nondestructive manner.

Nursing Diagnosis

Defensive Coping
Repeated projection of falsely positive self-evaluation based on a self-protective pattern that defends against underlying perceived threats to positive self-regard.

ASSESSMENT DATA

• Denial of problems
• Exaggeration of achievements
• Grandiose schemes, plans, or stated self-image
• Buying sprees
• Inappropriate, bizarre, or flamboyant dress or use of makeup or jewelry
• Flirtatious, seductive behavior
• Sexual acting-out

EXPECTED OUTCOMES

Immediate   The client will

• Demonstrate more appropriate appearance (dress, use of makeup, etc.) within 2 to 3 days
• Demonstrate increased feelings of self-worth within 4 to 5 days

Stabilization   The client will

• Verbalize increased feelings of self-worth
• Demonstrate appropriate appearance and behavior

Community   The client will

• Use internal controls to modify own behavior

IMPLEMENTATION

Nursing Interventions *denotes collaborative interventions	Rationale
Ignore or withdraw your attention from bizarre appearance and behavior and sexual acting-out, as much as possible.	Minimizing or withdrawing attention given to unacceptable behaviors can be more effective than negative reinforcement in decreasing unacceptable behavior.
Set and maintain limits regarding inappropriate behaviors. Convey expectations for appropriate behavior in a nonjudgmental, matter-of-fact manner.	The client needs to learn what is expected before he or she can meet expectations. Limits are intended to help the client learn appropriate behaviors, not as punishment for inappropriate behavior.
You may need to limit contact between the client and other clients or restrict visitors for a period of time. Discuss the situation with the client as tolerated.	The client may need to gain self-control before he or she can tolerate the presence of other people and behave in an appropriate manner.
Initially, give the client short-term, simple projects or activities. Gradually increase the number and complexity of activities and responsibilities. Give feedback at each level of accomplishment.	The client may be limited in the ability to deal with complex tasks. Any task that the client is able to complete provides an opportunity for positive feedback.
Give client positive feedback whenever appropriate.	Positive feedback provides reinforcement for the client's growth and can enhance self-esteem. It is essential to support the client in positive ways and not to give attention only for unacceptable behaviors.

Nursing Diagnosis

Disturbed Thought Processes*
Disruption in cognitive operations and activities.

*Note: This nursing diagnosis was retired in *NANDA-I Nursing Diagnoses: Definitions & Classification 2009–2011*, but the NANDA-I Diagnosis Development Committee encourages work to be done on retired diagnoses toward resubmission for inclusion in the taxonomy.

ASSESSMENT DATA

- Disorientation
- Decreased concentration, short attention span
- Loose associations (loosely and poorly associated ideas)
- Push of speech (rapid, forced speech)
- Tangentiality of ideas and speech
- Hallucinations
- Delusions

EXPECTED OUTCOMES

Immediate

The client will

- Demonstrate orientation to person, place, and time within 24 hours
- Demonstrate decreased hallucinations or delusions within 24 to 48 hours
- Demonstrate decreased push of speech, tangentiality, loose associations within 24 to 48 hours
- Demonstrate an increased attention span, for example, talk with staff about one topic for 5 minutes, or engage in one activity for 10 minutes, within 2 to 3 days
- Talk with others about present reality within 2 to 3 days

Stabilization	The client will

- Demonstrate orientation to person, place, and time
- Demonstrate adequate cognitive functioning

Community	The client will

- Sustain concentration and attention to complete tasks and function independently
- Be free of delusions or hallucinations

IMPLEMENTATION

Nursing Interventions *denotes collaborative interventions	Rationale
Set and maintain limits on behavior that is destructive or adversely affects others.	Limits must be established by others when the client is unable to use internal controls effectively. The physical safety and emotional needs of other clients are important.
See Care Plan 21: Delusions, Care Plan 22: Hallucinations, and Care Plan 46: Hostile Behavior.	
Initially, assign the client to the same staff members when possible, but keep in mind the stress of working with a client with manic behavior for extended periods of time.	Consistency can reassure the client. Working with this client may be difficult and tiring due to his or her agitation, hyperactivity, and so on.
See Care Plan 1: Building a Trust Relationship.	
Decrease environmental stimuli whenever possible. Respond to cues of increased agitation by removing stimuli and perhaps isolating the client; a private room may be beneficial.	The client's ability to deal with stimuli is impaired.
Reorient the client to person, place, and time as indicated (call the client by name, tell the client your name, tell the client where he or she is, etc.).	Repeated presentation of reality is concrete reinforcement for the client.
*Provide a consistent, structured environment. Let the client know what is expected of him or her. Set goals with the client as soon as possible.	Consistency and structure can reassure the client. The client must know what is expected before he or she can work toward meeting those expectations.
Spend time with the client.	Your physical presence is reality.
Show acceptance of the client as a person.	The client is acceptable as a person regardless of his or her behaviors, which may or may not be acceptable.
Use a firm yet calm, relaxed approach.	Your presence and manner will help to communicate your interest, expectations, and limits, as well as your self-control.
Make only promises you can realistically keep.	Breaking a promise will result in the client's mistrust and is detrimental to a therapeutic relationship.
Limit the size and frequency of group activities based on the client's level of tolerance.	The client's ability to respond to others and to deal with increased amounts and complexity of stimuli is impaired.
Help the client plan activities within his or her scope of achievement.	The client's attention span is short, and his or her ability to deal with complex stimuli is impaired.
Avoid highly competitive activities.	Competitive situations can exacerbate the client's hostile feelings or reinforce low self-esteem.
*Evaluate the client's tolerance for group activities, interactions with others, or visitors, and limit these accordingly.	The client is unable to provide limits and may be unaware of his or her impaired ability to deal with others.
Encourage the client's appropriate expression of feelings regarding treatment or discharge plans. Support any realistic plans the patient proposes.	Positive support can reinforce the client's healthy expression of feelings, realistic plans, and responsible behavior after discharge.
See Care Plan 18: Dual Diagnosis.	Substance abuse often is a problem in clients with bipolar disorder.

Nursing Diagnosis

Bathing Self-Care Deficit
Impaired ability to perform or complete bathing activities for self.

Dressing Self-Care Deficit
Impaired ability to perform or complete dressing activities for self.

Feeding Self-Care Deficit
Impaired ability to perform or complete self-feeding activities.

Toileting Self-Care Deficit
Impaired ability to perform or complete toileting activities for self.

ASSESSMENT DATA

- Inability to take responsibility for meeting basic health and self-care needs
- Inadequate food and fluid intake
- Inattention to personal needs
- Impaired personal support system
- Lack of ability to make judgments regarding health and self-care needs
- Lack of awareness of personal needs
- Hyperactivity
- Insomnia
- Fatigue

EXPECTED OUTCOMES

Immediate

The client will

- Participate in self-care activities, such as bathing, grooming, with nursing assistance, within 24 hours
- Establish adequate nutrition, hydration, and elimination, with nursing assistance, within 24 to 48 hours (e.g., eat at least 30% of meals)
- Establish an adequate balance of rest, sleep, and activity, within 48 to 72 hours (e.g., sleep at least 3 hours per night within 48 hours)

Stabilization

The client will

- Maintain adequate nutrition, hydration, and elimination, for example, eat at least 70% of meals by a specified date
- Maintain an adequate balance of rest, sleep, and activity, for example, sleep at least 5 hours by a specified date

Community

The client will

- Meet personal needs independently
- Recognize signs of impending relapse

IMPLEMENTATION

Nursing Interventions *denotes collaborative interventions	Rationale
Monitor the client's calorie, protein, and fluid intake. You may need to record intake and output.	The client may be unaware of physical needs or may ignore feelings of thirst and hunger.
The client may need a high-calorie diet and supplemental feedings.	The client's increased activity increases nutrition requirements.

(continued on page 194)

IMPLEMENTATION (continued)

Nursing Interventions *denotes collaborative interventions	Rationale
Provide foods that the client can carry with him or her (fortified milkshakes, sandwiches, "finger foods"). See Care Plan 52: The Client Who Will Not Eat.	If the client is unable or unwilling to sit and eat, highly nutritious foods that require little effort to eat may be effective.
Monitor the client's elimination patterns.	The client may be unaware of or ignore the need to defecate. Constipation is a frequent adverse effect of antipsychotic medications.
Provide time for a rest period during the client's daily schedule.	The client's increased activity increases his or her need for rest.
Observe the client for signs of fatigue and monitor his or her sleep patterns.	The client may be unaware of fatigue or may ignore the need for rest.
Decrease stimuli before bedtime (dim lights, turn off television).	Limiting stimuli will help encourage rest and sleep.
Use comfort measures or sleeping medication if needed.	Comfort measures and medications can enhance the ability to sleep.
Encourage the client to follow a routine of sleeping at night rather than during the day; limit interaction with the client at night and allow only a short nap during the day. See Care Plan 38: Sleep Disorders.	Talking with the client during night hours will interfere with sleep by stimulating the client and giving attention for not sleeping. Sleeping excessively during the day may decrease the client's ability to sleep at night.
If necessary, assist the client with personal hygiene, including mouth care, bathing, dressing, and laundering clothes.	The client may be unaware of or lack interest in hygiene. Personal hygiene can foster feelings of well-being and self-esteem.
Encourage the client to meet as many of his or her own needs as possible.	The client must be encouraged to be as independent as possible to promote self-esteem.

Nursing Diagnosis

Deficient Knowledge (Specify)

Absence or deficiency of cognitive information related to a specific topic.

ASSESSMENT DATA

- Inappropriate behavior related to self-care
- Inadequate retention of information presented
- Inadequate understanding of information presented

EXPECTED OUTCOMES

Immediate

The client will

- Acknowledge his or her illness and need for treatment within 48 hours
- Participate in learning about his or her illness, treatment, and safe use of medications within 4 to 5 days

Stabilization

The client will

- Verbalize knowledge of his or her illness
- Demonstrate knowledge of adverse and toxic effects of medications
- Demonstrate continued compliance with chemotherapy
- Verbalize knowledge and acceptance of the need for continued therapy, chemotherapy, regular blood tests, and so forth

Community   The client will

- Participate in follow-up care, for example, make and keep follow-up appointments
- Manage medication regimen independently

IMPLEMENTATION

Nursing Interventions *denotes collaborative interventions	Rationale
*Teach the client and family or significant others about manic behavior, bipolar disorder, and other problems as indicated.	The client and family or significant others may have little or no knowledge of disease processes or need for continued treatment.
*Teach the client and family or significant others about signs of relapse, such as insomnia, decreased nutrition, and poor personal hygiene.	If the client and his or her family or significant others can recognize signs of impending relapse, the client can seek treatment to avoid relapse.
*Inform the client and family or significant others about chemotherapy: dosage, need to take the medication only as prescribed, the toxic symptoms, the need to monitor blood levels, and other considerations.	Some medications, such as oxcarbazepine (Trileptal), lamotrigine (Lamictal), valproic acid (Depakote), and gabapentin (Neurontin) may be contraindicated in clients with impaired liver, renal, or cardiac functioning. Safe and effective use of medications may require maintenance and monitoring of therapeutic blood levels. When the therapeutic level is exceeded, toxicity can result. See Appendix E: Psychopharmacology for a listing of signs and symptoms that may indicate toxic or near-toxic blood levels.
*Stress to the client and family or significant others that medications must be taken regularly and continually to be effective; medications should not be discontinued just because the client's mood is level.	A relatively constant blood level, within the therapeutic range, is necessary for successful maintenance treatment with lithium and valproic acid.
*Explain information in clear, simple terms. Reinforce teaching with written material as indicated. Ask the client and significant others to state their understanding of the material as you explain. Encourage the client to ask questions and to express feelings and concerns.	The client and significant others may have little or no understanding of medications and toxicity. Asking for the client's perception of the material and encouraging questions will help to eliminate misunderstanding and miscommunication.

SECTION 7 REVIEW QUESTIONS

1. A client says to the nurse, "You are the best nurse I've ever met. I want you to remember me." What is the appropriate response by the nurse?

   a. "Thank you. I think you are special too."

   b. "I suspect you want something from me. What is it?"

   c. "You probably say that to all your nurses."

   d. "Are you thinking of suicide?"

2. A client with mania begins dancing around the dayroom. When she twirls her skirt in front of the male clients, it is obvious she is not wearing underwear. The nurse distracts her, and takes her to her room to put on underpants. The nurse acted as she did to:

   a. Minimize the client's embarrassment about her present behavior.

   b. Keep her from dancing with other clients.

   c. Avoid embarrassing the male clients who were watching.

   d. Teach the client about proper attire and hygiene.

3. The nurse is working with a client who is depressed, trying to engage him in interaction. The client does not respond. Which of the following responses by the nurse would be most appropriate?

   a. "I'll come back a little bit later to talk."

   b. "I'll find someone else for you to talk to."

   c. "I'll get you something to read."

   d. "I'll sit here with you for 10 minutes."

4. A client who is depressed tells the nurse she has lost her job. Which of the following responses by the nurse is best?

   a. "It must be very upsetting for you."

   b. "Tell me about your job."

   c. "You'll find another job when you feel better."

   d. "You're too depressed to be working now."

5. A client with mania is skipping in the hallway, bumping into other clients. Which of the following activities would be best for this client at this time?

   a. Leading a group activity

   b. Reading the newspaper

   c. Walking with the nurse

   d. Watching television

6. When developing a plan of care for a client with suicidal ideation, which of the following would be the priority?

   a. Coping skills

   b. Safety

   c. Self-esteem

   d. Sleep

SECTION 7 Recommended Readings

Bowers, L., Banda, T., & Nijman, H. (2010). Suicide inside: A systematic review of inpatient suicides. *The Journal of Nervous and Mental Disease, 198*(5), 315–328.

Pirruccello, L. M. (2010). Preventing adolescent suicide: A community takes action. *Journal of Psychosocial Nursing and Mental Health Services, 48*(5), 34–41.

Sherrod, T., Quinlan-Cowell, A., Lattimore, T. B., Shattell, M. M., & Kennedy-Malone, L. (2010). Older adults with bipolar disorder. *Journal of Gerontological Nursing, 36*(5), 20–27.

Weber, S., Puskar, K. R., & Ren, D. (2010). Relationships between depressive symptoms and perceived social support, self-esteem & optimism in a sample of rural adolescents. *Issues in Mental Health Nursing, 31*(9), 584–588.

SECTION 7 Resources for Additional Information

Visit thePoint (http://thePoint.lww.com/Schultz9e) for a list of these and other helpful Internet resources.

American Association of Suicidology
American Foundation for Suicide Prevention
Canadian Association for Suicide Prevention
CDC Violence Prevention Program Suicide Prevention
Depression and Bipolar Support Alliance
Johns Hopkins University Department of Psychiatry and Behavioral Sciences, Mood Disorders Program
Madison Institute of Medicine
Mental Health America
NARSAD: The Mental Health Research Association
National Center for Suicide Prevention Training
National Institute of Mental Health
National Mental Health Information Center
National Organization for People of Color Against Suicide
National Strategy for Suicide prevention
National Suicide Prevention Lifeline
Pendulum Resources
Suicide Action Prevention Network USA
Suicide Awareness Voices of Education
Suicide Prevention Resource Center
The Jason Foundation
The Jed Foundation
The Trevor Project

Anxiety Disorders

Anxiety is a common response to the stress of everyday life. Determinations about the existence of mental health or illness often are made based on a person's ability to handle stress and cope with anxiety. The overall goals of nursing care in working with anxiety and related disorders are to reduce the client's anxiety level to the point at which he or she can again become functional in daily life, and to help the client learn to deal with anxiety and stress more effectively in the future. The care plans in this section deal with the broad concept of anxious behavior as well as specific anxiety disorders.

CARE PLAN 28

Anxious Behavior

Anxiety is a feeling of apprehension or dread that develops when the self or self-concept is threatened. It is distinct from fear, which is a response to an identifiable, external threat. It is thought to be essential for human survival. The discomfort people feel when they are anxious provides the impetus for learning and change. Mild anxiety can cause a heightened awareness and sharpening of the senses and can be seen as constructive and even necessary for growth.

Anxiety that becomes severe can be destructive and cause an individual to become dysfunctional. Severe anxiety is believed by some theorists to be central to many psychiatric disorders, such as panic attacks, phobias, and obsessive-compulsive disorder, and is also frequently seen in conjunction with other psychiatric problems, such as depression, eating disorders, and sleep disturbances.

Individuals also may experience *separation anxiety,* in anticipation or at the time of separation from significant people or environments. Separation anxiety is seen as part of normal growth and development in toddlers and at other points in development, such as starting school, leaving home for the first time, and so forth. Separation anxiety becomes problematic when it is extended in length, is generalized to any changes in routine, or interferes with the person's ability to function. It may occur just before a client is discharged from treatment or an inpatient setting, as he or she prepares to return to more independent functioning without the structure and support of the therapeutic environment.

Peplau (1963) defined four levels of anxiety:

Mild. This is normal anxiety that results in enhanced motivation, learning, and problem-solving. Stimuli are readily perceived and processed.
Moderate. The individual's perceptual field is narrowed; he or she hears, sees, and grasps less. The individual may fail to attend to environmental stimuli but will notice things that are brought to his or her attention and can learn with the direction of another person.
Severe. The individual focuses on small or scattered details. The perceptual field is greatly reduced. The individual is unable to problem-solve or use the learning process.
Panic. The individual is disorganized, may be unable to act or speak, may be hyperactive and agitated, and may be dangerous to himself or herself.

Anxiety is observable through behavior and physiologic phenomena (e.g., elevated blood pressure, pulse, and respiratory rate; diaphoresis; flushed face; dry mouth; trembling; frequent urination; and dizziness). The client also may report nausea, diarrhea, insomnia, headaches, muscle tension, blurred vision, and palpitations or chest pain. Physiologic symptoms vary but usually become more intense as the level of anxiety increases.

Anxiety disorders are common in the United States and occur in men, women, and children, with prevalence rates and gender ratios varying according to the disorder. Factors underlying development of problematic anxiety and related disorders may include familial or genetic predisposition, excessive stress, exposure to traumatic events or situations, other psychiatric problems or disorders, biologic factors such as neurochemical alterations, or learned behavior. The onset, course, and duration of specific anxiety disorders vary with the disorder. Anxiety disorders are often chronic or long lasting, with fluctuations in severity over time.

Therapeutic goals in working with clients who exhibit anxious behavior include ensuring the client's safety, building a trust relationship, and fostering self-esteem. Medications, especially anxiolytics and antidepressants, may be used. Educating the client and significant others about anxiety and related disorders is important, because many clients have little or no understanding of these problems and may feel that they "should just be able to overcome" anxiety or related symptoms. The nurse also should collaborate with others on the treatment team to identify resources and make referrals for continued therapy or support.

NURSING DIAGNOSES ADDRESSED IN THIS CARE PLAN
Anxiety
Ineffective Coping
Ineffective Health Maintenance

RELATED NURSING DIAGNOSES ADDRESSED IN THE MANUAL
Risk for Injury
Impaired Social Interaction
Insomnia

Nursing Diagnosis

Anxiety

Vague uneasy feeling of discomfort or dread accompanied by an autonomic response (the source often nonspecific or unknown to the individual); a feeling of apprehension caused by anticipation of danger. It is an alerting signal that warns of impending danger and enables the individual to take measures to deal with threat.

ASSESSMENT DATA

- Decreased attention span
- Restlessness, irritability
- Poor impulse control
- Feelings of discomfort, apprehension, or helplessness
- Hyperactivity, pacing
- Wringing hands or other repetitive hand or limb movements
- Perceptual field deficits
- Decreased ability to communicate verbally

In addition, in panic anxiety:
- Inability to discriminate harmful stimuli or situations
- Disorganized thought processes
- Delusions

EXPECTED OUTCOMES

Immediate

The client will

- Be free from injury throughout hospitalization
- Discuss feelings of dread, anxiety, and so forth within 24 to 48 hours
- Participate in relaxation techniques with staff assistance and demonstrate a decreased anxiety level within 2 to 3 days

Stabilization

The client will

- Demonstrate the ability to perform relaxation techniques
- Reduce own anxiety level without staff assistance

Community

The client will

- Be free from anxiety attacks
- Manage the anxiety response to stress effectively

IMPLEMENTATION

Nursing Interventions *denotes collaborative interventions	Rationale
Remain with the client at all times when levels of anxiety are high (severe or panic).	The client's safety is a priority. A highly anxious client should not be left alone—his or her anxiety will escalate.
Move the client to a quiet area with minimal or decreased stimuli such as a small room or seclusion area.	Anxious behavior can be escalated by external stimuli. In a large area, the client can feel lost and panicked, but a smaller room can enhance a sense of security.
PRN medications may be indicated for high levels of anxiety, delusions, disorganized thoughts, and so forth.	Medication may be necessary to decrease anxiety to a level at which the client can feel safe.
Remain calm in your approach to the client.	The client will feel more secure if you are calm and if the client feels you are in control of the situation.
Use short, simple, and clear statements.	The client's ability to deal with abstractions or complexity is impaired.
Avoid asking or forcing the client to make choices.	The client may not make sound decisions or may be unable to make decisions or solve problems.
Be aware of your own feelings and level of discomfort.	Anxiety is communicated interpersonally. Being with an anxious client can raise your own anxiety level.
*Teach the client and his or her family or significant others about anxiety, treatment methods, ways in which others can be supportive of treatment and ongoing management, and medications, if any.	The client and his or her significant others may lack knowledge about anxiety and treatment; knowing how to support the client's self-management and avoid exacerbating anxiety will help the client after discharge from the treatment setting.
Encourage the client's participation in relaxation exercises such as deep breathing, progressive muscle relaxation, meditation, and imagining being in a quiet, peaceful place.	Relaxation exercises are effective, nonchemical ways to reduce anxiety.
Teach the client to use relaxation techniques independently.	Using relaxation techniques can give the client confidence in having control over anxiety.
Help the client see that mild anxiety can be a positive catalyst for change and does not need to be avoided.	The client may feel that all anxiety is bad and not useful.
*Encourage the client to identify and pursue relationships, personal interests, hobbies, or recreational activities that may appeal to the client. Consultation with a recreational therapist may be indicated.	The client's anxiety may have prevented him or her from engaging in relationships or activities recently, but these can be helpful in building confidence and having a focus on something other than anxiety.
*Encourage the client to identify supportive resources in the community or on the internet.	Supportive resources can assist the client in ongoing management of his or her anxiety and decrease social isolation.

Nursing Diagnosis

Ineffective Coping

Inability to form a valid appraisal of the stressors, inadequate choices of practiced responses, and/or inability to use available resources.

ASSESSMENT DATA

- Client-reported inability to deal with stress
- Overdependence on others
- Avoidance or escape patterns of behavior
- Ineffective expression of feelings
- Lack of coping resources (actual or perceived)
- Lack of confidence

EXPECTED OUTCOMES

Immediate	The client will
	• Verbalize feelings, for example, talk with staff about feelings for at least 15 minutes at least twice per day within 24 to 48 hours • Identify his or her behavioral response to stress, with staff assistance, within 2 to 3 days • Participate in realistic discussion of problems within 2 to 3 days
Stabilization	The client will
	• Demonstrate alternative ways to deal with stress, including problem-solving • Discuss future plans, based on realistic self-assessment
Community	The client will
	• Take action to deal with stress independently, for example, implement relaxation techniques or approach others for therapeutic interaction • Use community support to improve coping skills, for example, participate in a support group

IMPLEMENTATION

Nursing Interventions *denotes collaborative interventions	Rationale
Help the client recognize early signs of his or her anxious behavior.	The sooner the client recognizes the onset of anxiety, the more quickly he or she will be able to alter the response.
Talk with the client about his or her anxious behavior. Make observations to help the client see the relationship between what he or she thinks or feels and corresponding behavioral responses.	The client may be unaware of the relationship between emotional issues and his or her anxious behavior.
During times when the client is relatively calm, explore together ways to deal with stress and anxiety.	The client will be better able to problem-solve when anxiety is lower.
Encourage the client to express feelings and identify possible sources of anxiety. Encourage the client to be as specific as he or she can.	The more specific and concrete the client can be about anxiety-triggering stress, the better prepared he or she will be to deal with those situations.
Teach the client a step-by-step approach to solving problems: identifying problems, exploring alternatives, evaluating consequences of each alternative, and making a decision.	The client may be unaware of a logical process for examining and solving problems. Approaching a problem in an objective way can decrease anxiety and foster a feeling of control.
Encourage the client to evaluate the success of the chosen alternative. Help the client to continue to try alternatives if his or her initial choice is not successful.	The client needs to know that he or she can survive making a mistake and that making mistakes is part of the learning process.
Give the client support for viewing himself or herself and his or her abilities realistically.	Enhancing the client's confidence and abilities to self-evaluate promotes his or her sense of self-reliance.
Encourage the client to practice methods to reduce anxiety prior to approaching problems when possible.	The client will be able to better use problem-solving when anxiety is at lower levels.
Give the client positive feedback as he or she learns to relax, express feelings, problem solve, and so forth.	Positive feedback promotes the continuation of desired behavior.
Assist the client to anticipate future problems that may provoke an anxiety response. Role-playing may help the client to prepare to deal with anticipated difficulties.	Having a plan for managing anticipated difficulties may help reduce the client's anxiety and/or minimize separation anxiety.

Nursing Diagnosis

Ineffective Health Maintenance
Inability to identify, manage, and/or seek out help to maintain health.

ASSESSMENT DATA

- Frequent complaints regarding gastrointestinal distress, lack of appetite
- Sleep pattern disturbances
- Failure to manage stress and anxiety

EXPECTED OUTCOMES

Immediate

The client will

- Demonstrate decreased complaints of gastrointestinal distress within 2 to 3 days
- Obtain restful sleep, for example, sleep for at least 4 hours per night within 2 to 3 days
- Recognize related problems, for example, discuss the relationship between anxious feelings and lack of sleep, within 2 to 3 days

Stabilization

The client will

- Maintain adequate balanced physiologic functioning
- Verbalize intent to seek treatment for related problems, if indicated

Community

The client will

- Participate in follow-up care or support groups as needed
- Meet physiologic needs independently

IMPLEMENTATION

Nursing Interventions *denotes collaborative interventions	Rationale
Help the client channel energy constructively. Encourage activities using gross motor skills (e.g., walking, running, cleaning, exercising).	Physical activities provide an outlet for excess energy. Use of large muscles, followed by relaxation, also can facilitate sleep.
Encourage the client to have a bedtime routine that includes activities that have been successful for the client (e.g., warm milk, reading). See Care Plan 38: Sleep Disorders.	Relaxing, routine activities facilitate sleep and rest.
*Teach the client about healthful nutrition, especially regarding foods that can exacerbate gastrointestinal distress or difficulty sleeping, or that can cause anxiety-like symptoms (e.g., acidic or spicy foods, caffeine); Consultation with a dietitian may be helpful.	The client may be unaware of foods that can exacerbate anxiety-related symptoms. For example, caffeine can contribute to epigastric distress and insomnia, and can cause symptoms such as increased heart rate and feelings of nervousness.
Encourage the client to eat nutritious foods. Provide a quiet atmosphere at meal times. Avoid discussing emotional issues before, during, and immediately after meals.	Relaxation around meal times promotes digestion and avoids gastrointestinal distress. The client may have used eating (or not eating) as a way to deal with anxiety.
*Teach the client and his or her significant others to avoid discussing emotional topics at mealtimes.	The client's significant others may be unaware of the benefit of separating food from anxiety-provoking issues.
Encourage the client to develop a routine of daily physical activity after discharge.	Ongoing physical activity can be an effective tool in managing anxiety as well as increasing general health.
*Encourage continued treatment for any related problems (e.g., eating disorders, post-traumatic stress, abuse) or refer the client to support groups.	Anxiety and post-traumatic disorders often require long-term treatment and support.

CARE PLAN 29

Phobias

A *phobia* is an irrational, persistent fear of an event, situation, activity, or object. The client recognizes this fear as irrational but is unable to prevent it. Often, a client can avoid the source of the phobic response and does not seek treatment. When the phobic behavior is in response to something that is unavoidable or the avoidance behavior interferes with the client's daily life, the client usually seeks treatment.

Several types of phobias have been described, including the following:

Agoraphobia is a fear of being in places or situations in which the individual feels that he or she may be unable to escape or obtain help if needed. In severe cases, people may stay in their houses for months or even years, having food and other necessities delivered to them.

Social phobia is a person's fear that he or she will be publicly embarrassed by his or her own behavior. This may result in the individual's inability to eat in the company of others, engage in social conversation, and so forth.

Specific phobia is fear of a specific stimulus that is easily identifiable, for example, a fear of heights, animals, or water. With specific phobias, treatment may not be seen as necessary if it is easier to avoid the stimulus. Treatment is sought only if the phobia interferes with daily life or the person experiences a great deal of distress.

When phobic people are confronted with the object of the phobia, they experience intense anxiety and may have a *panic attack.* A *panic attack* is a "discrete period of intense fear or discomfort in the absence of real danger" and includes somatic or cognitive symptoms such as perspiring, shaking, feelings of choking, smothering, or lightheadedness, and "fear of losing control or 'going crazy'" (APA, 2000, p. 430). When the individual contemplates confronting the phobic situation, marked *anticipatory anxiety* also may occur and lead to avoidance of the situation.

Phobias are diagnosed more commonly in women than in men. In the United States, approximately 5% to 10% of the population suffers from specific or social phobia. The lifetime prevalence for specific phobia is 11%; estimates of prevalence for social phobia range from 3% to 13% (Sadock & Sadock, 2008). Phobias develop most commonly in childhood, adolescence, or early adulthood (APA, 2000). The onset may be acute (especially with panic attacks) or gradual, with levels of anxiety increasing to the point that the individual becomes sufficiently impaired or distressed to seek treatment. A phobia may be precipitated by a traumatic event or experience, especially with social phobias. The course of phobias is often chronic with variable severity of symptoms, although some people do experience remission as adults.

Typically, phobic behavior is treated with behavioral therapy, including *systematic desensitization,* which is most effective with clients who have specific phobias. Clients with agoraphobia who have panic attacks and severe functional impairment may need more complex and long-term treatment. Medications also may be used, especially with clients who have panic attacks.

NURSING DIAGNOSIS ADDRESSED IN THIS CARE PLAN
Fear

RELATED NURSING DIAGNOSES ADDRESSED IN THE MANUAL
Ineffective Coping
Ineffective Role Performance
Impaired Social Interaction
Anxiety

Nursing Diagnosis

Fear

Response to perceived threat that is consciously recognized as a danger.

ASSESSMENT DATA

- Anticipatory anxiety (when thinking about the phobic object)
- Panic anxiety (when confronted with the phobic object)
- Avoidance behaviors that interfere with relationships or functioning
- Recognition of the phobia as irrational
- Embarrassment over the phobic fear
- Sufficient discomfort to seek treatment

EXPECTED OUTCOMES

Immediate   The client will

- Verbalize feelings of fear and discomfort within 24 to 48 hours
- Perform relaxation techniques with staff assistance and respond with decreased anxiety within 2 to 3 days

Stabilization   The client will

- Effectively decrease own anxiety level, for example, using relaxation techniques without staff assistance
- Demonstrate decreased avoidance behaviors

Community   The client will

- Demonstrate effective functioning in social and occupational roles
- Manage the anxiety response effectively, for example, using relaxation techniques or initiating therapeutic interaction

IMPLEMENTATION

Nursing Interventions *denotes collaborative interventions	Rationale
Encourage the client to express feelings. Initially, it may be beneficial to focus only on the client's feelings without discussing the phobic situation specifically.	The client often experiences additional anxiety because he or she has been unable to handle the situation alone, especially because the client knows that the phobia is irrational.
*Teach the client and family or significant others about phobic reactions and dispel myths that may be troubling the client, such as that all he or she has to do is face up to [the phobic situation] and he or she will get over it.	The client and family or significant others may have little or no knowledge related to phobias or anxiety. Myths can be a barrier to successful treatment. Support from the client's significant others can enhance successful and lasting treatment.
Reassure the client that he or she can learn to decrease the anxiety and gain control over the anxiety attacks.	The client can feel greater self-confidence, which will enhance chances for success.
Reassure the client that he or she will not be forced to confront the phobic situation until prepared to do so.	The client can feel more comfortable knowing he or she will not be asked to confront a situation that produces extreme anxiety until equipped to handle it.
Assist the client to distinguish between the actual phobic trigger and problems related to avoidance behaviors.	The client may experience such pervasive anxiety that he or she is unclear about the specific phobic situation, which often has existed for some time before the client seeks treatment.
Instruct the client in progressive relaxation techniques, including deep breathing, progressive muscle relaxation, and imagining himself or herself in a quiet, peaceful place.	The client must have the ability to decrease anxiety to participate in treatment.

IMPLEMENTATION (continued)

Nursing Interventions *denotes collaborative interventions	Rationale
Encourage the client to practice relaxation until he or she is successful.	The client must feel well prepared with the techniques to be able to use them when anxiety does occur.
Explain systematic desensitization thoroughly to the client (see below).	Unknown situations can produce added anxiety.
Reassure the client that you will allow him or her as much time as needed at each step.	This will increase the client's sense of control and help lessen anxiety.
Have the client develop a hierarchy of situations that relate to the phobia by ranking from the least anxiety-producing to the most anxiety-producing situation. (For example, a client with a phobia of dogs might rank situations beginning with looking at a picture of a dog, up to actually petting a dog.)	Creating a hierarchy is the beginning step of systematic desensitization.
Beginning with the least anxiety-producing situation, have the client use progressive relaxation until he or she is able to decrease the anxiety. When the client is comfortable with that situation, go to the next item on the list, and repeat the procedure.	The client will be most successful initially in the least anxiety-producing situation. The client will be unable to progress to more difficult situations until he or she can master the current one.
If the client becomes excessively anxious or begins to feel out of control, return to the former step with which the client was successful; then proceed slowly to subsequent steps.	Staying too long with a step with which the client feels out of control will undermine his or her confidence. It is important for the client to feel confident in his or her ability to manage the anxiety.
Give positive feedback for the client's efforts at each step. Convey the idea that he or she is succeeding at each step. Avoid equating success only with mastery of the entire process.	This increases the number of times the client can experience success and gain self-confidence, which enhances the overall chance for mastery of the anxiety.
As the client progresses in systematic desensitization, ask the client if his or her avoidance behaviors are decreasing.	Avoidance behaviors should decrease as the client successfully copes with the phobia and resulting anxiety.
It may be necessary to address specific avoidance behavior(s) if any persist after the client has completed the desensitizing process.	Avoidance behaviors that interfere with daily life will require further work if they persist after the client masters the phobic situation. The client also may be experiencing difficulties that were not related to the phobic situation.
*Teach the client and significant others about continuing therapy and medications if appropriate.	The client's significant others can assist the client in managing his or her phobia outside the treatment setting.
*Help the client identify supportive resources in the community or on the internet.	Taking advantage of supportive resources can help the client progress with self management after discharge.

CARE PLAN 30

Obsessive-Compulsive Disorder

Obsessive thoughts are persistent, intrusive thoughts that are troublesome to the client, producing significant anxiety. *Compulsions* are ritualistic behaviors, usually repetitive in nature, such as excessive hand-washing or checking and rechecking behavior. *Obsessive-compulsive disorder* (OCD) is characterized by the presence of obsessions or compulsions that cause the client significant distress or impairment, and the adult client recognizes (at some time) as excessive and as produced by his or her own mind (APA, 2000).

Compulsive behavior is thought to be a defense that is perceived by the client as necessary to protect himself or herself from anxiety or impulses that are unacceptable (Sadock & Sadock, 2008). Specific obsessive thoughts and compulsive behaviors may be representative of the client's anxieties. Many obsessive thoughts are religious or sexual in nature and may be destructive or delusional. For example, the client may be obsessed with the thought of killing his or her significant other or may be convinced that he or she has a terminal illness. The client also may place unrealistic standards on himself or herself or others. Many people have some obsessive thoughts or compulsive behaviors but do not seek treatment unless the thoughts or behaviors impede their ability to function (Black & Andreasen, 2011).

Obsessive-compulsive disorder is equally common in adult men and women, though more boys than girls have onset in childhood; there is also some evidence of a familial pattern. In the United States, lifetime prevalence of OCD is fairly consistent at 2% to 3% (Sadock & Sadock, 2008). OCD can occur with other psychiatric problems, including depression, phobias, eating disorders, personality disorders, and overuse of alcohol or anxiolytic medications (APA, 2000). The onset of OCD is usually gradual, and the disorder is usually chronic, though the severity of symptoms fluctuates over time.

In early treatment, nursing care should be aimed primarily at safety concerns and reducing anxiety. Initial nursing care should allow the client to be undisturbed in performing compulsive acts or rituals (unless they are harmful), as drawing undue attention to or attempting to forbid compulsive behaviors increases the client's anxiety.

NURSING DIAGNOSES ADDRESSED IN THIS CARE PLAN
Anxiety
Ineffective Coping

RELATED NURSING DIAGNOSES ADDRESSED IN THE MANUAL
Ineffective Health Maintenance
Risk for Injury
Disturbed Thought Processes
Impaired Social Interaction

Nursing Diagnosis

Anxiety
Vague uneasy feeling of discomfort or dread accompanied by an autonomic response (the source often nonspecific or unknown to the individual); a feeling of apprehension caused by anticipation of danger. It is an alerting signal that warns of impending danger and enables the individual to take measures to deal with threat.

ASSESSMENT DATA

- Obsessive thoughts
- Compulsive, ritualistic behavior
- Self-mutilation or other physical problems (such as damage to skin from excessive washing)
- Overemphasis on cleanliness and neatness
- Fears
- Guilt feelings
- Denial of feelings

EXPECTED OUTCOMES

Immediate

The client will

- Be free from self-inflicted harm throughout hospitalization
- Demonstrate decreased anxiety, fears, guilt, rumination, or aggressive behavior within 2 to 3 days

Stabilization

The client will

- Verbalize feelings of fear, guilt, anxiety, and so forth, for example, talk with staff about feelings for 30 minutes twice a day by a specified date
- Express feelings nonverbally in a safe manner, for example, writing in a journal

Community

The client will

- Manage his or her anxiety response independently

IMPLEMENTATION

Nursing Interventions *denotes collaborative interventions	Rationale
The client may need to be secluded or restrained if he or she attempts self-mutilation or harm.	The client's physical safety, health, and well-being are priorities.
Try to substitute a physically safe behavior for harmful practices, even if the new behavior is compulsive or ritualistic. For example, if the client is cutting himself or herself, direct him or her toward tearing paper.	Substitute behaviors may satisfy the client's need for compulsive behaviors but protect the client's safety and provide a transition toward decreasing these behaviors.
If the client's behaviors are not harmful, try not to call attention to the compulsive acts initially.	Preventing or calling attention to compulsive acts may increase the client's anxiety.
At first, allow the client specific time periods, such as 10 minutes every hour, to focus on obsessive thoughts or ritualistic behaviors. Require the client to attend to other feelings or activities for the rest of the hour. Gradually decrease the time allowed (e.g., from 10 minutes per hour to 10 minutes every 2 hours).	Setting time limits recognizes the significance of these thoughts and acts in the client's life but still encourages a focus on other feelings or problems.
Encourage the client to verbally identify his or her concerns, life stresses, fears, and so forth.	Expressing feelings may help diminish the client's anxiety and thus diminish obsessive thoughts and compulsive acts.
Encourage the client to express his or her feelings in ways that are acceptable to the client (through talking, crying, physical activities, and so forth). Give the client positive feedback for expressing feelings in these ways.	The client may be uncomfortable with some ways of expressing emotions or find them unacceptable initially. Feelings are not inherently bad or good. Positive feedback conveys acceptance of the client as a person and recognizes the client's efforts.
Encourage the client to practice anxiety management techniques in the hospital.	If the client tries to build skills in the treatment setting, he or she can experience success and receive positive feedback for his or her efforts.

(continued on page 210)

IMPLEMENTATION (continued)

Nursing Interventions *denotes collaborative interventions	Rationale
If the client is ruminating (e.g., on his or her worthlessness), acknowledge the client's feelings, but then try to redirect the interaction. Discuss the client's perceptions of his or her feelings and possible ways to deal with these feelings. If the client continues to ruminate, withdraw your attention and state when you will return or will be available for interaction again.	Withdrawing attention may help decrease rumination by not reinforcing that behavior. Redirecting the client to focus directly on emotions may help diminish anxiety and rumination.
Do not argue with the client about the logic of delusional fears. Acknowledge the client's feelings, interject reality briefly (e.g., "Your tests show that you are not pregnant."), and move on to discuss a concrete subject. (See Care Plan 23: Delusional Disorder.)	Delusions are intense (though false) beliefs; clients often can give seemingly logical support for them. Arguing can reinforce delusional beliefs and may be futile. Providing a concrete subject for interactions can reinforce reality for the client.
Talk with the client about coping strategies he or she has used in the past that did not include compulsive behaviors.	The client may have had success using noncompulsive coping strategies in the past and may be able to re-establish and build on these to mitigate or replace compulsive behaviors.
*Teach the client and his or her family or significant others about coping strategies and anxiety management skills, such as increasing physical exercise, expressing feelings verbally or in a journal, or meditation techniques.	The client and his or her significant others may be unaware of specific techniques or may not have used positive techniques in the past.
*Help the client identify supportive resources in the community or on the internet.	Management of OCD may require long-term therapy and support.

Nursing Diagnosis

Ineffective Coping

Inability to form a valid appraisal of the stressors, inadequate choices of practiced responses, and/or inability to use available resources.

ASSESSMENT DATA

- Ambivalence regarding decisions or choices
- Disturbances in normal functioning due to obsessive thoughts or compulsive behaviors (loss of job, loss of or alienation of family members, and so forth)
- Inability to tolerate deviations from standards
- Rumination
- Low self-esteem
- Feelings of worthlessness
- Lack of insight
- Difficulty or slowness completing daily living activities because of ritualistic behavior

EXPECTED OUTCOMES

Immediate   The client will

- Talk with staff and identify stresses, anxieties, and conflicts within 2 to 3 days
- Verbalize realistic self-evaluation, for example, make a list of strengths and abilities, review list with staff within 3 to 4 days
- Establish adequate nutrition, hydration, and elimination within 4 to 5 days
- Establish a balance of rest, sleep, and activity, for example, sleep at least 4 hours per night within 4 to 5 days

Stabilization	The client will

- Identify alternative methods of dealing with stress and anxiety
- Complete daily routine activities without staff assistance or prompting by a specified date
- Verbalize knowledge of illness, treatment plan, and safe use of medications, if any

Community	The client will

- Demonstrate a decrease in obsessive thoughts or ritualistic behaviors to a level at which the client can function independently
- Demonstrate alternative ways of dealing with stress, anxiety, and life situations
- Maintain adequate physiologic functioning, including activity, sleep, nutrition
- Follow through with continued therapy if needed, for example, identify a therapist, make a follow-up appointment before discharge

IMPLEMENTATION

Nursing Interventions *denotes collaborative interventions	Rationale
Observe the client's eating, drinking, and elimination patterns, and assist the client as necessary.	The client may be unaware of physical needs or may ignore feelings of hunger, thirst, the urge to defecate, and so forth.
Assess and monitor the client's sleep patterns, and prepare him or her for bedtime by decreasing stimuli and providing comfort measures or medications. (See Care Plan 38: Sleep Disorders.)	Limiting noise and other stimuli will encourage rest and sleep. Comfort measures and sleep medications will enhance the client's ability to relax and sleep.
You may need to allow extra time, or the client may need to be verbally directed to accomplish activities of daily living (personal hygiene, preparation for sleep, and so forth).	The client's thoughts or ritualistic behaviors may interfere with or lengthen the time necessary to perform tasks.
Encourage the client to try to gradually decrease the frequency of compulsive behaviors. Work with the client to identify a baseline frequency and keep a record of the decrease.	Gradually reducing the frequency of compulsive behaviors will help diminish the client's anxiety and encourage success.
As the client's anxiety decreases and as a trust relationship builds, talk with the client about his or her thoughts and behavior and the client's feelings about them. Help the client identify alternative methods for dealing with anxiety.	The client may need to learn ways to manage anxiety so he or she can deal with it directly. This will increase the client's confidence in managing anxiety and other feelings.
Convey honest interest in and concern for the client. (Do not flatter the client or be otherwise dishonest.)	Your presence and interest in the client convey your acceptance of the client. Clients do not benefit from flattery or undue praise, but genuine praise that the client has earned can foster self-esteem.
Provide opportunities for the client to participate in activities that are easily accomplished or enjoyed by the client; support the client for participation.	The client may be limited in the ability to deal with complex activities or in relating to others. Activities that the client can accomplish and enjoy can enhance self-esteem.
Teach the client social skills, such as appropriate conversation topics and active listening. Encourage him or her to practice these skills with staff members and other clients, and give the client feedback regarding interactions.	The client may feel embarrassed by his or her OCD behaviors and may have had limited social contact. He or she may have limited social skills and confidence, which may contribute to the client's anxiety.
*Teach the client and family or significant others about the client's illness, treatment, or medications, if any.	The client and family or significant others may have little or no knowledge about these.
*Encourage the client to participate in follow-up therapy, if indicated. Help the client identify supportive resources in the community or on the internet.	Clients often experience long-term difficulties in dealing with obsessive thoughts.

CARE PLAN 31

Post-Traumatic Stress Disorder

Post-traumatic behavior occurs following the experience of an unusually traumatic event or situation that would be expected to produce significant distress in most people. The traumatic event may be due to natural causes or to human activity; distress related to human activity seems to be more severe than that following a natural event. *Post-traumatic stress disorder* (PTSD) is characterized by symptoms that occur after exposure to the traumatic event and last for at least 1 month. The symptoms include re-experiencing the event; avoiding stimuli associated with the event; decreased general responsiveness, such as feeling detached from others or being disinterested in activities; and increased arousal, such as hypervigilance and sleep difficulties (APA, 2000).

In the United States, the lifetime prevalence of PTSD is estimated between 9% and 15% (Sadock & Sadock, 2008), but the disorder is more prevalent among high risk groups such as rape, assault, terrorist attacks, combat, or genocide. Symptoms of PTSD can occur within 3 months of the traumatic event or may be delayed up to several years. Symptoms may resolve within 3 months or may persist for over a year, and may reappear with exposure to stimuli that recall the event (APA, 2000).

Experiences that evoke post-traumatic behavior include terrorist attacks, violent crimes, combat experiences, abuse, natural disasters, and major accidents. Post-traumatic behavior also is described in terms of specific traumas such as *rape trauma syndrome* following a rape, which has three stages: *acute, outward adjustment,* and *reorganization* (during which denial, fear, anger, guilt, and depression may occur). Post-traumatic behavior also is part of the *survivor theory,* which is based on the behaviors of survivors of the Hiroshima and Nagasaki bombings and of concentration camps. Post-traumatic behavior resembles a grief reaction and often can be described as delayed grief or a failure to grieve. As in grief, there may be a period of shock or denial immediately following the trauma.

Facilitation of the grief process is a major focus in working with clients who exhibit post-traumatic behavior. Other nursing goals include ensuring safety for the client and others, promoting the client's self-esteem, and helping the client develop skills in communicating his or her feelings to others.

It is important for the nurse to be aware of religious and cultural factors in working with these clients, as these factors may heavily influence the client's feelings regarding the trauma, especially guilt and shame. Anger often is a dominant symptom in post-traumatic behavior; it may occur overtly as violent or abusive behavior or covertly, internalized and manifested as depression. Recovery from trauma can require long-term therapy and support; assisting the client to identify and implement a realistic plan for continued help is a key part of acute intervention. Providing education to the client, family or significant others, and the community is also important, to dispel myths about the nature of such experiences as rape, incest, and combat, and about the responses and grief that follow them.

NURSING DIAGNOSES ADDRESSED IN THIS CARE PLAN
Post-Trauma Syndrome
Risk for Other-Directed Violence

RELATED NURSING DIAGNOSES ADDRESSED IN THE MANUAL
Complicated Grieving
Anxiety
Ineffective Coping
Insomnia
Ineffective Health Maintenance
Social Isolation
Situational Low Self-Esteem
Ineffective Role Performance
Risk for Suicide

Nursing Diagnosis

Post-Trauma Syndrome
Sustained maladaptive response to a traumatic, overwhelming event.

ASSESSMENT DATA

- Flashbacks or re-experiencing the traumatic event(s)
- Nightmares or recurrent dreams of the event or other trauma
- Sleep disturbances (e.g., insomnia, early awakening, crying out in sleep)
- Depression
- Denial of feelings or emotional numbness
- Projection of feelings
- Difficulty in expressing feelings
- Anger (may not be overt)
- Guilt or remorse
- Low self-esteem
- Frustration and irritability
- Anxiety, panic, or separation anxiety
- Fears—may be displaced or generalized (as in fear of men in rape victims)
- Decreased concentration
- Difficulty expressing love or empathy
- Difficulty experiencing pleasure
- Difficulty with interpersonal relationships, marital problems, divorce
- Abuse in relationships
- Sexual problems
- Substance use
- Employment problems
- Physical symptoms

EXPECTED OUTCOMES

Immediate

The client will

- Identify the traumatic event within 24 to 48 hours
- Demonstrate decreased physical symptoms within 2 to 3 days
- Verbalize need to grieve loss(es) within 3 to 4 days
- Establish a balance of rest, sleep, and activity, for example, sleep at least 4 hours per night within 3 to 4 days
- Demonstrate decreased anxiety, fear, guilt, and so forth, within 4 to 5 days
- Participate in treatment program, for example, join in a group activity or talk with staff for at least 30 minutes twice a day within 4 to 5 days

Stabilization	The client will

- Begin the grieving process, for example, talk with staff about grief-related feelings and acknowledge the loss or event
- Express feelings directly and openly in nondestructive ways
- Identify strengths and weaknesses realistically, for example, make a list of abilities and review with staff
- Demonstrate an increased ability to cope with stress
- Eliminate substance use
- Verbalize knowledge of illness, treatment plan, or safe use of medications, if any

Community	The client will

- Demonstrate initial integration of the traumatic experience into his or her life outside the hospital
- Identify support system outside the treatment setting, for example, identify specific support groups, friends, family, establish contact
- Implement plans for follow-up or ongoing therapy, if indicated, for example, identify a therapist and schedule an appointment before discharge

IMPLEMENTATION

Nursing Interventions *denotes collaborative interventions	Rationale
When you approach the client, be nonthreatening and professional.	The client's fears may be triggered by authority figures or other characteristics (e.g., gender, ethnicity).
Initially, assign the same staff members to the client if possible; try to respect the client's fears or feelings related to gender or other characteristics. Gradually increase the number and variety of staff members interacting with the client.	Limiting the number of staff members who interact with the client at first will facilitate familiarity and trust. The client may have strong feelings of fear or mistrust about working with staff members with certain characteristics. These feelings may have been reinforced in previous encounters with professionals and may interfere with the therapeutic relationship.
*Educate yourself and other staff members about the client's experience and about post-traumatic behavior.	Learning about the client's experience will help prepare you for the client's feelings and the details of his or her experience.
Examine and remain aware of your own feelings regarding both the client's traumatic experience and his or her feelings and behavior. Talk with other staff members to ventilate and work through your feelings.	Traumatic events engender strong feelings in others and may be quite threatening. You may be reminded of a related experience or of your own vulnerability, or issues related to sexuality, morality, safety, or well-being. It is essential that you remain aware of your feelings so that you do not unconsciously project feelings, avoid issues, or be otherwise nontherapeutic with the client.
Remain nonjudgmental in your interactions with the client.	It is important not to reinforce blame that the client may have internalized related to the experience.
Be consistent with the client; convey acceptance of him or her as a person while setting and maintaining limits regarding behaviors.	The client may test limits or the therapeutic relationship. Problems with acceptance, trust, or authority often occur with post-traumatic behavior.
*Assess the client's history of substance use (information from significant others might be helpful).	Clients often use substances to help repress (or release) emotions.
Be aware of the client's use or abuse of substances. Set limits and consequences for this behavior; it may be helpful to allow the client or group to have input into these decisions.	Substance use undermines therapy and may endanger the client's health. Allowing input from the client or group may minimize power struggles.
*If substance use is a major problem, refer the client to a substance dependence treatment program.	Substance use can inhibit the client's therapeutic progress and adversely affects other areas of the client's life.

IMPLEMENTATION (continued)

Nursing Interventions *denotes collaborative interventions	Rationale
Encourage the client to talk about his or her experience(s); be accepting and nonjudgmental of the client's accounts and perceptions.	Retelling the experience can help the client to identify the reality of what has happened and help to identify and work through related feelings.
Encourage the client to express his or her feelings through talking, writing, crying, or other ways in which the client is comfortable.	Identification and expression of feelings are central to the grieving process.
Especially encourage the expression of anger, guilt, and rage.	These feelings often occur in clients who have experienced trauma. The client may feel survivor's guilt that he or she survived when others did not or guilt about the behavior he or she undertook to survive (killing others in combat, enduring a rape, not saving others).
Give the client positive feedback for expressing feelings and sharing experiences. Remain nonjudgmental toward the client.	The client may feel that he or she is burdening others with his or her problems. It is important not to reinforce the client's internalized blame.
*Teach the client and the family or significant others about post-traumatic behavior and treatment.	Knowledge about post-traumatic behavior may help alleviate anxiety or guilt and may increase hope for recovery.
Help the client learn and practice stress management and relaxation techniques, assertiveness or self-defense training, or other skills as appropriate.	The client's traumatic experience may have resulted in a loss or decrease in self-confidence, sense of safety, or ability to deal with stress.
*As tolerated, encourage the client to share his or her feelings and experiences in group therapy, in a support group related to post-trauma, or with other clients informally.	The client needs to know that his or her feelings are acceptable to others and can be shared. Peer or support groups can offer understanding, support, and the opportunity for sharing experiences.
*If the client has a religious or spiritual orientation, referral to a member of the clergy or a chaplain may be appropriate.	Guilt and forgiveness often are religious or spiritual issues for the client.
Encourage the client to make realistic plans for the future, integrating his or her traumatic experience.	Integrating traumatic experiences and making future plans are important resolution steps in the grief process.
*Talk with the client about employment, job-related stress, and so forth. Refer the client to vocational services as needed.	Problems with employment frequently occur in clients with post-traumatic behavior.
*Help the client arrange for follow-up therapy as needed.	Recovering from trauma may be a long-term process. Follow-up therapy can offer continuing support in the client's recovery.
Encourage the client to identify relationships, social, or recreational situations that have been positive in the past.	The client may have withdrawn from social relationships and other activities following the trauma; social isolation and lack of interest in recreational activities are common problems following trauma.
*Encourage the client to pursue past relationships, personal interests, hobbies, or recreational activities that were positive in the past or that may appeal to the client. Consultation with a recreational therapist may be indicated.	The client may be reluctant to reach out to someone with whom he or she has had limited contact recently and may benefit from encouragement or facilitation. Recreational activities can serve as a structure for the client to build social interactions as well as provide enjoyment.
*Encourage the client to identify and contact supportive resources in the community or on the internet.	Many community or internet resources can be helpful to clients with PTSD and to their families and significant others.

Nursing Diagnosis

Risk for Other-Directed Violence

At risk for behaviors in which an individual demonstrates that he or she can be physically, emotionally, and/or sexually harmful to others.

RISK FACTORS

- Anger or rage (may be persistent, generalized, or sporadic; may not be overt)
- Hyperalertness, feelings of being endangered (may keep weapons)
- Paranoid behavior, suspiciousness, mistrust of others
- Abuse in relationships, especially with significant others (spouse or partner, or children)
- Hostility
- Verbal abuse
- Aggressive behavior
- Suicidal ideation or behavior
- Homicidal ideation
- Legal problems, criminal activity
- Difficulty with authority figures
- Substance use
- Lack of impulse control
- Thrill-seeking behavior

EXPECTED OUTCOMES

Immediate   The client will

- Be safe and free from injury throughout hospitalization
- Refrain from harming others throughout hospitalization
- Refrain from hostile, abusive, or violent behavior within 24 to 48 hours

Stabilization   The client will

- Verbalize recognition of risky or potentially dangerous behavior, for example, approach staff when feeling tense or angry, before feelings escalate to violent behavior
- Express feelings in a safe manner

Community   The client will

- Remain free of hostile, abusive, or violent behavior
- Participate in treatment for substance abuse, interpersonal, or relationship issues as indicated

IMPLEMENTATION

Nursing Interventions *denotes collaborative interventions	Rationale
Provide a safe environment for the client. Remove items that can be used to harm himself or herself or others. Ask the client if he or she has a weapon; it may be necessary to search the client or his or her belongings (with the client present).	The client's safety and the safety of others are priorities. The client may be mistrustful of others or feel so threatened that he or she keeps concealed weapons.
See Care Plan 26: Suicidal Behavior.	
Assure the client that staff members will provide control if he or she is not able to use internal controls effectively. Encourage the client to talk about feelings when he or she is not agitated.	The client may feel overwhelmed by the intensity of his or her feelings and may fear loss of control if he or she releases those feelings.

IMPLEMENTATION (continued)

Nursing Interventions *denotes collaborative interventions	Rationale
Be consistent and firm in setting and maintaining limits, enforcing policies, and so forth. Do not take the client's hostility personally. Protect other clients from abusive behaviors.	Clients who exhibit post-traumatic behavior may displace or act out anger in destructive ways.
Encourage the client to engage in physical exercise or to substitute safe physical activities for aggressive behaviors (e.g., punching bag, lifting weights).	Physical activity can help release aggression in a nondestructive manner and serve as a step in learning to express feelings verbally.
See Care Plan 47: Aggressive Behavior.	
*Talk with the client and the family or significant others about abusive behavior.	Abusive behavior occurs frequently in the relationships of clients with post-traumatic stress. The client may be too angry, overwhelmed, or ashamed to deal with these issues initially, but the client's significant others need attention immediately.
*Refer the client's family or significant others to a therapist, treatment center, or appropriate support groups. It may be necessary for the client's significant others to participate without the client initially.	Abuse in interpersonal relationships often requires long-term treatment. The client's significant others can begin therapy even if the client is not ready or able to participate immediately.
See Care Plan 49: Sexual, Emotional, or Physical Abuse.	

SECTION 8 REVIEW QUESTIONS

1. When assessing a client with anxiety, the nurse's questions should be:

   a. Avoided until the anxiety is gone

   b. Open-ended

   c. Postponed until the client volunteers information

   d. Specific and direct

2. The best outcome for a client learning a relaxation technique is that the client will:

   a. Confront the source of anxiety directly

   b. Experience anxiety without feeling overwhelmed

   c. Report no episodes of anxiety

   d. Suppress anxious feelings

3. The client with a phobia about eating in public places has just finished eating lunch in the dining area in the nurse's presence. Which of the following statements by the nurse would reinforce the client's positive action?

   a. "At dinner, I hope to see you eat with a group of peers."

   b. "It's a sign of progress to eat in the dining area."

   c. "Nothing happened to you while eating in the dining room."

   d. "That wasn't so hard, now was it?"

4. A newly admitted client with obsessive-compulsive disorder (OCD) has a ritual of making his bed 10 times before breakfast. This ritual caused him to miss breakfast yesterday. Which of the following interventions would the nurse use to help the client be on time for breakfast today?

   a. Advise the client to eat breakfast before he makes his bed.

   b. Stop the client's bed-making when it is time for breakfast.

   c. Tell the client to make his bed only once.

   d. Wake the client 1 hour earlier to perform the bed-making ritual.

SECTION 8 Recommended Readings

Berninger, A., Webber, M. P., Niles, J. K., Gustave, J., Lee, R., Cohen, H. W., … Prezant, D. J. (2010). Longitudinal study of probable post-traumatic stress disorder in firefighters exposed to the World Trade Center disaster. *American Journal of Industrial Medicine, 53*(12), 1177–1185.

Calleo, J. S., Bjorgvinsson, T., & Stanley, M. A. (2010). Obsessions and worry beliefs in an inpatient OCD population. *Journal of Anxiety Disorders, 24*(8), 903–908.

Pagura, J., Stein, M. B., Bolton, J. M., Cox, B. J., Grant, B., & Sareen, J. (2010). Comorbidity of borderline personality disorder and post-traumatic stress disorder in the U.S. population. *Journal of Psychiatric Research, 44*(16), 1190–1198.

Penas-Liedo, E., Jimenez-Murcia, S., Granero, R., Penelo, E., Aguera, Z., Alvarez-Moya, E., & Fernandez-Aranda, F. (2010). Specific eating disorder clusters based on social anxiety and novelty seeking. *Journal of Anxiety Disorders, 24*(7), 767–773.

Van Amerigen, M., Mancini, C., Simpson, W., & Patterson, B. (2010). Potential use of internet-based screening for anxiety disorders: A pilot study. *Depression and Anxiety, 27*(11), 1006–1010.

SECTION 8 Resources for Additional Information

Visit thePoint (http://thePoint.lww.com/Schultz9e) for a list of these and other helpful Internet resources.

American Academy of Experts in Traumatic Stress
American Professional Society on the Abuse of Children
American Psychiatric Association Healthy Minds
Anxiety Disorders Association of America
International OCD Foundation
International Society for Traumatic Stress Studies
Madison Institute of Medicine Obsessive-Compulsive Information Center
MedlinePlus
National Center for PTSD
National Center for Trauma-Informed Care
National Institute of Mental Health
National Mental Health Association
PILOTS (Published International Literature on Traumatic Stress) Database, National Center for PTSD
Sidran Institute

Somatoform and Dissociative Disorders

Some clients have difficulty expressing emotions and dealing with interpersonal conflict in a direct manner and may manifest various physical symptoms that are related to emotional or psychiatric problems. Although these symptoms do not have a demonstrable organic cause, they are nevertheless real to the client and should not be minimized or dismissed. Three care plans in this section address clients who manifest physical symptoms as a result of emotional difficulties: somatization disorder, conversion disorder, and hypochondriasis. The fourth care plan concerns dissociative disorders through which the client becomes detached from traumatic experiences (dissociation) when emotional trauma such as abuse is too painful to manage directly.

Somatization Disorder

Somatization disorder is characterized by a pattern of recurring, multiple physical complaints that results in seeking treatment or significant impairment in social, occupational, or other important areas of functioning (APA, 2000). The somatic complaints cannot be fully explained by any known medical condition, or if a medical condition exists, the reported symptoms or impairment are in excess of what would be expected from diagnostic tests, history, or physical assessment.

In somatization disorder, symptoms are present in the following areas (APA, 2000):

Pain: a history of pain in at least four different sites, such as head, back, extremities, chest, or rectum, or pain during intercourse or urination.

Gastrointestinal: a history of at least two symptoms other than pain, such as nausea, vomiting, diarrhea, or intolerance of several different foods.

Sexual: a history of one sexual or reproductive symptom other than pain, such as sexual indifference, erectile dysfunction, or irregular or excessive menstrual bleeding.

Pseudoneurologic: a history of at least one symptom or deficit suggesting a neurologic condition, not limited to pain; "conversion symptoms, such as impaired coordination or balance, paralysis or localized weakness … blindness, deafness, or seizures; dissociative symptoms such as amnesia; or loss of consciousness other than fainting" (APA, 2000, p. 486).

An important point is that these symptoms are not intentionally produced or feigned but are very real to the client and cause genuine distress. Clients with somatization disorder usually describe their complaints in exaggerated terms that lack specific information, tend to be poor historians, and seek treatment from a variety of providers, which sometimes results in potentially hazardous combinations of treatments.

Psychosocial theorists believe that clients with somatization disorder internalize feelings of anxiety or frustration and do not express these feelings directly. Instead, these feelings are expressed through physical symptoms when the client is in situations that are stressful or involve conflict with others. The physical symptoms provide relief from the stress or conflict (primary gain) and help the client meet psychological needs for attention, security, and affection (secondary gains) (Black & Andreasen, 2011).

Research about biologic causes of somatization disorder has shown that clients with this disorder cannot sort relevant from irrelevant stimuli and respond in the same way to all stimuli. In addition, somatic sensations are interpreted as intense, noxious, and disturbing. This means that a person may experience a normal sensation such as peristalsis and attach a pathologic meaning to it, or that minor discomfort, such as muscle tightness, is experienced as severe pain (Black & Andreasen, 2011).

Somatization disorder occurs in 0.2% to 2% of women in the general population and in less than 0.2% of men. It is reported in 10% to 20% of female first-degree biologic relatives of women with somatization disorder (APA, 2000). Symptoms of somatization disorder usually occur by the age of 25, but initial symptoms typically begin in adolescence. The course of this disorder is chronic, is characterized by remissions and exacerbations, and rarely remits completely (APA, 2000). Typically, symptoms are worse and impairment is more significant during times of emotional stress or conflict in the person's life.

Treatment is focused on managing symptoms and improving the client's quality of life. Showing sensitivity to the client's physical complaints and building a trust relationship will help keep the client with a single provider, which minimizes conflicting or unsafe combinations of treatments. Antidepressants, referral to a chronic pain clinic, and participation in cognitive-behavioral therapy groups may be helpful.

Clients with somatization disorder may have difficulty recognizing the emotional problems underlying their physical symptoms. Nursing goals include assisting the client to identify stress, decrease denial, increase insight, express feelings, participate in the treatment plan, and recognize and avoid seeking secondary gain.

NURSING DIAGNOSES ADDRESSED IN THIS CARE PLAN
Ineffective Coping
Ineffective Denial

RELATED NURSING DIAGNOSIS ADDRESSED IN THE MANUAL
Anxiety

Nursing Diagnosis

Ineffective Coping
Inability to form a valid appraisal of the stressors, inadequate choices of practiced responses, and/or inability to use available resources.

ASSESSMENT DATA

- Inadequate coping skills
- Inability to problem-solve
- Physical complaints or symptoms
- Resistance to therapy or to the role of a psychiatric client
- Anger or hostility
- Resentment or guilt
- Difficulty with interpersonal relationships
- Dependency needs
- Inability to express feelings
- Repression of feelings of guilt, anger, or fear
- Patterns of coping through physical illness with resulting secondary gains (attention, evasion of responsibilities) due to illness
- Anxiety or fear

EXPECTED OUTCOMES

Immediate

The client will

- Verbally express feelings of anxiety, fear, or anger within 2 to 3 days
- Acknowledge emotional or stress-related problems within 2 to 3 days
- Demonstrate increased willingness to relinquish the "sick role," for example, perform self-care and take part in activities rather than declining activities based on physical symptoms within 2 to 3 days
- Verbalize the relationship between emotional problems and physical symptoms within 4 to 5 days

Stabilization

The client will

- Verbalize an understanding of the relationship between emotional stress and physical symptoms
- Demonstrate appropriate use of medications
- Continue to verbally express feelings of anxiety, fear, or anger
- Verbalize knowledge of stress management techniques, therapeutic regimen(s), and medication use, if any

Community

The client will

- Demonstrate increased satisfaction in interpersonal relationships
- Verbalize or demonstrate use of the problem-solving process
- Verbalize or demonstrate alternative ways to deal with life stresses and the feelings that occur in response to them
- Be physically well or achieve management of physical symptoms

IMPLEMENTATION

Nursing Interventions *denotes collaborative interventions	Rationale
*Do a thorough initial assessment, including physical problems, complaints, history of diseases, treatment, surgeries, and hospitalizations. Obtaining the client's prior medical record(s) or interviewing family members or significant others may be helpful. Do not assume there is not a physiologic basis for the client's symptoms.	An adequate database is necessary to rule out pathophysiology. The client may be a poor historian. The client may have been seen in the treatment setting in the past (without evidence of pathophysiology), but may have developed a physiologic illness since that time.
Ask for the client's perceptions about physical problems, but do not argue or put the client on the defensive.	Arguing will damage your trust relationship. The client's symptoms are real to the client.
Ask the client to identify expectations of treatment, himself or herself, and the staff. Try to involve the client in identifying problems, goals, and actions to work toward goals.	If the client is involved and invests energy in his or her care, the chances for positive outcomes increase.
Develop and implement a nursing care plan regarding the client's physical health as soon as possible. Be matter-of-fact in your approach and treatment. Do not overemphasize physical problems or give undue attention to physical symptoms.	Optimal physical health facilitates achievement of emotional health. You must consider the client's physical care, but not as the primary focus. Remember that the client's problems are real to the client and not hypochondriacal or imaginary.
Talk with the client directly regarding a correlation between emotions, stress, and physical symptoms.	The client's chance for health is enhanced if the interrelatedness of physical and emotional health is recognized.
Assess the client's activities and interactions with others in the treatment setting and with visitors with regard to stress, support, dependency, and expressing feelings.	Stress-related factors are important in the dynamics of somatization disorder.
Talk with the client about your observations and ask for the client's perceptions regarding stress, sources of satisfaction and dissatisfaction, relationships, work, and so forth.	You are focusing on emotional issues. The client may have spent minimal time considering those aspects of health.
Give the client positive feedback for focusing on emotional and interpersonal issues rather than on physical symptoms.	Positive feedback increases the likelihood that the client will continue to express feelings and deal with interpersonal issues.
Without always connecting the client's physical problems with emotions, encourage the client to express feelings, by writing, in individual conversations, and in groups (start small and progress to larger).	It is less threatening for the client to begin expressing feelings to one person and work his or her way up to talking with more people about emotional issues.
Encourage the client to express feelings directly in relationships and stressful situations—especially feelings that are uncomfortable for the client. Role-play situations and give support for expressing feelings during and after role-playing. See "Key Considerations in Mental Health Nursing: Nurse–Client Interactions."	Role-playing allows the client to try out new behaviors in a nonthreatening situation.
Especially support the client for expressing feelings spontaneously or independently (e.g., writing, art work, or verbal expression).	True client change is best evidenced by spontaneous behavior.
*Teach the client and his or her family or significant others about physical symptoms, stress, and stress management skills.	The client may have little or no knowledge of stress or of stress management techniques.

IMPLEMENTATION (continued)

Nursing Interventions *denotes collaborative interventions	Rationale
Gradually attempt to identify with the client the connections between anxiety or stress and the exacerbation of physical symptoms.	Acknowledging the interrelatedness of physical health and emotional health will help the client recognize this and make changes in the future.
Encourage the client to identify his or her own strengths; making a written list may be helpful.	It may be difficult for the client to see his or her own strengths, but this can promote an increased sense of self-worth.
Teach the client about the problem-solving process: identify a problem, identify and evaluate possible solutions, choose and implement a solution, and evaluate its success.	The client may never have learned a logical, step-by-step approach to dealing with problems.
*Talk with the client and significant others about secondary gains. Identify the needs the client is attempting to meet (e.g., need for attention, means of dealing with perceived excess responsibilities). Help the client plan to meet these needs in more direct ways.	Significant others may be unaware of how they reward the client for physical symptoms. Their participation in treatment is essential so the client can give up the sick role and deal with emotional problems.
*Conferences with only the client's family or significant others may help increase their insight. For example, they unknowingly may be giving the client the message that emotional problems are a sign of weakness and that only physical illness is acceptable.	Unless significant others make changes in their relationships with the client, chances for positive client changes are diminished.
*Encourage the client to continue to identify stresses and attempt to deal with them directly. Encourage the client to continue therapy on an outpatient basis or refer to a chronic pain clinic if indicated.	Long-term change depends on how the client continues to progress after treatment.
*Encourage the client to develop an outside support system to continue to talk about feelings (e.g., significant others, support group, or group therapy).	The client needs to continue to express feelings to avoid returning to coping through physical symptoms.
*Teach the client and his or her family or significant others about treatment and medications for the client's physical symptoms, if any.	Clients need to have clear instructions regarding self-care and the safe use of medications if they require continued treatment.
Encourage the client to enhance his or her physical health (e.g., with regular exercise, good nutrition).	General physical wellness will facilitate management or control of illness.

Nursing Diagnosis

Ineffective Denial
Conscious or unconscious attempt to disavow the knowledge or meaning of an event to reduce anxiety and/or fear, leading to the detriment of health.

ASSESSMENT DATA

- Denial of emotional problems or stresses
- Lack of insight
- Resistance to therapy or to the role of a psychiatric client
- Inadequate coping skills
- Inability to express feelings
- Repression of feelings of guilt, anger, resentment, or fear
- Patterns of coping through physical symptoms with resulting secondary gains
- Discomfort with emotions
- Fear of intensity of feelings

EXPECTED OUTCOMES

Immediate	The client will
	• Participate in treatment program, for example, interact with staff for at least 30 minutes twice per day, within 2 to 3 days
	• Acknowledge emotional or stress-related problems within 4 to 5 days
	• Verbally express feelings of anxiety, fear, or anger within 4 to 5 days
Stabilization	The client will
	• Verbalize an understanding of the relationship between emotional stress and physical illness
	• Continue to verbally express feelings of anxiety, fear, or anger
Community	The client will
	• Report success in coping with conflict or stress without exacerbation of physical symptoms
	• Participate in ongoing therapy, if indicated, for example, identify a therapist and schedule an appointment prior to discharge
	• Demonstrate alternative ways to deal with life stresses and the anxiety or other feelings that occur in response to them, for example, use the problem-solving process

IMPLEMENTATION

Nursing Interventions *denotes collaborative interventions	Rationale
Assess the client's activities and interactions with others with regard to stress, support, dependency, and expression of emotions.	Stress-related factors are important in the dynamics of somatization disorder.
Ask for the client's perceptions about physical problems, but do not argue or put the client on the defensive.	Arguing will damage your trust relationship.
Talk with the client about your observations and ask for the client's perceptions regarding stress, sources of satisfaction and dissatisfaction, relationships, work, and so forth.	You are focusing on emotional issues. The client may have spent minimal time considering these aspects of health.
Talk with the client directly regarding a correlation between emotions, stress, and physical symptoms.	The client's chance for health is enhanced if the interrelatedness of physical and emotional health is recognized.
Give the client positive feedback for focusing on emotional and interpersonal issues rather than on physical symptoms.	Positive feedback increases the likelihood that the client will continue to express feelings and deal with interpersonal issues.
If the client denies experiencing stress or certain feelings, the discussion may need to be less direct. For example, point out apparent stresses or feelings and ask the client for feedback about them.	Directly confronting the client's denial can make the denial stronger if the client is not ready to deal with issues.
Without always connecting the client's physical problems with emotions, encourage the client to express feelings, by writing, in individual conversations, and in groups (start with small and progress to larger groups).	It is less threatening for the client to begin expressing feelings in writing or to one person and work his or her way up to talking with more people about emotional issues.
*Teach the client and family or significant others about the physical symptoms, stress, and stress management skills.	The client may have little or no knowledge of stress or stress management techniques.
Gradually attempt to identify with the client the connections between anxiety or stress and the exacerbation of physical symptoms.	Acknowledging the interrelatedness of physical health and emotional health provides a basis for the client's future lifestyle changes.
*Encourage the client to continue to identify stresses and attempt to deal with them directly. Encourage the client to continue therapy, if indicated.	Long-term change depends on how the client continues to progress after treatment.
*Encourage the client to develop an outside support system to continue to talk about feelings after discharge (e.g., significant others, a support group, or group therapy).	The client needs to continue to express feelings to avoid returning to coping through physical symptoms.

CARE PLAN 33

Conversion Disorder

Conversion disorder, also called *conversion reaction,* is characterized by physical symptoms or some loss of physical functioning, without a demonstrable organic problem. The client is not faking the physical symptoms and feels that symptoms are not in his or her control. Symptoms are usually manifested in sensory or motor function and suggest a neurologic or other medical condition, which cannot be demonstrated by medical tests or physical examination, or does not account for all of the symptoms. Common symptoms include blindness, deafness, loss of sensation or paralysis of the extremities, mutism, dizziness, ataxia, and seizures. Often, only a single physical symptom is present.

The physical symptoms manifested in a conversion reaction are considered to be an unconscious manifestation of a psychological stressor. The symptoms may be related to an underlying psychological conflict, as illustrated by the following situations.

The physical symptom may give the client a "legitimate reason" to avoid the conflict. For example, a young man wishes to attend college, but his father wants him to remain at home to help on the farm. The young man develops a paralysis of his legs, rendering him unable to do farm work and resolving the conflict with a physical disability beyond his control.

The physical symptom may represent perceived "deserved punishment" for behavior about which the client feels guilty. For example, a young woman gains pleasure from watching television, which is forbidden by her family's religious beliefs. She develops blindness, which she perceives as punishment and which relieves her guilt.

The type of conflict resolution demonstrated in the above examples is known as *primary gain*—the client gains a decrease in anxiety and awareness of the conflict by manifestation of physical symptoms or *somatization* of the conflict. In addition, the client may receive *secondary gains* related to the symptoms, including reduced responsibilities or increased attention from others. The client with a conversion disorder may be unconcerned about the severity of the symptom (called *la belle indifference*); unconsciously, the client may be relieved that the conflict is resolved.

Conversion disorder usually occurs between the ages of 10 and 35 and is diagnosed in less than 1% of the US population. It is more likely to occur in women and in clients from rural areas and lower socioeconomic levels, and who are less familiar with medical and psychological information (APA, 2000). Symptoms of conversion disorder usually appear suddenly and usually respond to treatment within a few weeks. However, the disorder may be chronic; 20% to 25% of clients with this disorder have a recurrence within 1 year (APA, 2000).

The focus of therapeutic work is on the resolution of the client's conflicting feelings, rather than on the physical symptom per se, even though the physical symptom is very real (e.g., the client actually cannot walk if paralysis is the symptom). Removal from the conflict (as occurs when the client is hospitalized) frequently produces gradual relief or remission of the physical symptom. In this situation, however, the physical symptom may return as the client approaches discharge.

Initial treatment goals include identifying the source of the conflict that forms the basis of the symptom(s) and preventing secondary gain. Then, treatment focuses on facilitating the client's recognition of the relationship between the conflict and the physical symptom and helping the client to resolve the conflict or deal with it in ways other than by developing physical symptoms.

NURSING DIAGNOSES ADDRESSED IN THIS CARE PLAN
Ineffective Coping
Ineffective Denial

RELATED NURSING DIAGNOSES ADDRESSED IN THE MANUAL
Ineffective Health Maintenance
Anxiety

Nursing Diagnosis

Ineffective Coping

Inability to form a valid appraisal of the stressors, inadequate choices of practiced responses, and/or inability to use available resources.

ASSESSMENT DATA

- Inability to identify and resolve conflict or ask for help
- Inability to meet role expectations
- Inability to cope with present life situation
- Inability to problem-solve
- Guilt and resentment
- Anxiety
- Feelings of inadequacy
- Difficulty with feelings of anger, hostility, or conflict
- Decreased ability to express needs and feelings
- Secondary gain related to the physical symptom or disability
- Unsatisfactory and inadequate interpersonal relationships
- Low self-esteem
- Physical limitation or disability (e.g., blindness, paralysis, loss of voice)
- Inability to perform self-care tasks or activities of daily living

EXPECTED OUTCOMES

Immediate

The client will

- Be free from injury throughout hospitalization
- Experience adequate nutrition, hydration, rest, and activity within 3 to 4 days
- Experience relief from acute stress or conflict within 4 to 5 days
- Identify the conflict underlying the physical symptom within 4 to 5 days
- Identify feelings of fear, anger, guilt, anxiety, or inadequacy within 4 to 5 days

Stabilization

The client will

- Verbalize feelings of fear, guilt, anxiety, or inadequacy
- Express anger in a direct, nondestructive manner, for example, initiate conversation with staff to verbalize angry feelings
- Be free from actual physical impairment
- Verbalize increased feelings of self-worth
- Verbalize knowledge of illness, including concept of secondary gain

Community

The client will

- Continue with therapy after discharge if indicated, for example, identify a therapist and make an initial appointment before discharge
- Cope successfully with conflict without recurrence of the conversion reaction
- Demonstrate interpersonal and intrapersonal strategies to deal with life stresses

IMPLEMENTATION

Nursing Interventions *denotes collaborative interventions	Rationale
Observe the client's ability to perform activities of daily living, ambulate independently, and so on. Intervene if the client is risking injury to himself or herself, but minimize attention given to the client's limitation and your supervision.	Often clients with histrionic types of behavior will not experience physical injuries.
*Obtain the client's thorough history on admission and request records from prior hospitalizations, if possible. Contact the family or significant others if necessary to complete the history.	A complete database is essential to the validity of the diagnosis.
Observe and document the client's behavior, especially in relation to the symptom, including precipitating events, the environment (such as the presence of others), and changes in the severity of the symptom(s).	Observational data will provide clues to the client's perception of stress and the relationship of the conversion symptom to that stress.
Assess the client's food and fluid intake, elimination, and amount of rest as unobtrusively as possible.	You must be aware of the client's physical status, without giving excessive attention to it.
Assist or prepare the client as necessary for any tests to rule out a physical (organic) basis of the symptom.	Organic pathology must be ruled out.
Approach the client with the attitude that you expect improvement in the physical symptom.	Communicating your expectation may help the client expect to improve. Hospitalization may relieve the conflict by removing the client from his or her usual environment.
Initially, avoid making demands on the client that are similar to the client's prehospitalization conflict or situation.	Such demands could intensify the client's conflict, resulting in exacerbation of the symptom.
Initially, if the conflict is related to a particular person in the client's life, visits from that person may need to be restricted or prevented.	Temporary limitations of visits may help alleviate the client's stress.
As the physical symptom improves, gradually allow stressful situations or increase visits, as tolerated; monitor the client's response.	The client can begin to tolerate increased stresses as his or her skills develop, but too much stress may exacerbate the symptom.
*Any intervention regarding the client's physical state (e.g., poor food or fluid intake) must be planned and consistently implemented by the treatment team.	A consistent team approach decreases opportunities for manipulation.
Provide nursing care in a matter-of-fact manner.	A matter-of-fact approach minimizes secondary gain and can help separate emotional issues from physical symptoms.
Talk with the client about his or her life, usual environment, work, significant others, and so forth.	General, leading questions or open discussion is a nonthreatening approach to discover the nature of the conflict.
Focus interactions on the client's feelings, home or work situation, and relationships.	Your consistent attention to emotional issues will help the client shift attention to these issues.
Encourage the client to express feelings directly, verbally, or in writing. Support the client's efforts to express feelings.	Direct expression of feelings can relieve tension and conflict, diminishing the need for physical symptoms.
Explore with the client his or her personal relationships and related feelings.	Conversion reaction symptoms often are related to interpersonal conflicts or situations.
*Teach the client and the family or significant others about conversion reaction, stress, stress management, interpersonal dynamics, and conflict resolution strategies.	The client and the family or significant others may have little or no knowledge of these areas. Increasing their knowledge can promote understanding, motivation for change, and support for the client.
Praise the client when he or she is able to identify the physical symptom as a method used to cope with conflict.	Positive feedback can reinforce the client's insight.
Explore alternative methods of expressing feelings related to the identified conflict.	The client has the opportunity to practice unfamiliar behavior with you in a nonthreatening environment.

(continued on page 228)

IMPLEMENTATION (continued)

Nursing Interventions *denotes collaborative interventions	Rationale
Provide opportunities for the client to succeed at activities, tasks, and interactions. Give positive feedback and point out the client's demonstrated strengths and abilities.	Activities within the client's abilities will provide opportunities for success. Positive feedback provides reinforcement for the client's growth and can enhance self-esteem.
Help the client set goals for his or her behavior; give positive feedback when the client achieves these goals.	Setting and achieving goals can foster the client's sense of control and self-esteem and teaches goal-setting skills.
Teach the client about the problem-solving process: identify the problem, examine alternatives, weigh the pros and cons of each alternative, select and implement an approach, and evaluate its success. Encourage him or her to use it to examine the conflict.	The client may have few or no problem-solving skills or knowledge of the problem-solving process.
Encourage the client to identify strategies to deal with the conflict and evaluate their effectiveness.	The client must actively explore new strategies because they are unfamiliar.
Give the client positive feedback for expressing feelings about the conflict and trying conflict resolution strategies.	Positive feedback can increase desired behavior.
*Refer the client and the family or significant others for continuing therapy if appropriate.	The client may need long-term therapy to deal with feelings, conflict, or relationships.
*Encourage the client to increase his or her support system outside the hospital. See Care Plan 2: Discharge Planning.	Extended support in the community strengthens the client's ability to cope more effectively.

Nursing Diagnosis

Ineffective Denial

Conscious or unconscious attempt to disavow the knowledge or meaning of an event to reduce anxiety and/or fear, leading to the detriment of health.

ASSESSMENT DATA

- Presence of physical limitation or disability with indifference to or lack of concern about the severity of the symptom
- Refusal to seek health care for the physical symptom
- Lack of insight into stresses, conflicts, or problematic relationships
- Difficulty with feelings of anger, hostility, or conflict
- Decreased ability to express needs and feelings
- Secondary gain related to the physical symptom or disability

EXPECTED OUTCOMES

Immediate   The client will

- Identify the conflict underlying the physical symptom within 4 to 5 days
- Identify feelings of fear, anger, guilt, anxiety, or inadequacy within 4 to 5 days
- Verbalize steps of the problem-solving process within 4 to 5 days

Stabilization   The client will

- Verbalize feelings of fear, guilt, anxiety, or inadequacy
- Verbalize knowledge of illness, including the concept of secondary gain
- Demonstrate use of the problem-solving process

Community   The client will

- Negotiate resolution of conflicts with family, friends, significant others

IMPLEMENTATION

Nursing Interventions *denotes collaborative interventions	Rationale
Involve the client in the usual activities, self-care, eating in the dining room, and so on as you would other clients.	Your expectation will enhance the client's participation and will diminish secondary gain.
After medical evaluation of the symptom, withdraw attention from the client's physical status except for necessary care. Avoid discussing the physical symptom; withdraw your attention from the client if necessary.	Lack of attention to expression of physical complaints will help minimize secondary gain and decrease the client's focus on the symptom.
Expect the client to participate in activities as fully as possible. Make your expectations clear and do not give the client special privileges or excuse him or her from all expectations due to physical limitations.	Granting special privileges or excusing the client from responsibilities are forms of secondary gain. The client may need to become more uncomfortable to risk relinquishing the physical conversion as a coping strategy.
Do not argue with the client. Withdraw your attention if necessary.	Arguing with the client undermines limits. Withdrawing attention may be effective in diminishing secondary gain.
Focus interactions on the client's feelings, home or work situation, and relationships.	Increased attention to emotional issues will help the client shift attention to these feelings.
Explore with the client his or her personal relationships and related feelings.	Conversion reaction symptoms often are related to interpersonal conflicts or situations. Talking about these things may help the client develop insight and additional coping mechanisms.
*Teach the client and the family or significant others about conversion reaction, stress management, interpersonal dynamics, coping, and conflict resolution strategies.	The client and the family or significant others may have little or no knowledge of these areas. Increasing their knowledge can promote understanding, motivation for change, and support for the client.
Talk with the client about coping strategies he or she has used in the past that did not include physical symptoms.	The client may have used coping strategies in the past that did not result in physical symptoms, perhaps for issues or conflicts that were less stressful for the client. The client may be able to build on these strategies in the future.
Teach the client about stress management skills, such as increasing physical exercise, expressing feelings verbally or in a journal, or meditation techniques. Encourage the client to practice this type of technique while in the hospital.	The client may have limited or no knowledge of or may not have used stress management techniques in the past. If the client begins to build skills in the treatment setting, he or she can experience success and receive positive feedback.
Teach the client the problem-solving process: identify the problem, examine alternatives, weigh the pros and cons of each alternative, select and implement an approach, and evaluate its success.	The client may not know the steps of a logical, orderly process to solve problems. Such a process can be helpful to the client in dealing with stressful situations in the future.
Praise the client when he or she is able to discuss the physical symptom as a method used to cope with conflict.	Positive feedback can reinforce the client's insight and help the client recognize physical symptoms as related to emotional issues in the future.
Give the client positive feedback for expressing feelings and trying conflict resolution strategies.	Positive feedback can increase desired behavior and help the client build confidence in preparation for discharge.

CARE PLAN 34

Hypochondriasis

Hypochondriasis is a preoccupation with or fear of a serious disease that is based on misinterpretation of signs or symptoms and cannot be fully accounted for by a demonstrable medical condition. The client's preoccupation with symptoms persists for at least 6 months despite medical testing, evaluation, and reassurance, but is not delusional in intensity (APA, 2000). The client with hypochondriasis may have learned to use somatic complaints as a way to deal with feelings, anxieties, or conflicts, and he or she may not be able to relinquish hypochondriasis behavior until his or her anxiety decreases or until he or she develops other behaviors to deal with these feelings (see Section 8: Anxiety Disorders). Hypochondriacal symptoms may be related to difficulty expressing anger satisfactorily and may be found in several types of psychiatric disorders, such as depression, schizophrenia, neurosis, or personality disorders.

Hypochondriasis can occur at any age, in both men and women, and is present in 1% to 5% of the US population (APA, 2000). It is usually chronic, and the prognosis may be poor because clients often deny emotional problems, exhibit other neurotic symptoms, and reject mental health treatment. The client may believe that he or she is receiving poor medical care or incorrect information and may change physicians frequently. It can be very frustrating to work with these clients if they are unwilling or unable to recognize the emotional aspects of this situation and continue to exhibit hypochondriacal behavior despite treatment efforts or as the client gets closer to being discharged from care. You must work through your own feelings while working with these clients to avoid acting out these feelings in nontherapeutic ways (such as avoiding the client).

The client may feel real symptoms (such as pain) even though an organic basis for the symptoms cannot be found; also, remember that even if a client's behavior may previously have been determined to be hypochondriacal, he or she may have a new complaint that is indeed based in organic pathology. Therefore, you must carefully assess the client's physical condition and refer all new somatic complaints to the medical staff for evaluation. Do *not* assume a complaint is hypochondriacal until after it has been evaluated medically.

Nursing goals related to hypochondriacal symptoms include decreasing complaints, ritualistic behaviors, excessive fears of disease, and reliance on medications or other treatments. It is especially important to help the client identify problems that may underlie hypochondriacal behavior and develop alternative ways of dealing with stress, anxiety, anger, and other feelings.

The client may be successfully avoiding responsibilities, receiving attention, or manipulating others by exhibiting hypochondriacal symptoms (all forms of *secondary gain*). Working with the client's family or significant others to decrease secondary gains and supporting the client's development of healthy ways to receive attention are other key interventions.

NURSING DIAGNOSES ADDRESSED IN THIS CARE PLAN
Ineffective Coping
Anxiety

RELATED NURSING DIAGNOSES ADDRESSED IN THE MANUAL
Ineffective Health Maintenance
Ineffective Denial

Nursing Diagnosis

Ineffective Coping

Inability to form a valid appraisal of the stressors, inadequate choices of practiced responses, and/or inability to use available resources.

ASSESSMENT DATA

- Denial of emotional problems
- Difficulty identifying and expressing feelings
- Lack of insight
- Self-preoccupation, especially with physical functioning
- Fears of or rumination on disease
- Numerous somatic complaints (may involve many different organs or systems)
- Sensory complaints (pain, loss of taste sensation, olfactory complaints)
- Reluctance or refusal to participate in psychiatric treatment program or activities
- Reliance on medications or physical treatments (such as laxative dependence)
- Extensive use of over-the-counter medications, home remedies, enemas, and so forth
- Ritualistic behaviors (such as exaggerated bowel routines)
- Tremors
- Limited gratification from interpersonal relationships
- Lack of emotional support system
- Anxiety
- Secondary gains received for physical problems
- History of repeated visits to physicians or hospital admissions
- History of repeated medical evaluations with no findings of abnormalities

EXPECTED OUTCOMES

Immediate

The client will

- Participate in the treatment program, for example, talk with staff for 15 minutes or participate in a group activity at least twice a day within 24 to 48 hours
- Demonstrate decreased physical complaints within 2 to 3 days
- Demonstrate compliance with medical therapy and medications within 2 to 3 days
- Demonstrate adequate energy, food, and fluid intake, for example, eat at least 50% of each meal within 3 to 4 days
- Identify life stresses and anxieties within 3 to 4 days
- Express feelings verbally within 3 to 4 days
- Identify alternative ways to deal with stress, anxiety, or other feelings, for example, talking with others, physical activity, keeping a journal, and so forth, within 3 to 5 days
- Identify the relationship between stress and physical symptoms within 4 to 5 days

Stabilization

The client will

- Demonstrate decreased ritualistic behaviors
- Demonstrate decreased physical attention-seeking complaints
- Verbalize increased insight into the dynamics of hypochondriacal behavior, including secondary gains
- Verbalize an understanding of therapeutic regimens and medications, if any

Community

The client will

- Eliminate overuse of medications or physical treatments
- Demonstrate alternative ways to deal with stress, anxiety, or other feelings

IMPLEMENTATION

Nursing Interventions *denotes collaborative interventions	Rationale
The initial nursing assessment should include a complete physical assessment, a history of previous complaints and treatment, and a consideration of each current complaint.	The nursing assessment provides a baseline from which to begin planning care.
*The nursing staff should note the medical staff's assessment of each complaint on the client's admission.	Genuine physical problems must be noted and treated.
*Each time the client voices a new complaint, the client should be referred to the medical staff for assessment (and treatment if appropriate).	It is unsafe to assume that all physical complaints are hypochondriacal—the client could really be ill or injured. The client may attempt to establish the legitimacy of complaints by being genuinely injured or ill.
*Work with the medical staff to limit the number, variety, strength, and frequency of medications, enemas, and so forth that are made available to the client.	A coordinated effort by the treatment team helps to prevent the client's manipulation of staff members to obtain additional medication. See Care Plan 48: Passive–Aggressive Behavior.
Observe and record the circumstances related to complaints; talk about your observations with the client.	Alerting the client to situations surrounding the complaint helps him or her see the relatedness of stress and physical symptoms.
Help the client identify and use nonchemical methods of pain relief, such as relaxation techniques.	Using nonchemical pain relief shifts the focus of coping away from medications and increases the client's sense of control.
When the client requests a medication or treatment, encourage the client to identify what precipitated his or her complaint and to deal with it in other ways.	If the client can obtain stress relief in a nonchemical, nonmedical way, he or she is less likely to use the medication or treatment.
*Minimize the amount of time and attention given to complaints. When the client makes a complaint, refer him or her to the medical staff (if it is a new complaint) or follow the team treatment plan; then tell the client you will discuss topics other than physical complaints. Tell the client that you are interested in the client as a person, not just in his or her physical complaints. If the complaint is not acute, ask the client to discuss the complaint during a regular appointment with the medical staff.	If physical complaints are unsuccessful in gaining attention, they should decrease in frequency over time. If medical attention to the complaint can be deferred until a regular appointment time, the client may be able to use a nonchemical method of addressing the problem, and it will minimize the secondary gain of receiving immediate medical attention.
Withdraw your attention if the client insists on making complaints the sole topic of conversation. Tell the client your reason for withdrawal and that you will return later to discuss other topics.	It is important to make clear to the client that attention is withdrawn from physical complaints, not from the client as a person.
Allow the client a specific time limit (such as 5 minutes per hour) to discuss physical complaints with one person. The remaining staff will discuss only other issues with the client.	Because physical complaints have been the client's primary coping strategy, it is less threatening to the client if you limit this behavior initially rather than forbid it. If the client is denied this coping mechanism before new skills can be developed, hypochondriacal behavior may increase.
Acknowledge the complaint as the client's perception and then follow the previous approaches; do not argue about the somatic complaints.	Arguing gives the client's complaints attention, albeit negative, and the client is able to avoid discussing feelings.
Use minimal objective reassurance in conjunction with questions to explore the client's feelings. ("Your tests have shown that you have no lesions. Do you still feel that you do? What are your feelings about this?") See Care Plan 30: Obsessive-Compulsive Disorder.	This approach helps the client make the transition to discussing feelings.
Reduce the benefits of illness as much as possible. Do not allow the client to avoid responsibilities or allow special privileges, such as staying in bed by voicing somatic discomfort.	If physical problems do not get the client what he or she wants, the client is less likely to cope in that manner.

IMPLEMENTATION (continued)

Nursing Interventions *denotes collaborative interventions	Rationale
Teach the client more healthful daily living habits, including diet, stress management techniques, daily exercise, rest, possible connection between caffeine and anxiety symptoms, and so forth.	Optimal physical wellness is especially important with clients who use physical symptoms as a coping strategy.
Initially, carefully assess the client's self-image, social patterns, and ways of dealing with anger, stress, and so forth.	This assessment provides a knowledge base regarding hypochondriacal behaviors.
Talk with the client about sources of satisfaction and dissatisfaction, relationships, employment, and so forth.	Open-ended discussion usually is nonthreatening and helps the client begin self-assessment.
After some discussion of the above and developing a trust relationship, talk more directly with the client and encourage him or her to identify specific stresses, recent and ongoing.	The client's perception of stressors forms the basis of his or her behavior and usually is more significant than others' perception of those stressors.
If the client is using denial of stress as a defense mechanism, point out apparent or possible stresses (in a nonthreatening way) and ask the client for feedback.	If the client is in denial, more direct approaches may produce anger or hostility and threaten the trust relationship.
Gradually, help the client identify possible connections between anxiety and the occurrence of physical symptoms, such as: What makes the client more or less comfortable? What is the client doing or what is going on around the client when he or she experiences symptoms?	The client can begin to see the relatedness of stress and physical problems at his or her own pace. Self-realization will be more acceptable to the client than the nurse telling the client the problem.
Encourage the client to keep a diary of situations, stresses, and occurrence of symptoms and use it to identify relationships between stresses and symptoms.	Reflecting on written items may be more accurate and less threatening to the client.
Encourage the client to discuss his or her feelings about fears or stresses rather than the fears themselves.	The focus is on feelings of fear, not fear of physical problems.
Help the client explore his or her feelings of lack of control over stress and life events.	The client may have helpless feelings but may not recognize this independently.
Talk with the client at least once per shift, focusing on the client's identifying and expressing feelings.	Demonstrating consistent interest in the client facilitates the relationship and can desensitize the discussion of emotional issues.
Encourage the client to ventilate feelings by talking or crying, through physical activities, and so forth.	The client may have difficulty expressing feelings directly. Your support may help him or her develop these skills.
Encourage the client to express feelings directly, especially feelings with which the client is uncomfortable (such as anger or resentment).	Direct expression of feelings will minimize the need to use physical symptoms to express them.
Notice the client's interactions with others and give positive feedback for self-assertion and expressing feelings, especially anger, resentment, and other so-called negative emotions.	The client needs to know that appropriate expressions of anger or other negative emotions are acceptable and that he or she can feel better physically as a result of these expressions.
Help the client plan to meet his or her needs in more direct ways. Show the client that he or she can gain attention when he or she does not exhibit symptoms, deals with responsibilities directly, or asserts himself or herself in the face of stress.	Positive feedback and support for healthier behavior tend to make that behavior recur more frequently.
*Talk with the client and significant others about secondary gains and together develop a plan to reduce those gains, including providing attention and caring when the client does not express or exhibit physical symptoms. Identify the needs the client is attempting to meet with secondary gains (such as attention or escape from responsibilities).	Maintaining limits to reduce secondary gain requires everyone's participation to be successful. The client's family and significant others must be aware of the client's needs if they want to be effective in helping to meet those needs. The client's family and significant others also must use positive reinforcement for healthy behaviors.
*Teach the client and his or her family or significant others about the dynamics of hypochondriacal behavior and the treatment plan, including plans after discharge.	The client and his or her family or significant others may have little or no knowledge of these areas. Knowledge of the treatment plan will promote long-term behavior change.

Nursing Diagnosis

Anxiety

Vague uneasy feeling of discomfort or dread accompanied by an autonomic response (the source often nonspecific or unknown to the individual); a feeling of apprehension caused by anticipation of danger. It is an alerting signal that warns of impending danger and enables the individual to take measures to deal with threat.

ASSESSMENT DATA

- Self-preoccupation, especially with physical functioning
- Fears of or rumination on disease
- History of repeated visits to physicians or hospital admissions
- Tremors
- Ineffective coping mechanisms
- Delusions
- Sleep disturbances
- Loss of appetite

EXPECTED OUTCOMES

Immediate

The client will

- Express feelings verbally, for example, talk with staff about feelings for at least 15 minutes at least twice per day within 2 to 3 days
- Identify life stresses and anxieties within 2 to 3 days

Stabilization

The client will

- Identify alternative ways to deal with stress, anxiety, or other feelings, for example, writing in a journal, talking with others, physical activity
- Communicate directly and assertively with others

Community

The client will

- Demonstrate alternative ways to deal with stress, anxiety, or other feelings
- Seek medical care only when indicated

IMPLEMENTATION

Nursing Interventions *denotes collaborative interventions	Rationale
Encourage the client to discuss his or her feelings about fears rather than the fears themselves.	The client needs to begin to focus on his or her feelings, not fear of physical problems.
Help the client explore his or her feelings of lack of control over stress and life events.	The client may have helpless feelings but may not recognize this independently.
Talk with the client at least once per shift, focusing on the identification and expression of the client's feelings.	Demonstrating consistent interest in the client facilitates the relationship and can desensitize discussion of emotional issues.
Encourage the client to ventilate feelings by talking or crying, through physical activities, and so forth.	The client may have difficulty expressing feelings directly. Your support may help the client develop these skills.
Encourage the client to express feelings, especially ones with which the client is uncomfortable (e.g., anger or resentment).	Direct expression of feelings will minimize the need to use physical symptoms to express them.
Notice the client's interactions with others and give positive feedback for self-assertion and expressing feelings, especially anger, resentment, and other so-called negative emotions.	The client needs to know that appropriate expressions of anger or other negative emotions are acceptable and that he or she can feel better physically as a result of those expressions.

IMPLEMENTATION (continued)

Nursing Interventions *denotes collaborative interventions	Rationale
Talk with the client about coping strategies he or she has used successfully in the past.	The client may have had success using coping strategies in the past but may have lost confidence in himself or herself or in his or her ability to cope with stressors and feelings.
Teach the client about positive coping strategies and stress management skills, such as increasing physical exercise, expressing feelings verbally or in a journal, or meditation techniques. Encourage the client to practice this type of technique while in the hospital.	The client may have limited or no knowledge of stress management techniques or may not have used positive techniques in the past. If the client's anxiety diminishes by practicing these within the treatment setting, he or she can build on these skills in the future.
Teach the client the problem-solving process: identify the problem, examine alternatives, weigh the pros and cons of each alternative, select and implement an approach, and evaluate its success.	The client may be overwhelmed by anxiety in response to problems and will benefit from knowing how to deal with problems by using a logical, orderly process.
*Encourage the client to pursue past relationships, personal interests, hobbies, or recreational activities that were positive in the past or that may appeal to the client. Consultation with a recreational therapist may be indicated.	Social isolation may contribute to anxiety and a focus on physical symptoms. Social contacts and recreational activities can serve as a structure for the client to receive attention and focus on relationships and enjoyment rather than physical problems.

Dissociative Disorders

Dissociative disorders are described in the *DSM-IV-TR* (APA, 2000) as having the essential feature of a "disruption in the usually integrated functions of consciousness, memory, identity or perception" (p. 519).

Dissociative disorders are diagnostically categorized as follows (APA, 2000, p. 519):

Dissociative amnesia is characterized by an inability to recall important personal information, usually of a traumatic or stressful nature, that is too extensive to be explained by ordinary forgetfulness.

Dissociative fugue is characterized by sudden, unexpected travel away from home or one's customary place of work, accompanied by an inability to recall one's past and confusion about personal identity or the assumption of a new identity.

Dissociative identity disorder (formerly called multiple personality disorder) is characterized by the presence of two or more distinct identities or personality states that recurrently take control of the individual's behavior, accompanied by an inability to recall important personal information that is too extensive to be explained by ordinary forgetfulness. It is a disorder characterized by identity fragmentation rather than a proliferation of separate personalities.

Depersonalization disorder is characterized by a persistent or recurrent feeling of being detached from one's mental processes or body that is accompanied by intact reality testing.

Clients with dissociative disorders, particularly dissociative identity disorder, commonly have been the victims of childhood abuse that may have been quite severe. Dissociation is a mechanism that protects the emotional self from the full impact of traumatic events, both during and after those events. As with other protective mechanisms, the individual's ability to dissociate becomes easier with repeated use. Dissociative experiences may begin to interfere with daily life, the individual's ability to function, and the ability to deal with the realities of the traumatic events.

Prevalence rates of the various types of dissociative disorders vary, but dissociative identity disorder is diagnosed more frequently in women than in men, and there may be a familial component to the disorder (APA, 2000). Dissociative disorders also vary greatly in intensity in different individuals. The onset of a dissociative disorder may be sudden or gradual, and the course episodic or chronic. Clients with dissociative disorders usually are engaged in long-term therapy in the community to deal with the myriad issues related to trauma and abuse. Some clients require hospitalization during times when their ability to function in daily life becomes so impaired that they need a protective environment. At these times, clients may have significant problems with eating, sleeping, overwhelming anxiety, and strong urges to harm themselves—ranging from risk-taking behavior and lack of care for safety, to self-mutilation, and even to suicide.

Survivors of rape, incest, or other trauma may experience physical pains, sleep and eating disturbances, and a variety of overwhelming feelings, such as shame, anxiety, depression, or no feelings at all. They also may "re-experience" the trauma, having both the feelings and the bodily sensations experienced at the time of the abuse, and often cope with these experiences by dissociating, as they did at the time of the trauma.

Often, a client may "block out" childhood abuse through dissociation and not report or deal with it until adulthood.

Controversy surrounds the accuracy of such reports, because childhood memories may be subject to distortion and some individuals with this disorder are highly hypnotizable and especially vulnerable to suggestive influences. However, reports by individuals with Dissociative Identity

Disorder of a past history of sexual or physical abuse are often confirmed by objective evidence. Furthermore, persons responsible for acts of physical and sexual abuse may be prone to deny or distort their behavior (APA, 2000, p. 527).

Dissociation often is portrayed in newspapers and other media in sensational ways, including stories of abuse allegations, which later are retracted, giving rise to doubts about the true existence of dissociative disorders. The Foundation of False Memory Syndrome in Philadelphia, Pennsylvania, was established to help combat what some people believe are false, damaging allegations of childhood abuse on family members or others by persons who are now adults.

Acute treatment for these clients focuses on safety and the improved ability to function in usual activities. It is not necessary or desirable for the nurse to become involved in long-term issues, and therapy sessions that deal with these issues often are modified or suspended during acute care episodes because the client's coping mechanisms are overwhelmed. When the client feels safe and is able to return to daily routines, therapy can resume if the client needs and wishes to continue.

NURSING DIAGNOSES ADDRESSED IN THIS CARE PLAN
Risk for Self-Mutilation
Ineffective Coping

RELATED NURSING DIAGNOSES ADDRESSED IN THE MANUAL
Anxiety
Bathing/Hygiene Self-Care Deficit
Dressing/Grooming Self-Care Deficit
Feeding Self-Care Deficit
Toileting Self-Care Deficit

Nursing Diagnosis

Risk for Self-Mutilation

At risk for deliberate self-injurious behavior causing tissue damage with the intent of causing nonfatal injury to attain relief of tension.

RISK FACTORS

- Self-harm urges (without lethal intent)
- Suicidal ideas, feelings, plans, attempts
- Inability to guarantee own safety
- Impulsivity
- Social isolation
- Anxiety
- Flashbacks
- Nightmares

EXPECTED OUTCOMES

Immediate

The client will

- Be safe and free from self-inflicted injury throughout hospitalization
- Agree to approach staff when feeling unsafe within 24 to 48 hours
- Be able to distinguish between ideas of self-harm and taking action on those ideas within 2 to 3 days
- Approach staff before acting on self-harm urges, by a specified date within 3 to 4 days

Stabilization

The client will

- Contract with himself or herself for safety
- Demonstrate use of alternative ways of dealing with stress and emotions
- Identify actions he or she can take to manage self-harm ideas or urges

Community   The client will

- Manage self-harm urges and ideas in nondestructive ways, for example, talk with others instead of acting on self-harm urges
- Continue with therapy after discharge if indicated

IMPLEMENTATION

Nursing Interventions *denotes collaborative interventions	Rationale
Determine the appropriate level of suicide or self-harm precautions for the client and explain the precautions fully to the client. See Care Plan 26: Suicidal Behavior.	Physical safety of the client is a priority.
Assess the client's suicide or self-harm potential, and evaluate the needed level of precautions at least daily.	The client's potential to harm himself or herself can vary; the risk may increase or decrease at any time.
Be alert to sharp objects and other potentially dangerous items (e.g., glass containers, lighters); these should not be in the client's possession when the client is not feeling safe.	Many common objects can be used in self-destructive ways. If the client lacks effective impulse control, he or she might use these objects if they are available.
If the client is at risk for serious self-harm, it may be necessary to use restraint or seclusion, with no objects that can be used for self-harm. If this is necessary, assure the client that he or she will be safe. Follow the facility's policies regarding seclusion and restraint, safety, and least restriction for the client.	Physical safety of the client is a priority. However, due to the history of trauma, the client may need to be reassured of his or her safety to minimize an increase in anxiety.
If the client is placed in seclusion or restraints, begin to talk to him or her about regaining internal control over his or her behavior as soon as possible.	To maximize the client's feelings of safety and control, it is especially important for the client to think about reassuming control of himself or herself at the onset of restraint or seclusion.
Discuss the client's ability to be safe openly and directly, in a matter-of-fact manner.	An open and nonjudgmental approach avoids conveying the message that the client is unworthy or bad, yet addresses the client's safety.
Initiate a "no self-harm" agreement as the client begins to manage his or her own safety. This contract is the client's agreement with himself or herself to avoid self-harm and keep himself or herself safe (as opposed to the client making this promise to the nurse).	Clients usually are able to be accurate and honest in reporting their ability to be safe. Because it is the client's responsibility to be safe, the agreement is with himself or herself. If a "promise" is made to the nurse, it may resemble a child's promise to a parent, which can undermine the client's self-reliance; then, if the client does engage in self-harm behaviors, he or she may have the added guilt of "letting down" another person.
Discuss the concept of having self-harm ideas as distinct from putting those ideas into action.	Many clients do not recognize the distinction between having ideas and urges of self-harm and acting out those ideas.
Tell the client that you believe he or she can gain control over self-harm behavior even if the urge for self-harm persists.	The client will benefit from knowing that the nurse believes he or she can gain control over self-harm behaviors.
Discuss activities or behaviors the client might use when self-harm urges are more intense, including contacting a friend, therapist, or significant other; physical activity; or other structured activity.	The client is less likely to act out self-harm ideas if he or she is otherwise occupied, or if he or she contacts someone and can express feelings verbally.
Talk with the client about coping strategies he or she has used successfully in the past.	The client may have had success using coping strategies in the past but may have lost confidence in himself or herself or in his or her ability to cope with stressors and feelings.
Teach the client about positive coping strategies and stress management skills, such as increasing physical exercise, expressing feelings verbally or in a journal, or meditation techniques. Encourage the client to practice this type of technique while in the hospital.	The client may have limited or no knowledge of stress management techniques or may not have used positive techniques in the past. If the client's anxiety diminishes by practicing these within the treatment setting, he or she can build on these skills in the future.

IMPLEMENTATION (continued)

Nursing Interventions *denotes collaborative interventions	Rationale
Teach the client the problem-solving process: identify the problem, examine alternatives, weigh the pros and cons of each alternative, select and implement an approach, and evaluate its success.	The client may be overwhelmed by anxiety in response to problems and will benefit from knowing how to deal with problems by using a logical, orderly process.
*Encourage the client to pursue interests, hobbies, volunteer work, or recreational activities that may appeal to the client. Consultation with a recreational therapist may be indicated.	Social isolation may contribute to anxiety and dissociation. Social contacts and recreational activities can serve as a structure for the client to experience positive relationships and enjoyment.

Nursing Diagnosis

Ineffective Coping

Inability to form a valid appraisal of the stressors, inadequate choices of practiced responses, and/or inability to use available resources.

ASSESSMENT DATA

- Feelings of being overwhelmed
- Feelings of worthlessness or hopelessness
- Guilt
- Difficulty identifying and expressing feelings
- Anxiety
- Lack of trust
- Social isolation
- Fatigue
- Low self-esteem
- Loss of personal control
- Feelings of helplessness
- Patterns of avoidance or escape behavior

EXPECTED OUTCOMES

Immediate

The client will

- Express feelings in a nondestructive manner, such as verbally, within 2 to 3 days
- Demonstrate decreased social isolation, for example, interact with staff or other clients at least twice per day within 2 to 3 days
- Focus on current functional abilities within 2 to 3 days

Stabilization

The client will

- Demonstrate alternative ways to deal with stress, including effective problem-solving
- Engage in social interaction about current topics at least four times per day by a specified date
- Assess own strengths and weaknesses realistically

Community

The client will

- Engage in productive activities such as school, work, recreation, and social events
- Report satisfying interpersonal experiences with others

IMPLEMENTATION

Nursing Interventions *denotes collaborative interventions	Rationale
Involve the client as much as possible in planning his or her own treatment.	The client's participation in his or her own plan of care can help to increase a sense of responsibility and control.
Approach the client for interaction. If the client says "I don't feel like talking," remain with the client in silence and indicate your willingness to sit together without talking; or state that you will be back at a later (specific) time.	Your presence demonstrates interest and caring, and promotes the building of trust. The client may be testing whether or not you are trustworthy, or may be attempting to remain isolated.
Give the client support for remaining out of his or her room, interacting with others, or attending activities.	The client's ability to interact with others is impaired. Positive feedback recognizes the client for his or her efforts.
Maintain the focus of care on the "here-and-now." Avoid the temptation to delve into therapy issues involving past abuse or trauma.	Treatment in the acute care setting is concerned with the client's safety and daily coping abilities. Therapy issues are long term and may be contributing to the client's feelings of being overwhelmed.
Encourage the client to identify and express fears and emotions; convey your acceptance of the client's feelings.	Discussion of feelings the client is experiencing at this time can help him or her work through these feelings and begin to distinguish between current and past feelings. Feelings are not inherently bad or good—they just are.
Help the client identify situations in which he or she is more comfortable expressing feelings; use role-playing to practice expressing emotions.	Expressing feelings can be helpful even if the feelings are uncomfortable for the client. Role-playing allows trying out new behaviors in a supportive environment.
Provide opportunities for the client to express emotions and release tension in a safe, nondestructive way, such as group discussion, activities, and physical exercise.	The client needs to develop skills with which to replace self-destructive behavior.
Help the client recognize early signs of anxiety.	The sooner the client recognizes the onset of anxiety, the more quickly he or she will be able to alter his or her response.
During the times the client is relatively calm, explore together ways in which he or she can deal with stress and anxiety.	The client will be better able to problem-solve when his or her anxiety level is lower.
Teach the client about the problem-solving process: identifying the problem, identifying and evaluating alternative solutions, choosing and implementing a solution, and evaluating its success.	The client may have never learned or may be neglecting to use a logical, step-by-step approach to problem resolution.
*Teach the client social skills, and encourage him or her to practice these skills with staff members and other clients. Give feedback regarding social interactions and discourage the client from discussing therapy, self-harm behaviors, and so forth in social situations.	The client may lack skills and confidence in social interactions, contributing to his or her isolation from others.
Encourage the client to pursue personal interests, hobbies, and recreational activities.	Recreational activities can help increase the client's social interaction and provide enjoyment. The client may have given up enjoyable activities or may have never learned to relax and have fun.
Give the client positive feedback as he or she begins to relax, express feelings, problem-solve, and so forth.	Positive feedback promotes the continuation of desired behavior.
Assist the client to identify specific community activities and make a written schedule to attend these events.	The client is more likely to follow through with community plans if he or she has a written plan.

SECTION 9 REVIEW QUESTIONS

1. Which of the following statements would indicate that teaching about somatization disorder has been effective?

   a. "The doctor believes I am faking my symptoms."

   b. "If I try harder to control my symptoms, I will feel better."

   c. "I will feel better when I start handling stress more effectively."

   d. "Nothing will help me feel better physically."

2. The nurse is caring for a client with a conversion disorder. Which of the following assessments will the nurse expect to see?

   a. Extreme distress over the physical symptom

   b. Indifference about the physical symptom

   c. Labile mood

   d. Multiple physical complaints

3. The nurse is caring for a client with a conversion disorder involving semi-paralysis of the lower extremities. The client has not come to the dining area for lunch.

Which of the following interventions would be most appropriate?

   a. Inform the client that he has 10 minutes to come to the dining room for lunch.

   b. Invite the client to lunch and accompany him to the dining room.

   c. Take the client's lunch tray to his room.

   d. Tell the client he'll have nothing to eat until dinner if he misses lunch.

4. A client with somatization disorder is referred to the outpatient clinic for problems with nausea, back pain, headaches, and problems with urination. The client tells the nurse that the nausea began when his wife asked him for a divorce. Which of the following would be most appropriate?

   a. Allowing the client to talk about his frustration with his symptoms

   b. Asking the client to describe his problem with nausea

   c. Directing the client to describe his feelings about the impending divorce

   d. Informing the client about medications used to treat nausea

SECTION 9 Recommended Readings

Asmundson, G. J., Abramowitz, J. S., Richter, A. A., & Whedon, M. (2010). Health anxiety: Current perspectives and future directions. *Current Psychiatric Reports, 12*(4), 306–312.

Conrado, L. A., Hounie, A. G., Diniz, J. B., Fossaluza, V., Torres, A. R., Miguel, E. C., & Rivitti, E. A. (2010). Body dysmorphic disorder among dermatologic patients: Prevalence and clinical features. *Journal of the American Academy of Dermatology, 63*(2), 235–243.

Schafer, I., Langeland, W., Hissbach, J., Luedecke, C., Ohlmeier, M. D., Chodzinski, C., … Driessen, M. (2010). Childhood trauma and dissociation in patients with alcohol dependence, drug dependence or both—A multi-center study. *Drug and Alcohol Dependence, 109*(1–3), 84–89.

Stone, J., Warlow, C., & Sharpe, M. (2010). The symptoms of functional weakness: A controlled study of 107 patients. *Brain: A Journal of Neurology, 133*(Pt. 5), 1537–1551.

Tocchio, S. L. (2009). Treatment of conversion disorder: A clinical and holistic approach. *Journal of Psychosocial and Mental Health Services, 47*(8), 42–49.

SECTION 9 Resources for Additional Information

Visit thePoint (http://thePoint.lww.com/Schultz9e) for a list of these and other helpful Internet resources.

Academy of Psychosomatic Medicine
American Professional Society on the Abuse of Children
American Psychosomatic Society
Foundation of False Memory Syndrome
International Society for the Study of Trauma and Dissociation
MedlinePlus
National Center for Trauma-Informed Care
Sidran Institute

Eating Disorders

The care plans in this section deal with maladaptive eating patterns that are long-term conditions: anorexia nervosa and bulimia nervosa. Clients with eating disorders are often mistakenly believed to be well adjusted, successful, and happy. Underlying that facade, however, the person attempts to deal with conflicts and emotions through destructive food-related behaviors. Eating disorders are complex problems that may require treatment in acute care settings, outpatient treatment, family or individual therapy, and years of work to overcome.

Behaviors and problems related to eating are seen in many different disorders and are briefly addressed in many of the care plans found in other sections of this *Manual*. The client's nutritional state is directly related to physical health and often influences, or is influenced by, emotional or psychiatric problems as well. Other types of problems related to nutritional intake are addressed in Care Plan 52: The Client Who Will Not Eat.

CARE PLAN 36

Anorexia Nervosa

Anorexia nervosa is an eating disorder "characterized by a refusal to maintain a minimally normal body weight" (i.e., the client weighs approximately 15% or more below ideal body weight), an intense fear of becoming obese, a distortion of body image, and amenorrhea (in postmenarchal women) (APA, 2000, p. 583). A number of characteristics have been noted in clients with anorexia, including depression, obsessive thoughts or compulsive behaviors, rigid thinking, and perfectionism. These clients have been said to lack a sense of identity and to feel helpless and ineffectual in their lives. They may be using weight loss as a means of controlling their bodies (which gives a sense of control in their lives) or avoiding maturity (Day, Ternouth, & Collier, 2009).

The cause of anorexia nervosa remains unknown, although biologic, psychological, familial, and sociocultural theories have been proposed. A precipitating factor sometimes can be identified that involves a major stress or change in the client's life related to maturing (e.g., puberty, first sexual encounter), leaving the family home (e.g., going to college), or loss. Obesity, real or perceived, and dieting at an early age are risk factors for anorexia nervosa (Day et al., 2009); however, it is much more complex than a diet taken too far.

Some evidence suggests both a familial pattern and a genetic component for anorexia nervosa (APA, 2000). Family dynamics appear to play a significant role in the development of anorexia nervosa; these families have been described as being enmeshed (having intense relationships and a lack of boundaries), overprotective, rigid, and lacking effective conflict resolution. In addition, a history of sexual abuse is reported in 30% of clients with anorexia (Ross, 2009).

In the United States, the lifetime prevalence of anorexia is reported as 0.9% in females and 0.3% in males (Hudson, Hiripi, Pope, & Kessler, 2006). Anorexia nervosa is more common in industrialized countries, and cultural factors may play a role in its development. Thinness, especially in women, is highly valued in some aspects of American culture, and women often internalize the societal message that they will be judged on their appearance rather than their abilities. The socialization of women may be confusing and overwhelming to adolescent and young adult women (e.g., conflicting messages regarding dependence versus independence, achieving in a career versus nurturing a family, etc.). Many characteristics noted in women with anorexia are ascribed to the female role in American society (dependency, pleasing others, helpfulness, and sensitivity).

More than 90% of clients with anorexia nervosa are female, though the disorder does occur in males. Prevalence in females has been estimated at 0.5% (APA, 2000) and as high as 1% in adolescent and young adult females (Black & Andreasen, 2011). Onset usually occurs in adolescence; it rarely occurs before puberty or after 40 years of age. This disorder may be a lifelong chronic illness or may be restricted to an acute episode; it also can occur with bulimia nervosa. An episode of anorexia nervosa may be described as *restricting* (if the client is using restriction of food or excess exercise to lose weight) or *binge eating/purging* (if the client is using purging behavior, with or without binging) (APA, 2000).

Anorexia nervosa can have grave physical consequences; mortality related to malnutrition, complications, and suicide has been reported as between 10% and 20%. Anorexia nervosa often requires long-term treatment and follow-up; success in treatment varies, but early recognition and treatment increase chances for recovery (Black & Andreasen, 2011).

During acute treatment episodes, nursing care is focused on keeping the client safe, facilitating or providing treatment for medical problems, and providing adequate nutrition and hydration. Other therapeutic goals include decreasing the client's withdrawn, depressive, manipulative, or regressive behavior, and preventing secondary gain. It is important to remain focused on the client's eventual discharge and to help the client build self-esteem, social skills, and non–food-related coping mechanisms. Because family dynamics are often a part of the client's illness, it is also important to assess the client's home environment, teach the client and family about the client's anorexia, and refer the client and family for continued treatment as indicated.

NURSING DIAGNOSES ADDRESSED IN THIS CARE PLAN
Imbalanced Nutrition: Less Than Body Requirements
Ineffective Coping

RELATED NURSING DIAGNOSES ADDRESSED IN THE MANUAL
Ineffective Denial
Chronic Low Self-Esteem
Disturbed Sensory Perception (Specify: Visual, Auditory, Kinesthetic, Gustatory,
    Tactile, Olfactory)
Noncompliance
Powerlessness
Ineffective Health Maintenance
Risk for Self-Mutilation
Risk for Suicide

Nursing Diagnosis

Imbalanced Nutrition: Less Than Body Requirements
Intake of nutrients insufficient to meet metabolic needs.

ASSESSMENT DATA

- Weight loss
- Body weight 15% or more under ideal body weight
- Refusal to eat
- Denial or loss of appetite
- Inability to perceive accurately and respond to internal stimuli related to hunger or nutritional needs
- Epigastric distress
- Vomiting
- Difficulty swallowing
- Use or abuse of laxatives
- Retaining feces and urine, eating large amounts of salt, or concealing weights on body to increase weight measurement
- Denial of illness or resistance to treatment
- Denial of being (too) thin
- Feelings of guilt, shame, or remorse after eating or eating certain foods
- Excessive exercise
- Physical problems or changes (may be life-threatening) that include malnutrition; starvation; pale, dry skin; poor skin turgor; little subcutaneous tissue; lanugo (soft, downy body hair); edema; constipation; amenorrhea, cardiac arrhythmias, bradycardia, or mitral and tricuspid valve prolapse; low basal metabolic rate; hypothermia; decreased mental acuity and concentration; hypotension; poor muscle tone and function; osteoporosis and fractures; absent secondary sexual characteristics; anemia and leukopenia; hypoglycemia; hypercholesterolemia; reduced serum immunoglobulins and increased susceptibility to infection and sepsis; impaired renal function; diabetes insipidus; decreased urinary 17-ketosteroids, estrogens, testosterone, and gonadotropins; fluid and electrolyte imbalance.

EXPECTED OUTCOMES

Immediate   The client will

- Increase caloric and nutritional intake, for example, will eat 30% of meals within 4 to 5 days
- Demonstrate improvement in physical status related to the physical complications of anorexia nervosa within 3 to 4 days
- Be free of complications of malnutrition within 6 to 8 days
- Maintain skin integrity throughout hospitalization
- Demonstrate weight gain, for example, will gain at least 2 pounds within 5 to 7 days

Stabilization   The client will

- Develop an adequate nutritional state, for example, fluid and electrolyte balance will be within normal range by a specified date
- Demonstrate regular, independent, nutritional eating habits
- Demonstrate continued improvement in physical status

Community   The client will

- Maintain a healthy weight level
- Meet nutritional goals independently

IMPLEMENTATION

Nursing Interventions *denotes collaborative interventions	Rationale
Note: It is especially important to use the following interventions selectively in developing an individual care plan for the client. There are several different kinds of interventions presented here that can be used with different approaches to the care of clients with anorexia. Some measures may be appropriate for clients whose nutritional state is severely compromised (total parenteral nutrition or nasoduodenal tube feedings), whereas others may be more effective in decreasing the attention given to food itself (e.g., to focus only on weight, not on intake and output) with a client whose nutritional state is not as severely compromised. You may want to develop a specific protocol for each client, with nursing interventions (e.g., tube feedings, supervision at and after meals) and client privileges based on compliance with calorie consumption or weight gain.	
If the client is critically malnourished:	
Parenteral nutrition through a central catheter may be indicated. Monitor the client closely for signs and symptoms of infection.	Adequate nutrition, electrolytes, and so forth can be provided parenterally. The client has no opportunity to vomit this kind of nutritive substance. The client's immune system may be compromised related to malnutrition and a central line catheter provides a portal for infection.
Tube feedings may be used alone or with oral or parenteral nutrition. Use of a feeding tube may be effective.	Fortified liquid diets can be provided through tube feedings. The use of a feeding tube decreases the chance of vomiting or siphoning feedings.
Supervise the client for a specified time (initially 90 minutes, decreasing gradually to 30 minutes) after tube feeding, or remove the tube after feeding.	Supervision decreases the client's opportunity to vomit or siphon feedings. Removing the tube prevents siphoning feedings.
Offer the client the opportunity to eat food orally. Use tube feedings if the client consumes insufficient calories or loses weight or if indicated by medical condition (electrolytes and acid–base balance). Decrease tube feedings as oral consumption becomes adequate.	The client may prefer to eat food orally rather than have a tube feeding; however, the client's physical health is a priority.

IMPLEMENTATION (continued)

Nursing Interventions *denotes collaborative interventions	Rationale
When tube feeding is indicated (see above), insert the tube immediately in a matter-of-fact, nonpunitive manner, and administer feeding. Do not use tube feeding as a threat or punishment, and do not allow bargaining.	Limits and consistency are essential in avoiding power struggles and decreasing manipulative behavior. Remember, tube feedings are medical treatment, not punishment.
Parenteral nutrition or tube feedings may be best administered at night.	Using these methods at night may decrease attention given to the client by others and will interfere less in the client's daytime activities.
General interventions (consider for any client):	
*Monitor the client's vital signs, electrolytes, acid–base balance, liver enzymes, albumin, and other medical measures as indicated and ordered by the physician.	The client's physical health is a priority. Information regarding the client's clinical state is necessary to plan effective nursing care.
Monitor the client's intake and output. Keep records at the nursing station (not at the client's bedside or room) and do not allow the client to complete records. Observations of intake and output should be made in an unobtrusive and matter-of-fact manner.	The client may provide inaccurate information on intake or output records. It is important to minimize direct attention given for eating and to remove emotional issues from food and eating.
Establish a contract with the client regarding treatment, if the client will agree.	Contracting can promote the client's sense of control and self-responsibility and help establish goals, but is ineffective if the client is not in agreement with its terms.
Initially, do not allow the client to eat with other clients or visitors.	Other clients may repeat family patterns by urging the client to eat or giving attention to the client for not eating.
Provide a structure to the client's mealtimes. Tell the client when it is time to eat, present the food, and state limits in a consistent matter-of-fact manner.	Clear limits let the client know what is expected.
Do not bribe, coax, or threaten the client or focus on eating at all; withdraw your attention if the client refuses to eat. When the mealtime is over, remove food without discussion.	It is important to minimize the client's secondary gain from not eating. Issues of control (especially regarding eating) are central to the client's problem and must not be reinforced.
Supervise the client during and after meals (initially for 90 minutes, then decrease gradually). Do not allow the client to use the bathroom until at least 30 minutes after each meal.	The client may spill, hide, or discard food. The client may use the bathroom to vomit or dispose of concealed foods.
Provide a pleasant, relaxing environment for eating, and minimize distractions. Encourage the use of relaxation techniques, rest, and quiet before and after meals.	The client may have significant anxiety and guilt about eating, making mealtime very stressful.
Encourage the client to seek out a staff member after eating to talk about feelings of anxiety or guilt or if the client has the urge to vomit.	Talking with a staff member promotes a focus on emotional issues rather than on food. The client may feel guilt, remorse or shame after eating or eating certain foods (e.g., foods perceived as fattening by the client).
Allow the client increasing choices regarding food, mealtime, and so forth.	The client needs to develop independence in eating habits.
Grant and restrict privileges based on weight gain (or loss) and do not focus on eating, mealtimes, calorie counts, or physical activity. If weight loss occurs, decrease privileges and talk with the client to explore the circumstances and feelings involved.	Decreasing direct attention given to food and eating encourages the client to focus on emotional issues instead.
Weigh the client daily, after the client has voided and before the morning meal, with the client wearing only a hospital gown. Measure weight in a matter-of-fact manner; do not approve or disapprove of weight gain or loss.	Consistency is necessary for accurate comparison of weight over time. The client may retain urine or conceal weights on his or her body to increase weight measurement. Weight gain or loss is a measure of health, not of success or failure. A matter-of-fact attitude will help separate emotional issues from the client's eating (or noneating) behaviors.

(continued on page 248)

IMPLEMENTATION (continued)

Nursing Interventions *denotes collaborative interventions	Rationale
Monitor the client's elimination patterns. The client's diet should include sufficient fiber and adequate amounts of fluids.	The client may be constipated or have less frequent stools. Bulk and fluid promote adequate elimination.
Discourage the client's use of enemas, laxatives, or suppositories.	The client may abuse laxative preparations as a means of controlling weight.
Observe and record the client's physical activity; be aware that this may be covert (e.g., jogging in the shower, doing calisthenic exercises in bed).	The client may exercise to excess to control weight.
You may need to structure exercise activities into the client's treatment plan. Do not forbid all physical exercise unless the client is critically ill and exercise would be truly harmful or unsafe.	Restricting physical activity too severely may greatly increase the client's anxiety (see Care Plan 30: Obsessive-Compulsive Disorder). Also, moderate exercise is a valuable long-term health behavior and should not be discouraged.
Provide skin care, especially over bony prominences.	The client is at risk for skin breakdown due to diminished nutrition and lack of muscle and subcutaneous tissue.
Encourage the client to use a shower for bathing.	Sitting in a bathtub may be uncomfortable for the client due to bony prominences and lack of muscle or subcutaneous tissue.
Provide warm bedding. Be aware of room air temperatures.	The client is especially apt to feel cold because of decreased fat and subcutaneous tissue.
*Provide or encourage dental hygiene. Referral to a dentist may be appropriate.	The client's teeth or gums may be in poor condition due to the effects of vomiting (decreased tooth enamel from contact with gastric fluids) and malnutrition.
Gradually decrease limits on meals and snacks, and allow the client more control over food intake, choice of foods, preparation, and so forth.	The client needs to develop independent eating habits.
Give positive feedback for healthy eating behaviors.	Positive support tends to reinforce desired behaviors.
Be aware of your role in modeling healthy behavior.	You are a role model for the client.
*Assess the client's knowledge of weight, nutrition, and so forth. Client teaching may be indicated; this should be done in factual and unemotional terms and should be limited in frequency and duration. Refer the client to a dietitian for detailed instruction if appropriate.	The client may have false ideas about food, weight, and nutrition. The client needs to decrease his or her emotional investment in food or eating. Areas outside the nursing area of expertise are best referred to other health professionals.
Do not engage in nonteaching interactions with the client on topics of food and eating.	This allows you to focus on emotional issues with the client and limits focusing on food and eating.
Discharge should not occur until the client has reached a healthy weight, as agreed in the treatment plan. This limit should be maintained without bargaining after the goal has been set (although the client may have initial input into the goal).	The client's physical health is a priority. Bargaining may undermine the limit. Allowing the client's input in the treatment plan can encourage cooperation and enhance the client's sense of control.

Nursing Diagnosis

Ineffective Coping

Inability to form a valid appraisal of the stressors, inadequate choices of practiced responses, and/or inability to use available resources.

ASSESSMENT DATA

- Denial of illness or resistance to treatment
- Inability to ask for help
- Inability to problem-solve
- Inability to meet basic needs
- Inability to meet role expectations
- Feelings of helplessness or powerlessness
- Depressive behavior
- Anxiety
- Guilt
- Anger
- Suicidal ideas or feelings
- Manipulative behavior
- Regressive behavior
- Hyperactivity
- Sleep disturbances, such as early awakening
- Social isolation
- Decreased sexual interest
- Rumination
- Refusal to eat
- Dread of certain foods or types of foods (such as carbohydrates)
- Disgust at the thought of eating
- Preoccupation with food
- Hiding or hoarding food
- Preoccupation with losing weight
- Unceasing pursuit of thinness
- Intense fear of becoming obese
- Family problems
- Low self-esteem
- Problems with sense of identity
- Delusions
- Body image distortions

EXPECTED OUTCOMES

Immediate

The client will

- Be free from self-inflicted injury throughout hospitalization
- Participate in treatment program, for example, participate in at least one activity per shift or two interactions per shift within 2 to 3 days
- Demonstrate decreased manipulative, depressive, or regressive behavior and suicidal ideas and feelings within 3 to 4 days
- Demonstrate beginning trust relationships with others within 3 to 4 days
- Verbalize recognition of perceptual distortions (e.g., distorted body image) within 4 to 5 days
- Identify non–food-related coping mechanisms, for example, talking with others about feelings, keeping a journal within 4 to 5 days
- Interact with others in non–food-related ways within 3 to 4 days
- Demonstrate increased social skills, for example, approach others for interaction, make eye contact, and so forth within 3 to 4 days

Stabilization

The client will

- Demonstrate more effective interpersonal relationships with family or significant others
- Exhibit age-appropriate behavior, for example, complete school assignments on time without prompting by staff

- Demonstrate change in attitudes about food and eating
- Verbalize increased feelings of self-worth
- Demonstrate non–food-related coping mechanisms
- Demonstrate decreased associations between food and emotions
- Verbalize knowledge of illness and medications, if any

Community

The client will

- Participate in continuing therapy after discharge, if appropriate
- Demonstrate independence and age-appropriate behaviors
- Verbalize a realistic perception of body image

IMPLEMENTATION

Nursing Interventions *denotes collaborative interventions	Rationale
Assess and observe the client closely for self-destructive behavior or suicidal intent. See Care Plan 26: Suicidal Behavior.	Clients with anorexia nervosa are at risk for self-destructive behaviors. The client's safety is a priority.
Initially, limit the number of staff assigned to and interacting with the client, then gradually increase the variety of staff interacting with the client. See Care Plan 1: Building a Trust Relationship, Care Plan 25: Major Depressive Disorder, and Care Plan 45: Withdrawn Behavior.	Initially limiting the number of staff can build trust, maximize consistency, and minimize manipulation.
*Maintain consistency of treatment. One staff member per shift should be identified to have the final word on all decisions (although other staff members and the client may have input).	Consistency minimizes the possibility of manipulation of staff members by the client.
Supervise or remain aware of the client's interactions with others and intervene as appropriate.	Other clients or visitors, especially family members, may reinforce manipulative behavior or provide secondary gain for the client's not eating.
Do not restrict the client to his or her room as a restriction of privileges.	Social isolation may be something the client desires or may be part of the client's disorder.
Remember the client's age, and relate to the client accordingly. Expect age-appropriate behavior from the client.	The client may appear to be younger than his or her actual age and may want to be dependent and avoid maturity and responsibility.
Expect healthy behavior from the client.	When a client is diagnosed with an illness, you may expect and inadvertently reinforce behaviors characteristic of the disorder.
Encourage the client to do schoolwork while in the hospital if the client is missing school due to hospitalization.	Schoolwork is a normal part of an adolescent's life. The client may receive a secondary gain from not being expected to do schoolwork or by falling behind in school.
Give the client positive support and honest praise for accomplishments. Focus attention on the client's positive traits and strengths (not on feelings of inadequacy).	Positive support tends to provide reinforcement for desired behaviors.
Do not flatter or be dishonest in interactions with or feedback to the client.	The client will not benefit from dishonest praise or flattery. Honest, positive feedback can help build self-esteem.
Foster successful experiences for the client. Arrange for the client to help other clients in specific ways, and suggest activities to the client that are within his or her realm of ability, then increase complexity as appropriate.	Any activity that the client is able to complete provides an opportunity for positive feedback.
*Use group therapy and role-playing with the client. Give the client feedback on his or her behaviors and the reactions of others.	The client can share feelings and try out new behaviors in a supportive, nonthreatening environment. The client may lack insight into his or her behaviors and their consequences or effects on others.

IMPLEMENTATION (continued)

Nursing Interventions *denotes collaborative interventions	Rationale
*Be aware of your own feelings about the client and his or her behaviors. Express your feelings to other staff members rather than to the client.	You may have strong feelings of helplessness, frustration, and anger in working with this client. Working through your feelings will decrease the possibility of acting them out in your interactions with the client.
Be nonjudgmental in your interactions with the client. Do not express approval or disapproval or be punitive to the client.	Issues of control, approval, and guilt often are problems with the client. Nonjudgmental nursing care decreases the possibility of power struggles.
Remain aware of your own behavior with the client. Be consistent, truthful, and nonjudgmental.	Staff members are the client's role models for appropriate behavior and self-control.
*Make referrals for recreational and occupational therapy as appropriate.	The client may need to learn non–food-related ways to relax, spend leisure time, and so forth.
Allow the client food only at specified snack and meal times. Do not talk with the client about emotional issues at these times. Encourage the client to ventilate his or her feelings at other times in ways not associated with food.	It is important for the client to separate emotional issues from food and eating.
Withdraw your attention if the client is ruminating about food or engaging in rituals with food or eating.	Minimizing attention given to these behaviors may help decrease them.
Observe and record the client's responses to stress. Encourage the client to approach the staff at stressful times.	The client may be unaware of his or her responses to stress and may need to learn to identify stressful situations.
Help the client identify others in the home environment with whom the client can talk and who can be supportive. Identify non–food-related activities that may decrease stress or anxiety (e.g., hobbies, writing, drawing).	The client needs to learn new skills to deal with stress.
As tolerated, encourage the client to express his or her feelings regarding achievement, family issues, independence, social skills, sexuality, and control.	These issues often are problem areas for clients with anorexia.
See Care Plan 28: Anxious Behavior.	
*Assess the client's home environment. Interview the client's family, make a home visit if possible, or observe the family's behavior at mealtime. Encourage the family's participation in family therapy if indicated.	Family dynamics are often involved in the development and progression of anorexia nervosa, and family therapy can be successful in treating the disorder.
Encourage the client to ventilate his or her feelings about family members, family dynamics, family roles, and so forth.	Ventilation of feelings can help the client identify, accept, and work through feelings, even if these are painful or uncomfortable for the client.
Send the client home for a specified, limited period of time, then evaluate the success of this trial period with the client in the hospital before discharge. Observe and record the client's feelings, mood, and activities before and after time at home.	Hospitalization may decrease pressure for the client by removing the client from home and by interrupting family dynamics. Returning home may increase the client's stress and result in weight loss or other anorexic behaviors.
*Include the client's family or significant others in teaching, treatment, and follow-up plans. Teaching should include dynamics of illness, nutrition, and medication use, if any.	Family dynamics may play a significant role in anorexia nervosa.
*Assist the client and the family to arrange for follow-up therapy. Encourage contact with the follow-up therapist before discharge.	Follow-up and long-term therapy for the client and the family can be effective in preventing future weight loss. Meeting the therapist prior to discharge can help lessen the client's anxiety.

(continued on page 252)

IMPLEMENTATION (continued)

Nursing Interventions *denotes collaborative interventions	Rationale
*Refer the client and family to support groups in the community or via the internet (e.g., the National Anorexic Aid Society for Anorexia Nervosa and Associated Disorders). However, caution the client and family about internet groups that encourage anorexia and provide guidance regarding evaluation of online resources.	Support groups sponsored by professional organizations can offer support, education, and resources to clients and their families. Some internet groups, however, encourage eating-disordered behavior and unhealthy weight loss and can undermine therapeutic goals.
See Care Plan 2: Discharge Planning.	

CARE PLAN 37

Bulimia Nervosa

Bulimia nervosa, or *bulimia,* is an eating disorder characterized by recurrent episodes of binge eating and the use of inappropriate activities (e.g., self-induced vomiting, laxative misuse) to prevent weight gain (APA, 2000). During binge eating, the client rapidly consumes very large amounts of food at one time; these episodes may occur from two times a week to several times a day.

Clients with bulimia, especially those who use purging and fasting as weight-control measures, may be at, near, or under their ideal body weight. Clients with bulimia often experience a distortion of body image (perceiving themselves as fat even when thin) and body image dissatisfaction; their level of self-esteem often is strongly related to their perception of their weight. These clients often are ashamed of their eating behaviors and try to keep them secret. During binge eating, the client may experience feelings of being out of control or of dissociation. Clients with bulimia may be severely malnourished and often experience medical complications, such as fluid and electrolyte imbalances, which can be severe and life threatening.

Some evidence indicates that clients with bulimia have an increased risk for mood disorders and substance abuse, and their family members have an increased risk for bulimia (APA, 2000). These clients often have histories or family histories of substance abuse, impulsive behavior (e.g., shoplifting and promiscuity), affective disorders (e.g., major depressive disorder, self-mutilation, or suicidal behavior), anxiety disorders, or personality disorders (Black & Andreasen, 2011). Many clients with bulimia report a history of dieting behavior and of having been overweight before developing bulimia.

Clients with bulimia are usually female (at least 90%). In the United States, lifetime prevalence of bulimia and binge-eating in females is reported to be 1.5% and 3.5%, respectively, and 0.5% and 2%, respectively, in males (Hudson et al., 2006). Onset usually occurs in late adolescence or the early twenties. The course of this disorder often is long term, with intermittent or chronic symptoms.

Treatment of clients with bulimia often is long term and can involve both medications and psychotherapy; antidepressant medications have been effective in bulimia (Black & Andreasen, 2011). Periods of hospitalization, if they occur, are relatively short and may occur only during medical or psychiatric crises. These clients may be seen initially on a medical unit due to physical complications from binge–purge behaviors, malnutrition, and so forth. It is important to identify these eating-disordered clients, refer them for therapy, and encourage them to follow through with treatment for the eating disorder.

Nursing goals with clients in treatment for bulimia or excessive eating involve working with the client to meet both physiologic and psychological needs. These goals include:

- Providing a safe environment
- Promoting adequate nutritional intake and retention
- Providing or facilitating treatment for associated physical problems (e.g., constipation, dental problems, fluid and electrolyte imbalance, etc.)
- Encouraging the client's participation in treatment
- Decreasing the client's anxiety
- Decreasing perceptual distortions
- Promoting the client's sense of control regarding himself or herself, relationships, and life situation
- Promoting the client's understanding of and insight into his or her behavior or disorder
- Promoting the client's self-esteem and ability to assess self realistically
- Promoting the client's development of coping skills, supportive relationships, and resources for continued therapy

NURSING DIAGNOSES ADDRESSED IN THIS CARE PLAN
Imbalanced Nutrition: Less Than Body Requirements
Imbalanced Nutrition: More Than Body Requirements
Ineffective Coping

RELATED NURSING DIAGNOSES ADDRESSED IN THE MANUAL
Ineffective Denial
Noncompliance
Chronic Low Self-Esteem
Disturbed Sensory Perception (Specify: Visual, Auditory, Kinesthetic, Gustatory,
    Tactile, Olfactory)
Anxiety

Nursing Diagnosis

Imbalanced Nutrition: Less Than Body Requirements
Intake of nutrients insufficient to meet metabolic needs.

Imbalanced Nutrition: More Than Body Requirements
Intake of nutrients that exceeds metabolic needs.

ASSESSMENT DATA

- Weight gain or loss
- Overuse of laxatives, diet pills, or diuretics
- Dysfunctional eating patterns
- Binge eating
- Compulsive eating
- Feelings of guilt, remorse, or shame after eating
- Diuretic use
- Laxative use
- Inadequate nutritional intake
- Excessive caloric intake
- Secrecy regarding eating habits or amounts eaten
- Recurrent vomiting after eating
- Physical signs and symptoms: ulceration or scarring on dorsal surface of hand or finger calluses (from manually stimulating vomiting), hypertrophy of salivary or parotid glands, erosion of dental enamel (from acidity of emesis), ulcerations around mouth and cheeks (from emesis splashback)
- Physical problems or changes (may be life-threatening): fluid and electrolyte imbalances, including dehydration and volume depletion, hypokalemia, hyponatremia, hypomagnesemia, and hypocalcemia; cardiac problems, including electrocardiogram disturbances, heart failure, and myopathy; metabolic alkalosis or acidosis; seizures; hypotension; elevated aldosterone level; edema of hands and feet; fatigue; muscle weakness, soreness, or cramps; headache; nausea; laxative dependence; gastrointestinal problems, including constipation, colitis, malabsorption disorders, delayed gastric emptying, gastric bleeding, ulcers, or rupture; sore throat; emetine toxicity (from ipecac misuse); elevated serum amylase; esophagitis, esophageal erosions, bleeding, stricture, or perforation; pancreatitis; hypoglycemia; disturbance in hormone levels; irregular menses.

EXPECTED OUTCOMES

Immediate

The client will

- Interrupt binge (binge–purge) eating patterns within 24 to 48 hours
- Be free from use of diuretics, laxatives, or diet pills throughout hospitalization
- Evidence improvement in physical status related to complications of bulimia or excessive eating, for example, the client's fluid and electrolyte levels will be within normal limits within 5 to 7 days
- Demonstrate regular (adequate, not excessive) nutritional eating behavior within 5 to 7 days

Stabilization

The client will

- Maintain normal bowel elimination without laxatives
- Eliminate binge (binge–purge) eating patterns
- Continue to evidence improvement in physical status related to complications of bulimia or excessive eating
- Establish regular (adequate, not excessive) nutritional eating patterns

Community

The client will

- Maintain regular (adequate, not excessive) nutritional eating patterns
- Verbalize acceptance of stable body weight within 10% of ideal body weight

IMPLEMENTATION

Nursing Interventions *denotes collaborative interventions	Rationale
Monitor the client's laboratory values for electrolyte imbalance.	Persistent vomiting, diuretic use, or use of laxatives can result in hypokalemia, hyponatremia, dehydration, and metabolic alkalosis or acidosis.
Spend time with the client after meals. Avoid letting the client go to the bathroom or to an isolated area unaccompanied.	Vomiting behavior usually is secretive. The client may feel guilty and anxious about having eaten, and your presence can deter vomiting and be supportive to the client.
*Help the client determine a daily meal plan that contains an appropriate number of calories, includes all food groups, and provides adequate nutrition. Consultation with a dietitian is helpful.	A meal plan provides a structure for the client's eating behavior. Though the client may be preoccupied with food, he or she may not know about the type and amounts of food that constitute a healthful diet.
Initially, allow the client to avoid some foods the client fears or sees as bad, as long as he or she gets adequate nutrition.	The client's anxiety may be increased if he or she is unable to avoid certain foods, and he or she can exercise some control by being allowed to avoid certain foods.
Gradually include foods that the client has avoided as forbidden or fattening or has come to fear (e.g., carbohydrates).	Gradual introduction of feared foods will help minimize the client's anxiety and help the client learn that these foods are not harmful.
When the client feels the urge to binge, go on a walk with the client or engage in other distracting activities. Encourage the client to use physical activity to deal with the urge to binge but not to use excessive exercise as a weight control measure.	Physical activity can provide a release for feelings that promote binge behavior. It also is a way to postpone eating until mealtime.
Have the client measure and record weight daily. Avoid letting the client weigh more than once a day or skip daily weight measures.	The client may have avoided weight measurement because he or she is convinced of being overweight. Clients may binge or purge based on feeling fat rather than on actual weight.
Discourage the client's use of diuretics, diet pills, or laxatives. Ask the client to relinquish these items. You may need to search the client's belongings, with the client's permission.	Continued use of diuretics, diet pills, or laxatives reinforces bulimic behavior and can have severe medical consequences.

(continued on page 256)

IMPLEMENTATION (continued)

Nursing Interventions *denotes collaborative interventions	Rationale
Discontinue laxative use. The client's diet should have adequate fiber to promote normal elimination. If the client is constipated, use glycerin suppositories to stimulate evacuation.	Laxative dependence must be eliminated. Judicious use of glycerin suppositories will not foster dependence as do laxatives.
*Be alert to the possibility of the client asking friends or family to smuggle food, laxatives, or other drugs to him or her. Talk with the client and his or her visitors if necessary.	The client may feel out of control or panicked when binge foods, laxatives, or other drugs are not available. The client's significant others can be supportive of the client's health by not reinforcing bulimic behaviors.
Be nonjudgmental and matter of fact in your approach to the client and his or her behavior.	This approach will not reinforce the client's already excessive feelings of guilt and shame.

Nursing Diagnosis

Ineffective Coping
Inability to form a valid appraisal of the stressors, inadequate choices of practiced responses, and/or inability to use available resources.

ASSESSMENT DATA

- Inability to meet basic needs
- Inability to ask for help
- Inability to problem-solve
- Inability to change behaviors
- Self-destructive behavior
- Suicidal thoughts or behavior
- Inability to delay gratification
- Poor impulse control
- Stealing or shoplifting behavior
- Desire for perfection
- Feelings of worthlessness
- Feelings of inadequacy or guilt
- Unsatisfactory interpersonal relationships
- Self-deprecatory verbalization
- Denial of feelings, illness, or problems
- Anxiety
- Sleep disturbances
- Low self-esteem
- Excessive need to control
- Feelings of being out of control
- Preoccupation with weight, food, or diets
- Distortions of body image
- Overuse of laxatives, diet pills, or diuretics
- Secrecy regarding eating habits or amounts eaten
- Fear of being fat
- Recurrent vomiting
- Binge eating
- Compulsive eating
- Substance use

EXPECTED OUTCOMES

Immediate	The client will

- Be free from self-inflicted harm throughout hospitalization
- Identify non–food-related methods of dealing with stress or crises, for example, initiate interaction with others or keep a journal, within 2 to 3 days
- Verbalize feelings of guilt, anxiety, anger, or an excessive need for control within 3 to 4 days

Stabilization	The client will

- Demonstrate more satisfying interpersonal relationships
- Demonstrate alternative methods of dealing with stress or crises
- Eliminate shoplifting or stealing behaviors
- Express feelings in non–food-related ways
- Verbalize understanding of disease process and safe use of medications, if any

Community	The client will

- Verbalize more realistic body image
- Follow through with discharge planning, including support groups or therapy as indicated
- Verbalize increased self-esteem and self-confidence

IMPLEMENTATION

Nursing Interventions *denotes collaborative interventions	Rationale
Ask the client directly about thoughts of suicide or self-harm. See Care Plan 26: Suicidal Behavior.	The client's safety is a priority. You will not give the client ideas about suicide by addressing the issue directly.
Set limits with the client about eating habits, for example, food will be eaten in a dining room setting, at a table, only at conventional mealtimes. Convey the expectation that the client will eat three meals per day; do not allow the client to skip meals.	Setting and maintaining limits on eating behaviors will discourage binge behavior, such as hiding, sneaking, and gulping food, and help the client return to normal eating patterns. Eating three meals a day will prevent self-starvation during the day and subsequent overeating in the evening.
Encourage the client to eat with other clients, when tolerated.	Eating with other people will discourage secrecy about eating, though initially the client's anxiety may be too high to join others at mealtime.
Encourage the client to express feelings, such as anxiety and guilt about having eaten.	Expressing feelings can help decrease the client's anxiety and the urge to engage in purging behaviors.
Encourage the client to use a diary to write types and amounts of foods eaten and feelings that occur before, during, and after eating, especially related to urges to engage in binge or purge behavior.	A diary can help the client explore food intake, feelings, and relationships among these feelings and behaviors. Initially, the client may be able to write about these feelings and behaviors more easily than talk about them.
Discuss the types of foods that are soothing to the client and that relieve anxiety.	You may be able to help the client see how he or she has used food to deal with feelings.
Maintain a nonjudgmental approach when discussing the client's feelings.	Being nonjudgmental gives the client permission to discuss feelings that may be negative or unacceptable to him or her without fear of rejection or reprisal.
Encourage the client to describe and discuss feelings verbally. However, avoid discussing food-related feelings during mealtimes and begin to separate dealing with feelings from eating or purging behaviors.	Separating feelings from food-related behaviors will help the client identify non–food-related ways to express and deal with feelings.
Help the client explore ways to relieve anxiety, express feelings, and experience pleasure that are not related to food or eating.	It is important to help the client separate emotional issues from food and eating behaviors.

(continued on page 258)

IMPLEMENTATION (continued)

Nursing Interventions *denotes collaborative interventions	Rationale
Give positive feedback for the client's efforts to discuss feelings.	Your sincere praise can promote the client's attempts to deal openly and honestly with anxiety, anger, and other feelings.
Encourage the client to express his or her feelings about family members and significant others, their roles and relationships.	Expressing feelings can help the client to identify, accept, and work through feelings in a direct manner.
*Teach the client and significant others about bulimic behaviors, physical complications, nutrition, and so forth. Refer the client to a dietitian if indicated.	The client and significant others may have little knowledge of the illness, food, and nutrition. Factual information can be useful in dispelling incorrect beliefs and in separating food from emotional issues.
*Encourage the client and significant others to discuss feelings and interpersonal issues in non–food-related settings (i.e., discourage discussion of family problems at mealtimes). Referral for family therapy may be indicated.	The client's significant others may not understand the importance of separating emotional issues from foods and food-related behaviors.
*Teach the client and significant others about the purpose, action, timing, and possible adverse effects of medications, if any.	Antidepressant and other medications may be prescribed for bulimia. Remember some antidepressant medications may take several weeks to achieve a therapeutic effect.
Teach the client about the use of the problem-solving process: identify the problem, examine alternatives, weigh the pros and cons of each alternative, select and implement an approach, and evaluate its success.	Successful use of the problem-solving process can help increase the client's self-esteem and confidence.
Explore with the client his or her personal strengths. Making a written list is sometimes helpful.	You can help the client discover his or her strengths, but it will not be useful for you to make a list for him or her. The client needs to identify his or her own strengths for this to be most effective.
Discuss with the client the idea of accepting a less than "ideal" body weight.	The client's previous expectations or perception of an ideal weight may have been unrealistic, and even unhealthy.
Encourage the client to incorporate fattening (or "bad") foods into his or her meals as tolerated.	This will enhance the client's sense of control of overeating.
*Refer the client to assertiveness training books or classes if indicated.	Many clients with bulimia are passive in interpersonal relationships. Assertiveness training may foster a sense of increased confidence and healthier relationship dynamics.
*Refer the client to long-term therapy if indicated. Contracting with the client may be helpful to promote follow through with continuing therapy.	Treatment for eating disorders often is a long-term process. The client may be more likely to engage in ongoing therapy if he or she has contracted to do this.
*Ongoing therapy may need to include significant others to sustain the client's non–food-related coping skills.	Dysfunctional relationships with significant others often are a primary issue for clients with eating disorders.
*Refer the client and family and significant others to support groups in the community or via the internet (e.g., Anorexia Nervosa and Associated Disorders, Overeaters Anonymous). Provide guidance regarding identification and use of internet sites.	Support groups sponsored by professional organizations can offer support, education, and resources to clients and their families or significant others. Some internet groups, however, encourage eating-disordered behavior and can undermine therapeutic goals.
*Refer the client to a substance dependence treatment program or substance dependence support group (e.g., Alcoholics Anonymous), if appropriate. See Care Plan 17: Substance Dependence Treatment Program.	Substance use is common among clients with bulimia.
See Care Plan 2: Discharge Planning.	

SECTION 10 REVIEW QUESTIONS

1. The nurse is caring for a client with anorexia nervosa. Even though the client has been eating all her meals and snacks, her weight has remained unchanged for 1 week. Which of the following interventions is indicated?

   a. Supervise the client closely for 2 hours after meals and snacks.

   b. Increase the daily caloric intake from 1,500 to 2,000 calories.

   c. Increase the client's fluid intake.

   d. Request an order from the physician for an anti-anxiety medication.

2. The nurse is evaluating the progress of a client with bulimia. Which of the following behaviors would indicate that the client is making positive progress?

   a. The client can identify the calorie content for each meal.

   b. The client identifies healthy ways of coping with anxiety.

   c. The client spends time resting in her room after meals.

   d. The client verbalizes knowledge of former eating patterns as unhealthy.

3. A client diagnosed with bulimia tells the nurse that she eats excessively when she is upset and then vomits so she won't gain weight. Which of the following nursing diagnoses would be most appropriate for this client?

   a. Anxiety

   b. Disabled Family Coping

   c. Imbalanced Nutrition: More Than Body Requirements

   d. Ineffective Coping

4. When teaching a group of adolescents about anorexia nervosa, the nurse would describe this disorder as being characterized by which of the following?

   a. Excessive fear of becoming obese, near-normal weight, and a self-critical body image

   b. Extreme concern about dieting, calorie-counting, and an unrealistic body image

   c. Intense fear of becoming obese, emaciation, and a disturbed body image

   d. Obsession with the weight of others, chronic dieting, and an altered body image

SECTION 10 Recommended Readings

Feldman, M. B., & Meyer, I. H. (2010). Comorbidity and age of onset of eating disorders in gay men, lesbians, and bisexuals. *Psychiatry Research, 180*(2–3), 126–131.

Fitzsimmons, E. E., & Bardone-Cone, A. M. (2010). Differences in coping across stages of recovery from and eating disorder. *International Journal of Eating Disorders, 43*(8), 689–693.

Hartmann, A., Zeeck, A., & Barrett, M. S. (2010). Interpersonal problems in eating disorders. *International Journal of Eating Disorders, 43*(7), 619–627.

Roberto, C. A., Grilo, C. M., Masheb, R. M., & White, M. A. (2010). Binge eating, purging, or both: Eating disorder psychopathology findings from an internet community survey. *International Journal of Eating Disorders, 43*(8), 724–731.

Segura-Garcia, C., Ammendolia, A., Procopio, L., Papaianni, M. C., Sinopoli, F., Bianco, C., … Capranica, L. (2010). Body uneasiness, eating disorders, and muscle dysmorphia in individuals who overexercise. *Journal of Strength and Conditioning Research, 24*(11), 3098–3104.

Tury, F., Gulec, H., & Kohls, E. (2010). Assessment methods for eating disorders and body image disorders. *Journal of Psychosomatic Research, 69*(6), 601–611.

SECTION 10 Resources for Additional Information

Visit thePoint (http://thePoint.lww.com/Schultz9e) for a list of these and other helpful Internet resources.

Academy for Eating Disorders
American Dietetic Association
Eating Disorder Referral and Information Center
Eating Disorders Anonymous
Eating Disorders Association of Canada
Eating Disorders Coalition for Research, Policy, & Action
Eating Disorders Treatment Help: A Toolkit
International Association of Eating Disorders Professionals Foundation
National Association of Anorexia Nervosa and Associated Disorders
National Eating Disorder Information Centre
National Eating Disorders Association
National Women's Health Information Center
Overeaters Anonymous
The Renfrew Center Foundation

Sleep Disorders and Adjustment Disorders

Clients with sleep disorders and adjustment disorders are rarely seen in the acute care setting for these diagnoses alone. These clients may be encountered in a variety of other health care settings, such as clinics, outpatient settings, or in the office of their primary care provider. Nursing care is focused on assisting the client to re-establish healthful patterns of physiologic functioning and more effective methods of coping with stress and life events.

CARE PLAN 38

Sleep Disorders

Sleep disturbances are a common complaint that can be associated with a variety of emotional or physical disorders or that can occur as a primary symptom. Transient sleep disturbances can be a normal part of life, sometimes associated with an identifiable psychosocial stressor. According to the *DSMIVTR* (APA, 2000), *sleep disorders* are categorized as primary, related to another mental disorder, due to a general medical condition, or substance-induced. When a sleep problem is substance-induced or related to another mental disorder, specific criteria must be met to diagnose a sleep disorder. This care plan presents information related to clients with sleep disturbances or sleep disorders; those problems usually found in mental health and substance abuse clients include both *insomnia* (difficulty falling asleep, staying asleep, or experiencing a restful sleep) and *hypersomnia* (excess sleep).

Sleep disturbances are commonly seen in major depressive disorder, bipolar disorder, anxiety disorders, schizophrenia, adjustment disorders, post-traumatic stress disorder, somatoform disorders, and personality disorders (APA, 2000). Problems with sleep may also be related to excess caffeine intake, alcohol or substance use or abuse, or as an effect of certain medications.

Sleep problems are seen in both men and women and at any age. Insomnia occurs more commonly than hypersomnia in clients with other mental disorders. The onset of sleep problems may occur in concert with other mental health problems, for example, insomnia during a manic episode. Or sleep difficulties may be chronic and long term, for example, in a client with post-traumatic stress disorder. It is common for people to attempt self-medication with prescription or over-the-counter drugs or alcohol. Though this may have a beneficial effect temporarily, prolonged use of these remedies may result in further sleep problems.

When sleep disturbances are related to an identifiable cause, such as manic behavior, treatment will be directed primarily toward that cause. However, assisting the client with other measures to facilitate restful sleep can enhance the therapeutic effects of treatment or help the client rest when an underlying cause cannot be identified or the client fails to respond fully to treatment. Teaching the client and family or significant others about sleep and the effects of chemicals, foods, and fluids on sleep, facilitating relaxation, and establishing and practicing a bedtime routine are other valuable interventions.

NURSING DIAGNOSIS ADDRESSED IN THIS CARE PLAN
Insomnia

RELATED NURSING DIAGNOSIS ADDRESSED IN THE MANUAL
Anxiety

Nursing Diagnosis

Insomnia
A disruption in amount and quality of sleep that impairs functioning.

ASSESSMENT DATA

- Inadequate amount of sleep
- Unrefreshing sleep
- Difficulty falling asleep
- Periods of wakefulness during desired hours of sleep
- Fragmented sleep pattern
- Nightmares, night terrors
- Preoccupation with not obtaining restful sleep

EXPECTED OUTCOMES

Immediate

The client will

- Identify factors that facilitate sleep within 24 to 48 hours
- Eliminate or minimize factors that inhibit restful sleep within 2 to 4 days
- Establish regular hours for sleeping within 2 to 4 days
- Verbalize decreased anxiety about sleep difficulties within 2 to 4 days

Stabilization

The client will

- Fall asleep within 30 minutes after going to bed
- Sleep an adequate number of hours (considering age, activity level, previous sleeping patterns) each night
- Report feeling refreshed when awakening
- Verbalize diminished fatigue, anxiety

Community

The client will

- Participate in or verbalize plans for treatment of related problems
- Verbalize knowledge about sleep disturbance and effects of activity, medications, or chemicals on sleep

IMPLEMENTATION

Nursing Interventions *denotes collaborative interventions	Rationale
Substitute decaffeinated products for coffee, tea, or soda. Discourage use of chocolate and cocoa products.	Chemical stimulants, such as caffeine, will interfere with sleep.
Offer a limited amount of milk as a substitute for other bedtime beverages.	Milk products contain L-tryptophan, which is a natural sedative.
Avoid full meals and foods that cause gastric distress at least 3 hours prior to bedtime.	After 3 hours the stomach has emptied, and the client will not feel uncomfortable. Gastric distress interferes with relaxation.
Provide a light bedtime snack (small amounts of well-tolerated food) for the client.	Hunger can awaken people if they sleep lightly or have difficulty sleeping.
Limit fluid intake for 4 to 5 hours before bedtime.	Limiting fluid intake can eliminate awakening due to a full bladder.
If the client smokes, advise him or her to have the last cigarette at least 30 minutes before bedtime.	Nicotine is a central nervous system stimulant.

(continued on page 264)

IMPLEMENTATION (continued)

Nursing Interventions *denotes collaborative interventions	Rationale
Encourage the client to increase physical activity during waking hours, even though he or she may feel fatigued. However, limit vigorous physical activity for 2 hours prior to bedtime.	The client may avoid physical activity due to a lack of energy, but activity during the day will promote a feeling of physical "tiredness," which can facilitate sleep. The stimulating effects of physical activity last for several hours and interfere with efforts to relax prior to bedtime.
*Teach the client about the effects of alcohol on sleep. The client should refrain from alcohol intake until restful sleep patterns are established.	Although alcohol can produce initial drowsiness, when the initial effects wear off, fragmented sleep results. The greater the alcohol intake, the more fragmented the sleep will be.
*Educate the client about the effects of sleeping medications. If the client has been using sleep medications regularly, it may be best to decrease the frequency and dosage of such medications gradually.	Sleep-inducing medications can become ineffective when used regularly, or the client may feel unrefreshed after sleep due to a decrease in rapid eye movement (REM) sleep resulting from some medications. Abrupt cessation of sleep medications may increase sleep difficulties.
Assist the client to determine the desired number of sleeping hours each night, then designate times to retire and to rise to obtain that amount of sleep.	Regular hours help establish a routine. If the client waits to go to bed until he or she "feels sleepy," sleep patterns may be erratic.
Encourage the client to avoid naps, unless indicated by age or physical condition.	Daytime napping may interfere with the ability to sleep an adequate number of hours at night, unless there is a physiologic need for additional sleep.
Limit the client's attempts to sleep to his or her bed rather than on the couch or in a recliner. The client should use the bed only for sleep-related activities, rather than to talk on the telephone or work and so forth.	These actions will enhance the client's expectation that going to bed facilitates sleep and ability to sleep.
Provide an atmosphere conducive to sleep (e.g., dim light, quiet).	External stimuli or disturbances interfere with sleep.
Assist the client to identify factors that induce relaxation, either former habits that were effective or new behaviors.	The client may not have experience in purposeful relaxation before retiring.
*Teach the client progressive relaxation techniques and encourage practice. The use of an audio relaxation program may be helpful.	Relaxation techniques frequently are helpful in facilitating sleep, but need to be practiced to be fully effective.
Suggest that the client try a warm bath, reading, or other nonstimulating activities for relaxation.	The client may have to try several activities to determine which ones are effective.
If the client does not feel drowsy 20 minutes after retiring, suggest that he or she get up and engage in 20 minutes of a quiet activity that is boring for the client (e.g., reading or knitting), then return to bed. This should be repeated until the client begins to feel ready for sleep.	Lying in bed for extended periods can increase the client's focus on and frustration with sleeping difficulties. Monotonous activities can facilitate drowsiness.
Encourage the client to practice these techniques and maintain the bedtime routine consistently for a minimum of 2 weeks, even if there seems to be no benefit.	A minimum of 2 weeks may be needed to fully evaluate the effectiveness of newly initiated sleep-promoting activities.
*Educate the client's family or significant others about sleep, relaxation, and the need for bedtime routines. Enlist their support for the client's efforts.	The client's family or significant others may have little or no knowledge about these areas and may unwittingly interfere with the client's sleep.
*Encourage the client to seek treatment for problems that may adversely affect sleep.	Sleep disturbances are associated with many physical and psychiatric problems and may not entirely be resolved without treatment of the associated problem.

CARE PLAN 39

Adjustment Disorders of Adults

An *adjustment disorder* involves a maladaptive reaction to an identified psychosocial stressor or change. The severity of the client's reaction may be described as excessive in that the client experiences greater distress and impairment in social or occupational functioning than would be expected from the observed severity of the stressor.

Adjustment disorders are further specified according to the primary feature, such as adjustment disorders with anxious mood, depressed mood, withdrawal, and so forth. Although these features may be similar to other diagnoses, they are not severe enough to be diagnosed as anxiety, depression, or other such disorders.

An adjustment disorder may be related to developmental milestones, such as graduation, marriage, retirement, and so forth. Not all stressors are "negative" life events; some are generally perceived as happy occasions and many have been awaited with great anticipation, such as the birth of a child.

Clients who experience adjustment disorders typically cope with day-to-day life effectively, provided there are no major changes in their roles or in the expectations placed on them. However, major life changes or the culmination of several smaller stressors results in the client's inability to deal with the change.

Adjustment disorders can occur at any age. More adult women than men are diagnosed with adjustment disorders, though prevalence rates vary. Between 2% and 8% of the elderly and over 10% of medical inpatients referred for mental health services are diagnosed with adjustment disorders (APA, 2000). An adjustment disorder occurs within 3 months after the onset of a stressor and is expected to remit within 6 months after the stressor is no longer present or when the client reaches a new level of adaptation (APA, 2000).

Nursing care includes facilitating the client's expression of feelings associated with the stressor and helping the client build coping skills to successfully adapt to stressors. Also, it is important for the nurse to work with the interdisciplinary treatment team to identify resources for continued treatment and support.

NURSING DIAGNOSIS ADDRESSED IN THIS CARE PLAN
Ineffective Coping

RELATED NURSING DIAGNOSES ADDRESSED IN THE MANUAL
Situational Low Self-Esteem
Ineffective Role Performance
Anxiety

Nursing Diagnosis

Ineffective Coping
Inability to form a valid appraisal of the stressors, inadequate choices of practiced responses, and/or inability to use available resources.

ASSESSMENT DATA

- Feelings of inadequacy or being overwhelmed
- Difficulty with problem-solving
- Loss of control over life situation

- Mild mood alterations
- Low self-esteem
- Emotional reactions that are disproportional to life stressors
- Difficulty fulfilling occupational or social role expectations
- History of successful coping skills
- Imminent or recent change in life status
- Occurrence of a significant life event within the past 3 months

EXPECTED OUTCOMES

Immediate   The client will

- Identify difficulties of current life change or stress within 24 to 48 hours
- Express relief from feelings of anxiety, fear, or helplessness within 2 to 4 days
- Identify personal strengths within 3 to 5 days

Stabilization   The client will

- Verbalize feelings of self-worth, for example, verbally identify areas of strength or capabilities
- Demonstrate the ability to solve problems effectively

Community   The client will

- Demonstrate successful resolution of the current crisis
- Demonstrate integration of the change into day-to-day functioning

IMPLEMENTATION

Nursing Interventions *denotes collaborative interventions	Rationale
Assist the client to identify aspects of the change that he or she likes and dislikes.	The client may need help viewing the change as having both positive and negative aspects. Identifying dislikes may be particularly important if the change is supposed to be a happy one, such as retirement.
Have the client make a written list of the aspects identified.	A written list may provide a more concrete way of specifying positive and negative aspects. Once a negative aspect is written, the client can move on to identify others, rather than dwelling on one particular aspect.
Explore with the client ways in which he or she might view the change more constructively, such as "It sounds like you have more time with your son away at college. What are some things you always wanted to do if you had more time?"	Many times the client is focused on the change or loss. Exploring positive alternatives can help broaden the client's perspective.
Avoid giving the client specific suggestions, such as "Wouldn't you like to…" or "How about trying…."	If the client is having negative feelings, he or she may respond to your suggestions with reasons why they won't work. Allowing the client to identify suggestions gives the client the responsibility for ideas.
Encourage the client to express feelings and explore vague feelings. For example, if the client feels overwhelmed, ask if he or she is scared, angry, and so forth.	Outward expression of feelings is a way of acknowledging and beginning to deal with them. The more specific the feelings, the easier it is for the client to deal with them.
Give positive feedback for expressing feelings, particularly negative ones.	Your acceptance helps the client see that negative feelings are normal, not necessarily "good" or "bad."
Help the client identify his or her strengths and difficulties in dealing with changes. Have the client make written lists.	The client may have difficulty recognizing strengths. Written lists provide a concrete method for seeing assets.
Help the client identify past ways of coping that were successful and encourage him or her to apply them to the present situation.	The client can build on his or her successful coping skills to deal with the current situation.

IMPLEMENTATION (continued)

Nursing Interventions *denotes collaborative interventions	Rationale
Teach the client the problem-solving process: identify the problem, examine alternatives, weigh the pros and cons of each alternative, select and implement an approach, and evaluate its success.	The client may not know the steps of a logical, orderly process to solve problems.
Help the client evaluate the success or failure of a new approach and encourage him or her to try another if the first was unsuccessful.	The client needs to know that he or she can make a mistake without it being a tragedy and needs support to try again.
*Encourage the client to ask for the help of family or significant others in dealing with aspects of the change.	The help of family or significant others enhances the chance for likelihood of success.
*Help the client and significant others to anticipate future changes. Encourage them to talk about ways to deal with changes before they occur, when possible.	Once the client identifies that change is difficult for him or her, it is helpful to preplan for dealing with future changes.

SECTION 11 REVIEW QUESTIONS

1. Which of the following interventions would the nurse implement for the client who is having difficulty sleeping?

   a. Allow the client to stay up until he or she is sleepy.

   b. Engage the client in physical activity.

   c. Invite the client to play a game of cards with the nurse.

   d. Teach the client to use relaxation exercises before bedtime.

2. A client is diagnosed with an adjustment disorder. He tells the nurse, "I just can't get over being laid off. I've talked to family and friends, but nothing helps. No one really understands. I don't know what to do." Which of the following would be most beneficial for this client initially?

   a. Managing feelings and emotions

   b. Referral for vocational counseling

   c. Support system assessment

   d. Unemployment assistance

3. A client comes to the mental health clinic. She says she has been "going downhill" since her youngest child went off to college. She adds that her husband and friends are no help because they keep telling her how wonderful it must be to finally have time for herself. Which of the following is the best initial response by the nurse?

   a. "Describe the angry feelings you're having toward your family and friends."

   b. "Do you have any plans about how to spend your free time?"

   c. "Tell me about the positive and negative aspects of this change in your life."

   d. "What would you identify as the underlying cause for your problems?"

4. A client tells the nurse, "I think I'll have some wine before bed each night to help me sleep." Which of the following would be the best response by the nurse?

   a. "Alcohol can be helpful since it makes you drowsy."

   b. "Alcohol can often increase problems with sleeping."

   c. "Drinking wine every night can lead to alcoholism."

   d. "You can try that and see if it's helpful for you."

SECTION 11 Recommended Readings

Edge, L. C. (2010). The role of brain processing during sleep in depression. *Journal of Psychiatric and Mental Health Nursing, 17*(10), 857–861.

Engin, E., Keskin, G., Dulgerler, S., & Bilge, A. (2010). Anger and alexithymic characteristics of the patients diagnosed with insomnia: A control group study. *Journal of Psychiatric and Mental Health Nursing, 17*(8), 692–699.

Garms-Homolova, V., Flick, U., & Rohnsch, G. (2010). Sleep disorders and activities in long term care facilities—A vicious cycle? *Journal of Health Psychology, 15*(5), 744–754.

Roustit, C., Renahy, E., Guermec, G., Lesieur, S., Parizot, I., & Chauvin, P. (2009). Exposure to interparental violence and psychosocial maladjustment in the adult life course: Advocacy for early prevention. *Journal of Epidemiology and Community Health, 63*(7), 563–568.

Sacker, A., & Cable, N. (2010). Transitions to adulthood and psychological distress in young adults born 12 years apart: Constraints on and resources for development. *Psychological Medicine, 40*(2), 301–313.

SECTION 11 Resources for Additional Information

Visit thePoint (http://thePoint.lww.com/Schultz9e) for a list of these and other helpful Internet resources.

American Academy of Sleep Medicine
Anxiety Disorders Association of America
Associated Professional Sleep Societies
National Guidelines: Insomnia, Narcolepsy
National Institute of Mental Health: Anxiety Disorders
National Sleep Foundation
Sleep Research Society

Personality Disorders

A personality disorder is evidenced by a client's enduring pattern of thinking, believing, and behaving that deviates markedly from the expectations of his or her culture (APA, 2000). The individual has difficulties with impulse control, interpersonal functioning, cognition, or affect. These maladaptive coping patterns and skewed perceptions of self or others are long-standing and are present in many life situations even though they are ineffective or cause significant distress or impaired functioning.

Clients with borderline personality disorder or antisocial personality disorder may be encountered in mental health or other health care settings for difficulties associated with these diagnoses or as they seek treatment for medical conditions unrelated to emotional or mental health problems. Clients with other psychiatric diagnoses may also have a personality disorder that makes their care more complex.

CARE PLAN 40

Paranoid Personality Disorder

Paranoid behavior is characterized by lack of trust, suspicion, grandiose or persecutory delusions, and hostility. A number of psychiatric disorders may include paranoid behavior, for example, paranoid schizophrenia, delusional disorder, depression, dementia, sensory or sleep deprivation, and substance use. *Paranoid personality disorder* is a specific disorder in which a client has persistent personality traits comprising a pattern of thought, emotions, and behavior reflecting consistent distrust of others (APA, 2000).

In addition to a pervasive mistrust of others, clients with paranoid personality disorder may have fantasies or even delusions that are *grandiose* (e.g., he or she is a prominent religious or political figure), *destructive* (e.g., getting even with tormentors), or *conspiratorial* (e.g., groups of people are watching, following, torturing, or controlling the client). This may involve *ideas of reference*—the client thinks that statements by others or events are caused by or specifically meant for him or her (e.g., that a television program was produced to send the client a message). Many clients with paranoid behavior have above-average intelligence, and their delusional systems may be very complex and appear to be logical.

No clear etiology has been identified for paranoid personality disorder, but both environmental and hereditary factors may play roles in its development. The psychodynamics of paranoid behavior may be rooted in an earlier experience of loss or disappointment that is unconsciously denied by the client. The client uses the defense mechanism of projection to ascribe to others the feelings he or she has (as a result of those earlier experiences and denial) and attempts to protect himself or herself with suspiciousness. The client may have extremely low self-esteem or feel powerless in life and compensate with delusions to mitigate those feelings.

Paranoid personality disorder is diagnosed more often in men than in women, and its prevalence in the United States has been estimated at 0.5% to 2.5% (Sadock & Sadock, 2008). These clients are at increased risk for other mental health problems, including psychotic episodes, delusional disorder, substance abuse, and other personality disorders. Paranoid personality disorder usually develops early in life, often in adolescence or early adulthood, and persists over time as a chronic disorder.

Treatment focuses on managing symptoms (e.g., aggression, depression) and often includes medication management and limit setting. It is especially important for the nurse to ensure a safe environment, be consistent, and remain aware of any of his or her own behaviors that may be perceived as threatening or as a basis for mistrust, such as inconsistency, secretiveness, and not keeping one's word. Misperceptions may also include culturally based perceptions of humiliation, embarrassment, or behaviors deemed inappropriate in the client's culture that may be acceptable in the nurse's culture.

Nursing goals include ensuring the client's ingestion of medications and promoting trust. Although full trust may not be possible to achieve with clients whose mistrust is severe, consistency and reliability will help ensure the maximum level of trust. Also, because the mistrust in paranoid behavior often leads to social isolation, facilitating successful interactions between the client and others is an important goal that can enhance the client's success after discharge.

NURSING DIAGNOSES ADDRESSED IN THIS CARE PLAN
Disturbed Thought Processes
Defensive Coping
Impaired Social Interaction
Ineffective Self-Health Management

RELATED NURSING DIAGNOSES ADDRESSED IN THE MANUAL
Ineffective Health Maintenance
Insomnia
Risk for Other-Directed Violence
Anxiety

Nursing Diagnosis

Disturbed Thought Processes
Disruption in cognitive operations and activities.

*Note:** This nursing diagnosis was retired in *NANDA-I Nursing Diagnoses: Definitions & Classification 2009–2011*, but the NANDA-I Diagnosis Development Committee encourages work to be done on retired diagnoses toward resubmission for inclusion in the taxonomy.

ASSESSMENT DATA

- Non–reality-based thinking
- Disorganized, illogical thoughts
- Impaired judgment
- Impaired problem solving
- Alterations in perceptions (hallucinations, ideas of reference)
- Delusions, especially grandiose and persecutory
- Sensory deprivation or overload
- Suicidal ideation
- Rumination
- Hostility, aggression, or homicidal ideation

EXPECTED OUTCOMES

Immediate

The client will

- Be free from self-inflicted harm throughout hospitalization
- Refrain from harming others throughout hospitalization
- Demonstrate decreased psychotic symptoms, for example, be free of hallucinations within 3 to 4 days

Stabilization

The client will

- Verbalize recognition that others do not share his or her paranoid ideas
- Demonstrate reality-based thinking, for example, talk with others about events without expressing paranoid ideas

Community

The client will

- Demonstrate recognition of paranoid ideas as distinct from reality
- Act on reality-based thinking, not paranoid ideas
- Validate ideas with a trusted person, such as a significant other or case manager, prior to acting on ideas

IMPLEMENTATION

Nursing Interventions *denotes collaborative interventions	Rationale
Search the client's belongings carefully for weapons; also search the client's vehicle, if at the facility.	Clients with paranoid behavior may carry or conceal weapons.
Be calm and nonthreatening in all your approaches to the client, using a quiet voice; do not surprise the client.	If the client is feeling threatened, he or she may perceive any person or stimulus as a threat.
Note environmental factors (e.g., noise level, the number of other people) that precipitate or exacerbate symptoms, and try to decrease these factors (see Care Plan 47: Aggressive Behavior).	Assessment provides information on which to base interventions. The client's ability to deal with stimuli or other people is impaired.
Observe the client closely for agitation, and decrease stimuli or move the client to a less stimulating area or secluded area if indicated.	Whenever possible, it is best to intervene before the client loses control. The client's ability to deal with stimuli may be impaired.
Be aware of PRN medication orders and prepare to administer them if needed.	The client's agitation may require medication if he or she becomes dangerous to others or to himself or herself.
Administer medications in liquid or injectable form as needed to ensure ingestion.	The client may hide an oral medication in his or her mouth, then discard when not being observed. *Note:* some oral medications are irritating to mucous membranes; observe precautions as indicated.
Observe the client's interactions with visitors. The length, number, or frequency of visits may need to be limited.	The client's ability to deal with other people may be impaired.
Do not argue with the client about delusions or ideas of reference, but interject reality when appropriate (you might say, "I don't see it that way."). Do not give any indication that you believe as the client does.	Introducing and reinforcing reality may help diminish psychotic symptoms.
Do not joke with the client regarding his or her beliefs.	The client's ability to understand and use abstractions, such as humor, is impaired.
Do not enter into political, religious, or other controversial discussions with the client.	Controversial discussions may precipitate arguments and increase hostility or aggression.
Encourage the client to discuss topics other than delusions such as home life, work, or school.	Concrete or familiar topics may be helpful in directing the client's attention to reality.
Do not allow the client to ruminate about delusions; if the client refuses to discuss other topics, talk with the client about his or her feelings regarding the delusions or withdraw your attention, stating your intent to return.	It is important to minimize reinforcement of psychotic symptoms. Talking about feelings may help the client begin to deal with emotional issues. It must be clear that you accept the client as a person even if you reject his or her behavior.
*If the client has religious delusions, referral to the facility chaplain may be indicated (if the chaplain has education or experience in this area).	Areas beyond nursing's scope require referral to appropriate people or agencies.
You may need to reassure the client that his or her fears are internal and not based on external reality.	Reassurance of the safety of his or her environment may help diminish the client's fears.

Nursing Diagnosis

Defensive Coping

Repeated projection of falsely positive self-evaluation based on a self-protective pattern that defends against underlying perceived threats to positive self-regard.

ASSESSMENT DATA

- Lack of trust, suspicion
- Low self-esteem
- Fears
- Feelings of powerlessness
- Projection of blame on others
- Rationalization
- Superior attitude toward others
- Ineffective interpersonal relationships

EXPECTED OUTCOMES

Immediate

The client will

- Demonstrate decreased fears within 24 to 48 hours
- Demonstrate decreased suspicious behavior within 2 to 3 days

Stabilization

The client will

- Verbalize realistic feelings of self-worth
- Verbalize realistic self-assessment

Community

The client will

- Demonstrate more direct, constructive ways to deal with stress, loss, feelings of powerlessness, and so forth

IMPLEMENTATION

Nursing Interventions *denotes collaborative interventions	Rationale
Introduce and identify yourself as a staff member on your first approach to the client (and thereafter if necessary). Be nonthreatening in all your approaches to the client.	The client may be fearful, suspicious, or not in contact with reality.
Assure the client that the environment is safe and protective, that the staff will help him or her maintain control, and that he or she will not be "in trouble" for having feelings.	The client may fear that personal feelings may be overwhelming or unacceptable, or that experiencing feelings may cause him or her to lose control.
Give the client clear information regarding his or her safety, confidentiality, identity and function of staff members, and so forth.	Giving matter-of-fact information will help to reassure and reorient the client.
If the client is pacing, walk with the client to converse if necessary.	You must meet the client at his or her level of functioning. Your willingness to walk with the client indicates caring and can interrupt ruminating or other symptoms.
If the client is experiencing hallucinations or illusions, try to talk with him or her in an area of decreased stimuli.	External stimuli may be misperceived by the client, and he or she is unable to deal with excess stimuli.
Let the client see the notes that you take during interviews. Answer questions honestly with little or no hesitation.	Open and direct behavior on your part may help decrease suspicion.
Include the client in the formulation of the treatment plan when possible and appropriate.	Including the client may help build trust and decrease suspicion and feelings of powerlessness.
Do not be secretive or whisper to others in the presence of the client.	Secretive behavior will reinforce the client's suspicion.
Approach the client at least once per shift and encourage him or her to express feelings. Determine the length of interactions by the client's tolerance.	Expressing feelings can help the client identify, accept, and work through feelings, even if they are painful or otherwise uncomfortable.

(continued on page 274)

IMPLEMENTATION (continued)

Nursing Interventions *denotes collaborative interventions	Rationale
If the client seems to be experiencing intense emotions, point this out and explain what leads you to think this (e.g., the client's facial expression). Ask for the client's perceptions.	The client may be unaware of emotions he or she is experiencing. Giving the client feedback in a nonthreatening way may help him or her recognize emotional cues.
Encourage the client to express feelings verbally or in other outward ways (such as physical activity).	Physical exercise and talking about feelings can help the client decrease tension and deal with feelings directly.
Use role-playing to elicit the expression of feelings ("Pretend that I'm your [husband, wife, etc.]. What would you like to say to me?").	Role-playing allows the client to explore feelings and try out new behaviors in nonthreatening situations.
Demonstrate honest interest in and concern for the client; do not flatter the client or be otherwise dishonest.	Clients with low self-esteem do not benefit from flattery or undue praise. These can be seen as dishonest and belittling.
Support the client for his or her participation in activities, treatment, and interactions.	Positive feedback can reinforce desired behaviors.
Provide opportunities for the client to perform activities that are easily accomplished or that the client likes to do. Provide recognition and support for their completion or success.	The client's abilities to deal with complex tasks may be impaired. Any task that the client can complete provides an opportunity for positive feedback to the client.

Nursing Diagnosis

Impaired Social Interaction
Insufficient or excessive quantity or ineffective quality of social exchange.

ASSESSMENT DATA

- Avoidance of others
- Limited verbal responses
- Discomfort around others
- Refusal to communicate with others
- Mistrust of others
- Social isolation
- Hostile or aggressive behavior

EXPECTED OUTCOMES

Immediate   The client will

- Interact with staff, for example, for 15 minutes at least twice per day within 24 to 48 hours
- Attend small group activities, for example, for at least 15 minutes at least twice per day within 2 to 3 days

Stabilization   The client will

- Express personal feelings directly by talking with staff, family, or significant others
- Express own needs

Community   The client will

- Communicate effectively with family or significant others
- Demonstrate ability to interact with others for brief periods or for basic purposes of daily living

IMPLEMENTATION

Nursing Interventions *denotes collaborative interventions	Rationale
Initially, the staff may need to protect the client from other clients' responses to his or her paranoid or grandiose behavior.	The client may be hostile or abusive to other clients who may not recognize this as the client's illness.
Initially, limit the number of different staff members assigned to interact with the client.	Limiting the number of new contacts initially will provide consistency and promote trust.
After the client's initial days on the unit, begin assigning different staff members to him or her and encourage other staff members to approach him or her for brief interactions.	The number of people interacting with the client should increase as soon as possible to facilitate communication and relationships with a variety of people.
*Help the client make individual contacts with staff members and other clients; progress to small groups, then larger groups as the client tolerates.	The client's ability to respond to others may be impaired, so it is best to begin with a single person, then progress to more difficult situations as the client's comfort and skills increase.
Observe the client's interactions with other clients, and encourage the development of appropriate relationships with others. Give the client feedback on his or her interactions and relationships.	The client may be unaware of interpersonal dynamics. Feedback can help increase insight and give support to the client's efforts to develop relationships.
Give the client support for any attempts to interact with others.	Positive feedback may reinforce desired behaviors.
*Involve the client in activities that are noncompetitive at first, then progress to more competitive activities as tolerated.	Competition may reinforce the client's low self-esteem or hostile feelings.
*Help the client build social skills through leisure-time counseling and referral to community resources (e.g., occupational or recreational therapy, outpatient social groups).	The client's relationships with others in the community may be limited or impaired and need to be re-established.

Nursing Diagnosis

Ineffective Self-Health Management

Pattern of regulating and integrating into daily living a therapeutic regimen for treatment of illness and its sequelae that is unsatisfactory for meeting specific health goals.

ASSESSMENT DATA

- Reluctance or refusal to take medications
- Inability to carry out responsibilities at work, home, and so forth
- Inadequate attention to need for nutrition, rest, or sleep
- Inability to carry out activities of daily living

EXPECTED OUTCOMES

Immediate

The client will

- Ingest medications as given within 12 to 24 hours
- Establish an adequate balance of nutrition, hydration, and elimination, for example, eat at least 40% of meals within 24 to 48 hours
- Establish an adequate balance of rest, sleep, and activity, for example, sleep at least 4 hours per night within 24 to 48 hours

Stabilization	The client will
	• Demonstrate ability to carry out activities of daily living, for example, bathing and hygiene, without assistance from staff
Community	The client will
	• Maintain adequately balanced physiologic functioning independently
	• Comply with continuing therapy, including medications

IMPLEMENTATION

Nursing Interventions *denotes collaborative interventions	Rationale
Give the liquid form of a medication when possible if the client is reluctant to take medication or if there is a question whether the client is ingesting medication.	Giving liquid medications helps ensure that the client ingests the medication. *Note:* Some liquid medications are irritating to oral membranes; observe precautions as indicated.
Tell the client that the medications are a part of the treatment plan and you expect him or her to take them as prescribed. Check the client's mouth if necessary after giving oral medications (have the client open mouth, raise tongue, etc.).	It is important to know if the client is ingesting medications. Being direct with the client will help him or her know what is expected.
Be straightforward with the client when giving information about medications, including the name and desired effects (e.g., "to help clear your thinking" or "to make the voices go away").	Clear information will help build trust and decrease suspicion.
Observe the client's eating, drinking, and elimination patterns, and assist the client as necessary (see Care Plan 52: The Client Who Will Not Eat).	The client may be unaware of physical needs or may ignore feelings of thirst, hunger, the urge to defecate, and so forth.
If the client is overactive, offer juice, milk, or finger foods that can be ingested while walking.	If the client is unable to sit and eat, providing nutritious foods that require little effort to eat may be effective.
Assess and record the client's caffeine intake and limit it if necessary.	Caffeine consumption, especially in large amounts, may increase anxiety or paranoid feelings.
Monitor the client's sleep patterns, and prepare him or her for bedtime by decreasing stimuli and administering comfort measures or medications (see Care Plan 38: Sleep Disorders).	Limiting noise and other stimuli will encourage rest and sleep. Comfort measures and sleeping medications will enhance the client's ability to relax and sleep.

CARE PLAN 41

Schizotypal Personality Disorder

The client with a *schizotypal personality disorder* exhibits a pervasive pattern of peculiarities of ideation, appearance, and behavior and deficits in interpersonal relatedness (APA, 2000).

Clients with a schizotypal personality disorder frequently are isolated but not by their own choice. They become very uncomfortable in social situations, so even though they may wish to meet others and make friends, they are unable to do so successfully. Therefore, the majority of their interactions are often limited to the nuclear family or one person outside the family, and even these relationships are characterized by an aloof, somewhat distant participation on the part of the client.

The client with a schizotypal personality disorder displays a great deal of anxiety when social situations with unfamiliar people are unavoidable. He or she generally appears eccentric in a variety of ways, including magical thinking; unusual perceptual experiences; inappropriate facial expressions; beliefs in superstition, clairvoyance, or telepathy (when these beliefs are inconsistent with subcultural norms); and an unkempt, frequently unusual manner of dress (APA, 2000). Clients with this personality disorder do not exhibit symptoms severe enough to support a diagnosis of schizophrenia, but under extreme stress, they may experience a psychotic episode, and up to 10% may develop schizophrenia (Sadock & Sadock, 2008).

Schizotypal personality disorder occurs in about 3% of the population and may occur slightly more often in men than in women (APA, 2000). These clients are at increased risk for depression and for other personality disorders. Symptoms are evident in childhood and persist through adulthood. These clients may have problems holding a job, but may be able to sustain employment of a routine, repetitive nature. Often, these clients stay with the nuclear family or live alone if forced to leave the family. It is thought that many homeless people have these types of personality disorders.

It is important for the nurse to be realistic in setting goals for these clients. Nursing care focuses on maximizing the client's independence and facilitating necessary interaction with others.

NURSING DIAGNOSIS ADDRESSED IN THIS CARE PLAN
Ineffective Role Performance

RELATED NURSING DIAGNOSES ADDRESSED IN THE MANUAL
Bathing Self-Care Deficit
Dressing Self-Care Deficit
Feeding Self-Care Deficit
Toileting Self-Care Deficit
Ineffective Self-Health Management

Nursing Diagnosis

Ineffective Role Performance
Patterns of behavior and self-expression that do not match the environmental context, norms, and expectations.

ASSESSMENT DATA

- Flat or inappropriate affect
- Lack of success in social interaction
- Inability to conform behavior to social expectations
- Magical thinking
- Belief in telepathy, clairvoyance, and superstition
- Vague, digressive, or abstract speech
- Unkempt appearance
- Bizarre mannerisms

EXPECTED OUTCOMES

Immediate   The client will

- Identify his or her basic needs within 24 to 48 hours
- Participate in a treatment plan, for example, interact with staff or participate in group activities for at least 15 minutes twice a day within 24 to 48 hours
- Verbalize preferences, interests, or desires within 2 to 3 days
- Express bizarre ideas and beliefs only to therapeutic staff within 4 to 5 days

Stabilization   The client will

- Communicate needs appropriately to others
- Demonstrate adequate hygiene and grooming

Community   The client will

- Participate in vocational planning or training
- Meet needs in community setting to maintain independence

IMPLEMENTATION

Nursing Interventions *denotes collaborative interventions	Rationale
Direct care toward changing essential behaviors that have brought negative attention to the client.	The client has limited interest or desire for behavioral changes.
Give the client honest feedback about those behaviors that draw negative attention to him or her.	The client needs to know the behaviors that cause uncomfortable consequences for him or her.
Explain to the client that the reason to make changes is to avoid hospitalization and maximize his or her freedom. Do not give rationale for change based on what is socially acceptable.	The client will be indifferent to others' reactions to his or her behavior, but it is possible to engage the client in behavioral changes if he or she perceives a concrete benefit to himself or herself.
Be specific in giving feedback to the client (e.g., identify the problem as talking about telepathic beliefs).	The client lacks the ability or desire to interpret concepts or abstract ideas.
Do not expect the client to develop the ability to respond to subtleties or social cues.	The client may be unable or lack the desire to develop these social abilities.
Encourage the client to make a list of people with whom communication is required, such as a store clerk and landlord.	A written list is easier to manage because the client's abstract thinking abilities are impaired.
*If possible, identify one community person to coordinate services for the client over time, such as a social worker or case manager.	The fewer the people the client is required to interact with, the more successful he or she will be.
*Involve the community contact person as soon as possible in the client's care.	Contact before discharge facilitates transferring the therapeutic relationship to the community person.
Encourage the client to write or use the telephone or Internet to request or purchase what is needed.	Written requests allow the client to avoid the displeasure of interaction. Telephone or Internet contact is less threatening than face-to-face interaction.

IMPLEMENTATION (continued)

Nursing Interventions *denotes collaborative interventions	Rationale
*If face-to-face contact is required, it may help to have a family member or the community contact person accompany the client.	The contact person or family member can serve as a buffer for the client if needed.
Expect only those client interactions necessary to obtain services that he or she truly wants or needs.	The client has a greater chance for success if he or she values the need for the service.
*Assist the client's family or significant others to focus on realistic expectations for the client.	Significant others may base their expectations on what they desire, rather than the client's ability, which is impaired.
Encourage the client to establish a daily routine for completion of hygiene.	Repetitive simple tasks and routines have a greater chance of success than changing expectations.
*If the client lives with someone else, include that person in developing daily routine expectations for room care, hygiene, and so forth, that can be continued at home.	The client will be more successful in transferring skills and behaviors if they are similar to those expected or needed in the community.
Assist the client to explore any interests or activities that do not involve much contact with other people.	This type of activity is most likely to appeal to the client.
*Assist the client to explore alternative living arrangements if indicated. These might include a "board and care" type of facility, where meals and laundry service are provided, but little interaction is required.	If the client lives with his or her family, it is likely he or she will need to live elsewhere as family members become unable to care for the client at home. The client is most likely to succeed in a living situation that provides services that meet basic needs but requires little social participation.
*Refer the client to vocational services if the client is able to develop a vocational interest.	It is possible for the client to use intellectual abilities to increase independence and meet basic needs.

CARE PLAN 42

Antisocial Personality Disorder

The client with *antisocial personality disorder* frequently is in conflict with society's social, moral, or legal norms and demonstrates behaviors that show a disregard for and violate others' rights, such as lying, manipulating others, and breaking the law. In addition, these clients are reckless, irresponsible, and show little or no remorse for harm they do to others (APA, 2000).

The client with antisocial behavior may be charming, entertaining, and persuasive in interpersonal interactions. He or she usually has the ability to succeed, is of average or above-average intelligence, and creates a good first impression. This client rarely sees himself or herself as having difficulties and usually does not seek help voluntarily, unless it is to avoid unpleasant consequences such as jail and debts. These clients may return to jail or hospitals repeatedly.

Clients with antisocial personality disorder have a history of behavior problems, including symptoms of conduct disorder in early adolescence (see Care Plan 10: Conduct Disorders). These clients' problems include truancy, poor grades, disruptive behavior in class, and fighting with other children throughout their school years. There is evidence for both genetic and environmental factors in the development of antisocial personality disorder, including a history of having been abused or neglected as a child (APA, 2000).

Men are three times more likely than women to have antisocial personality disorder; its prevalence is approximately 1% in women and 3% in men in the general population (Sadock & Sadock, 2008). These clients are also likely to have one or more of the following: substance abuse, anxiety, depression, somatization, or other personality disorders (APA, 2000). Antisocial personality disorder is chronic, but some symptoms may diminish as the client ages, especially after age 40. Although symptoms may be evident in childhood or adolescence, the disorder per se is not diagnosed (by definition) until age 18 (APA, 2000).

Nursing interventions focus primarily on managing symptoms such as aggressive behavior, setting and maintaining limits, or managing medications. It is important to remember that the client with an antisocial personality disorder will not develop insight into his or her behavior that leads to lasting change. Remember that these clients can be very persuasive and manipulative, and they may convince others, including staff, that they have changed or will change. However, the client's behavior is self-centered and based on desires of the moment, with little consideration for consequences or the feelings of other people, and these clients can be frustrating for staff members.

NURSING DIAGNOSIS ADDRESSED IN THIS CARE PLAN
Ineffective Coping

RELATED NURSING DIAGNOSES ADDRESSED IN THE MANUAL
Risk for Other-Directed Violence
Noncompliance
Risk for Self-Mutilation

Nursing Diagnosis

Ineffective Coping

Inability to form a valid appraisal of the stressors, inadequate choices of practiced responses, and/or inability to use available resources.

ASSESSMENT DATA

- Low frustration tolerance
- Impulsive behavior
- Inability to delay gratification
- Poor judgment
- Conflict with authority
- Difficulty following rules and obeying laws
- Lack of feelings of remorse
- Socially unacceptable behavior
- Dishonesty
- Ineffective interpersonal relationships
- Manipulative behavior
- Failure to learn or change behavior based on past experience or punishment
- Failure to accept or handle responsibility

EXPECTED OUTCOMES

Immediate

The client will

- Refrain from harming self or others throughout hospitalization
- Identify behaviors leading to hospitalization within 24 to 48 hours
- Function within limits of therapeutic milieu, for example, follow no-smoking rules, participate in group activities within 2 to 3 days

Stabilization

The client will

- Demonstrate nondestructive ways to deal with stress and frustration
- Identify ways to meet own needs that do not infringe on the rights of others

Community

The client will

- Achieve or maintain satisfactory work performance
- Meet own needs without exploiting or infringing on the rights of others

IMPLEMENTATION

Nursing Interventions *denotes collaborative interventions	Rationale
Encourage the client to identify the actions that precipitated hospitalization (e.g., debts, law violation).	These clients frequently deny responsibility for consequences to their own actions.
Give positive feedback for honesty. The client may try to avoid responsibility by acting as though he or she is "sick" or "helpless."	Honest identification of the consequences for the client's behavior is necessary for future behavior change.
Identify unacceptable behaviors, either general (stealing others' possessions) or specific (embarrassing Ms. X by telling lewd jokes).	You must supply clear, concrete limits when the client is unable or unwilling to do so.
Develop specific consequences for unacceptable behaviors (e.g., the client may not watch television).	Unpleasant consequences may help decrease or eliminate unacceptable behaviors. The consequence must be related to something the client enjoys to be effective.

(continued on page 282)

IMPLEMENTATION (continued)

Nursing Interventions *denotes collaborative interventions	Rationale
Avoid any discussion about why requirements exist. State the requirement in a matter-of-fact manner. Avoid arguing with the client.	The client may attempt to bend the rules "just this once" with numerous excuses and justifications. Your refusal to be manipulated or charmed will help decrease manipulative behavior.
Inform the client of unacceptable behaviors and the resulting consequences in advance of their occurrence.	The client must be aware of expectations and consequences.
*Communicate and document in the client's care plan all behaviors and consequences in specific terms.	The client may attempt to gain favor with individual staff members or play one staff member against another. ("Last night the nurse told me I could do that."). If all team members follow the written plan, the client will not be able to manipulate changes.
Avoid discussing other staff members' actions or statements unless the other staff member is present.	The client may try to manipulate staff members or focus attention on others to decrease attention to himself or herself.
*Be consistent and firm with the care plan. Do not make independent changes in rules or consequences. Any change should be made by the staff as a group and conveyed to all staff members working with this client. (You may designate a primary staff person to be responsible for minor decisions and refer all questions to this person.)	Consistency is essential. If the client can find just one person to make independent changes, any plan will become ineffective.
Avoid trying to coax or convince the client to do the "right thing."	The client must decide to accept responsibility for his or her behavior and its consequences.
When the client exceeds a limit, provide consequences immediately after the behavior in a calm, firm, matter-of-fact manner.	Consequences are most effective when they closely follow the unacceptable behavior. Do not react to the client in an angry or punitive manner. If you are angry, the client may take advantage of it. It is better to get out of the situation if possible and let someone else handle it.
Point out the client's responsibility for his or her behavior in a nonjudgmental manner.	The client needs to learn the connection between behavior and consequences, but blame and judgment are not appropriate.
Provide immediate positive feedback or reward for acceptable behavior.	Immediate positive feedback may help increase acceptable behavior. The client must receive attention for positive behaviors, not just unacceptable ones.
Gradually, require longer periods of acceptable behavior and greater rewards, and inform the client of changes as decisions are made. For example, at first the client must demonstrate acceptable behavior for 2 hours to earn 1 hour of television time. Gradually, the client could progress to 3 days of acceptable behavior and earn a 4-hour pass.	This gradual progression will help develop the client's ability to delay gratification. This is necessary if the client is to function effectively in society.
Encourage the client to identify past sources of frustration, how he or she dealt with it previously, and any unpleasant consequences that resulted.	This may facilitate the client's ability to accept responsibility for his or her own behavior.
Explore alternative, socially and legally acceptable methods of dealing with identified frustrations.	The client has the opportunity to learn to make alternative choices.
Help the client try alternatives as situations arise. Give positive feedback when the client uses alternatives successfully.	The client can role-play alternatives in a nonthreatening environment.
*Discuss job seeking, work attendance, court appearances, and so forth when working with the client in anticipation of discharge.	Dealing with consequences and working are responsible behaviors. The client may have had little or no successful experience in these areas and may benefit from assistance.

CARE PLAN 43

Borderline Personality Disorder

The client with a *borderline personality disorder* exhibits a multitude of problems in many different areas of life, including problems found in other personality disorders, as well as a pervasive pattern of instability that encompasses self-image, interpersonal relationships, mood, and behavior (APA, 2000). These clients can be described as socially contrary, pessimistic, demanding, and self-destructive. Clients with this disorder may also have other mental health problems, including mood or eating disorders, substance abuse, and other personality disorders.

These clients' interpersonal relationships are characterized by alternating periods of clinging dependency and hostile rejection. A friend or significant other may be idolized, then devalued for no apparent reason. Relationships are very intense, and the client will go to extremes to avoid feeling bored or abandoned, both of which are frequent complaints.

Clients with a borderline personality disorder have a persistent identity disturbance, which can include uncertainty about sexual orientation, values or belief systems, goals, self-image, and other major life issues. Mood swings (e.g., from anger to anxiety to elation) are common. When these clients' desires are not fulfilled immediately, they can react with intense emotions, such as rage; excessive drinking episodes; or aggressive, self-destructive, self-mutilating, or suicidal behavior. Approximately 8% to 10% of clients with this disorder successfully commit suicide (APA, 2000).

These clients are impulsive and unable to delay gratification or tolerate frustration; under extreme stress, they can display psychotic symptoms of brief duration, commonly seeking hospitalization. Some clients are not as severely impaired, and although they experience many dissatisfactions, they are intermittently capable of moderate moods, an absence of outbursts, and employment. Participation in community support services frequently is helpful for these clients.

There is evidence of a familial component in the development of this disorder, as well as a number of other risk factors, including a history of childhood physical or sexual abuse, neglect, or loss of a parent (APA, 2000). Borderline personality disorder occurs in 1% to 2% of the population and is twice as common in women than in men (Sadock & Sadock, 2008). This disorder is usually evident by early adulthood when problems usually are most severe. Many characteristics of this disorder are chronic, but the severity of symptoms diminishes in many clients in middle age or after therapy (APA, 2000).

Because clients with borderline personality disorder are at increased risk for suicide and self-injury, ensuring the client's safety is a key nursing goal. Consistency and limit setting are also important to build a trust relationship and minimize manipulative behavior. These clients can be frustrating for the treatment team because they may engage in behaviors that can create conflict among staff members, and may try to influence other clients to join them in their negative feelings toward the staff. They may also attempt to form personal relationships with staff members or exhibit flirtatious or dependent behavior; it is vitally important to maintain your professional nursing role with these clients.

NURSING DIAGNOSES ADDRESSED IN THIS CARE PLAN
Risk for Self-Mutilation
Ineffective Coping
Social Isolation

RELATED NURSING DIAGNOSES ADDRESSED IN THE MANUAL
Noncompliance
Chronic Low Self-Esteem
Risk for Other-Directed Violence
Risk for Suicide

Nursing Diagnosis

Risk for Self-Mutilation
At risk for deliberate self-injurious behavior causing tissue damage with the intent of causing nonfatal injury to attain relief of tension.

RISK FACTORS

- Impulsive behavior
- Displays of temper
- Inability to express feelings verbally
- Physically self-damaging acts
- Attention-seeking behavior
- Ineffective coping skills

EXPECTED OUTCOMES

Immediate

The client will

- Be safe and free from injury throughout hospitalization
- Refrain from harming others or destroying property throughout hospitalization
- Respond to external limits within 24 to 48 hours
- Participate in a treatment plan, for example, talk with staff or participate in group activities for at least 30 minutes twice a day within 24 to 48 hours

Stabilization

The client will

- Eliminate acting-out behaviors (temper tantrums, self-harm, suicidal threats)
- Develop a schedule or daily routine that includes socialization and daily responsibilities

Community

The client will

- Independently control urges for self-harming behavior
- Demonstrate alternative ways of expressing feelings, such as contact with a therapist or significant other

IMPLEMENTATION

Nursing Interventions *denotes collaborative interventions	Rationale
In your initial assessment of the client, find out if he or she has any history of suicidal behavior or present suicidal ideation or plans.	The client's physical safety is a priority. Although absence of a suicidal history does not preclude risk, presence of a suicidal history increases risk. The client with a history of self-harm can also be at risk for suicide. Do not underestimate the suicidal risk for the client by focusing only on self-harm behaviors.
Place the client in a room near the nursing station or where the client can be observed easily, rather than in a room near an exit or stairwell, and so forth.	The client is easier to observe and has less chance to leave the area undetected.
See Care Plan 26: Suicidal Behavior and Care Plan 47: Aggressive Behavior.	
Assess the client for the presence of self-harm urges and history of scratching, cutting, or burning behaviors.	The client has a pattern of injurious behavior and is likely to engage in similar self-harm behaviors when stressed.

IMPLEMENTATION (continued)

Nursing Interventions *denotes collaborative interventions	Rationale
Closely supervise the client's use of sharp or other potentially dangerous objects.	The client may use these items for self-destructive acts.
Be consistent with the client. Set and maintain limits regarding behavior, responsibilities, rules, and so forth.	Consistent limit setting is essential to decrease negative behaviors.
Withdraw your attention as much as possible if the client acts out (if the client's safety is not at risk).	Withdrawing your attention will tend to decrease acting-out behaviors.
Encourage the client to identify feelings that are related to self-mutilating or self-destructive behaviors. Encourage the client to express these feelings directly (see "Nursing Diagnosis: Ineffective Coping").	The client may be unaware of feelings or experiences that trigger self-destructive behavior and needs to develop more effective skills to avoid self-destructive behavior in the future.

Nursing Diagnosis

Ineffective Coping

Inability to form a valid appraisal of the stressors, inadequate choices of practiced responses, and/or inability to use available resources.

ASSESSMENT DATA

- Inconsistent behavior
- Uncertainty about identity (e.g., role, self-image, career choices, loyalties)
- Poor impulse control
- Inability to delay gratification
- Inability to tolerate frustration, anxiety
- Dissatisfaction with life
- Mood swings
- Alcohol or drug use
- Frequent somatic complaints

EXPECTED OUTCOMES

Immediate

The client will

- Participate in treatment plan, for example, participate in group activities for at least 30 minutes at least twice per day within 24 to 48 hours
- Ask for what he or she needs in an acceptable manner within 24 to 48 hours
- Demonstrate resolution of the crisis that precipitated hospitalization within 4 to 5 days.

Stabilization

The client will

- Demonstrate diminished efforts to manipulate staff or other clients
- Demonstrate impulse control
- Delay gratification of needs and requests without acting out
- Verbalize plans for moderation of lifestyle

Community

The client will

- Eliminate the need for inpatient hospitalization
- Demonstrate effective problem solving in the community

IMPLEMENTATION

Nursing Interventions *denotes collaborative interventions	Rationale
Do not assume that physical complaints are not genuine or that the client is just manipulating or seeking attention.	The client may be physically ill. This must be validated or ruled out.
*The medical staff should investigate each physical complaint within a certain time period or at a structured time. Then, withdraw attention from conversation about physical complaints.	After the medical staff evaluates physical problems, you can focus on interpersonal issues and not allow the client to use physical symptoms to avoid dealing with emotional problems.
Assess the extent of the client's substance use. Interview the client's significant others if necessary.	If substance use exists, it needs to be identified and addressed.
Give the client support for direct communication and for fulfilling responsibilities.	Positive support tends to increase positive behaviors.
It may be helpful to assign the responsibility for decisions regarding the client to one staff member.	If only one person makes final decisions, there is less opportunity for manipulation by the client.
When talking with the client, focus on self-responsibility and active approaches that the client can take. Avoid reinforcing the client's passivity, feelings of hopelessness, and so forth.	If the client is blaming others for his or her problems, it is unlikely the client will accept responsibility for making changes.
Encourage the client to express feelings or concerns, including identity questions and uncertainties. Remain nonjudgmental and assure the client that you will not reject or ridicule him or her or take concerns lightly.	A nonjudgmental attitude will help the client feel safe in sharing concerns. It is unlikely that the client has relationships that allow discussing personal concerns without fear of rejection.
Encourage the client to identify a problem or life situation that precipitated hospitalization, including his or her role in the situation.	The client may have difficulty identifying his or her role in the situation that has led to hospitalization.
Teach the client the problem-solving process: identifying problems, exploring alternatives, making a decision, and evaluating its success.	The client may be unaware of a logical process for solving problems.
Ask for the client's perceptions of his or her skills, level of functioning, and independence.	The client's perception of self is an essential component of baseline data.
Help the client identify strengths and successful coping behaviors that he or she has used in the past. It may help to have the client make a written list. Encourage the client to try to use these coping behaviors in present and future situations.	The client's self-perception may be one of hopelessness or helplessness. The client needs your assistance to recognize strengths.
Teach the client additional positive coping strategies and stress management skills, such as increasing physical exercise, expressing feelings verbally or in a journal, or meditation techniques. Encourage the client to practice these skills while in the hospital.	The client may have limited or no knowledge of stress management techniques or may not have used positive techniques in the past. If the client tries to build skills in the treatment setting, he or she can experience success and receive positive feedback for his or her efforts.
Observe how the client functions in various situations. How does the client interact with peers? With authority figures? How does the client function during structured activities? Unstructured time?	You need to assess what the client can do and what skills he or she needs to develop.
Give the client feedback regarding your observations; involve the client in identifying realistic goals and plans to work on deficient areas or to use and augment strengths. Use written lists, priority schedules, and so forth.	Involving the client facilitates his or her acceptance of responsibility. Using schedules and lists provides structure and helps achieve an independent lifestyle.
*Work with professionals in other disciplines (vocational rehabilitation, education, psychology) for client testing and specific training (e.g., job interviewing).	Using other health professionals for areas beyond nursing's scope enhances the client's chance for success.

IMPLEMENTATION (continued)

Nursing Interventions *denotes collaborative interventions	Rationale
*Help the client obtain resources, such as social services or vocational rehabilitation, as appropriate.	The client may need these resources to live in the community but may be unaware of how to obtain services.
*Refer the client to professionals in other disciplines (e.g., social work or law) if the client has legal problems. Take care to promote the client's autonomy; do not reinforce the client's pattern of dependence on others.	Legal difficulties are beyond the scope of nursing. Your responsibility is appropriate referral.
Discuss discharge planning in a positive manner throughout hospitalization, beginning with the initial interview.	The client receives the message that he or she can be independent and that hospitalization is temporary.

Nursing Diagnosis

Social Isolation

Aloneness experienced by the individual and perceived as imposed by others and as a negative or threatening state.

ASSESSMENT DATA

- Intolerance of being alone
- Chronic feelings of boredom or emptiness
- Alternate clinging and avoidance behavior in relationships
- Excessive dependency needs
- Manipulation of others for own needs
- Sense of entitlement
- Lack of insight

EXPECTED OUTCOMES

Immediate

The client will

- Interact appropriately with staff, visitors, and other clients, for example, initiate interactions with others at least four times per day within 2 to 3 days
- Engage in leisure activities, for example, participate in a group activity, read, or do a hobby activity at least once per day within 2 to 3 days

Stabilization

The client will

- Participate in relationships without excessive clinging or avoidance
- Meet dependency needs in a socially acceptable manner

Community

The client will

- Develop a social support group outside the hospital
- Initiate leisure activities that he or she enjoys

IMPLEMENTATION

Nursing Interventions *denotes collaborative interventions	Rationale
With the client, establish acceptable limits in relationships; provide limits for the client if he or she is unable to do so.	Limits must be supplied by you until the client is able to control his or her own behavior. The client may not recognize nor have experienced relationships with appropriate limits and needs help to develop awareness and skills in building appropriate relationships.

(continued on page 288)

IMPLEMENTATION (continued)

Nursing Interventions *denotes collaborative interventions	Rationale
Be aware of the client's interactions and intervene when necessary to prevent the client's manipulating staff, other clients, or visitors.	Other clients' needs for protection must be considered and may require your intervention.
Remember: Although the client must feel that the staff members care about him or her as a person (therapeutically), do not undermine the client's independence by encouraging dependence on the staff or agency.	Sympathy and friendship are only appropriate to personal or social relationships. The client's independence is a goal of a therapeutic relationship. Reliance on staff may be flattering to you but is nontherapeutic for the client.
Help the client recognize feelings of boredom and identify activities that diminish these feelings. It may be helpful to use a written schedule.	The client needs to see that boredom is his or her problem and that it is his or her responsibility to resolve it. A written schedule can help the client structure his or her time.
Help the client see that manipulating others results in the loss of their company, then boredom and loneliness.	If the client dislikes boredom and loneliness, he or she may diminish manipulative behavior to avoid these feelings.
Help the client determine appropriate people and times to discuss personal issues.	Due to the client's dependency needs and poor impulse control, he or she may disclose intimate issues to casual acquaintances or strangers, which can lead to rejection.
Talk with the client about his or her interactions and give the client feedback about interpersonal dynamics.	Sharing observations and providing feedback allows the client to develop awareness of interpersonal relationships and express his or her feelings in a therapeutic setting.
*Encourage the client to meet others in his or her community or to contact support groups before discharge.	The client needs to meet relationship needs with others outside the hospital or agency. Increasing the client's support system by establishing new relationships within an appropriate context may help decrease future difficulties.

CARE PLAN 44

Dependent Personality Disorder

Clients with *dependent personality disorder* are excessively, consistently dependent on other people, and they are passive, clinging, and submissive in relationships. They rely on others for basic decision making and help in day-to-day living and have strong fears of being alone or losing the support of others. These clients may not have developed basic independent living skills, and they lack confidence in their own abilities (APA, 2000).

Clients who are very dependent or who lack adequate skills for daily living may be repeatedly admitted to a hospital with varying complaints and complex problems related to inadequate coping skills, such as a poor job history or legal problems from writing bad checks.

Dependent personality disorder is more common in women than in men and represents 2.5% of all personality disorders (Sadock & Sadock, 2008). Clients with dependent personality disorder may survive adequately in the community until faced with a crisis or the loss of a significant other, which precipitates their admission to a hospital. No etiology for this disorder has been identified, but risk factors include an early history of a chronic medical condition or separation anxiety disorder. These clients are also at increased risk for mood, anxiety, or adjustment disorders, or other personality disorders (APA, 2000).

When deprived of others to depend on, these clients can be at risk for acting-out or self-destructive behaviors. The client's safety is always a primary nursing goal.

These clients may transfer their excessive dependency needs to staff members or a therapist. It is important for the nurse to minimize opportunities for the client to develop dependency on the staff and to foster the development of basic skills and confidence in the client. However, these clients may not be able to recognize their abilities, and their behaviors and lack of insight can be frustrating for the staff. Using limit setting and communicating clear, consistent expectations can be helpful, but remember to keep expectations within the client's abilities.

NURSING DIAGNOSES ADDRESSED IN THIS CARE PLAN
Ineffective Coping
Powerlessness

RELATED NURSING DIAGNOSES ADDRESSED IN THE MANUAL
Impaired Social Interaction
Social Isolation
Hopelessness
Chronic Low Self-Esteem
Risk for Self-Mutilation

Nursing Diagnosis

Ineffective Coping
Inability to form a valid appraisal of the stressors, inadequate choices of practiced responses, and/or inability to use available resources.

ASSESSMENT DATA

- Inadequate skills for daily living or to meet changes and crises
- Low frustration tolerance
- Poor impulse control
- Poor judgment
- Anxiety
- Anger or hostility (often covert)

EXPECTED OUTCOMES

Immediate

The client will

- Be free from injury throughout hospitalization
- Demonstrate decreased manipulative, attention-seeking behavior within 2 to 3 days
- Verbally express feelings, especially anger within 2 to 3 days

Stabilization

The client will

- Discuss relationship of physical complaints, legal difficulties, or substance use to ineffective coping
- Verbalize adequate skills to deal with life changes or crises

Community

The client will

- Demonstrate adequate daily living skills
- Make decisions and solve problems independently

IMPLEMENTATION

Nursing Interventions *denotes collaborative interventions	Rationale
Assess the client's immediate environment, possessions, and hospital room for potentially dangerous objects.	The client's safety is a priority. The client is at risk for self-destructive behavior.
Provide adequate supervision while the client is involved in activities, with other clients or off the unit.	Self-destructive acting out is more likely to occur during unsupervised times.
Treat self-mutilating acts in a matter-of-fact manner. Provide any physical treatment needed, then try to interact with the client about how he or she is feeling rather than about the act itself.	The more attention the client receives for these behaviors, the more likely the client is to repeat the behaviors.
In the event of destructive behavior, take the client to a secluded, physically safe area without delay.	Immediate isolation minimizes the attention the client receives. The client is removed from the audience.
Withdraw your attention from the client when nondestructive acting-out behavior occurs.	Decreased attention tends to decrease the behavior.
Encourage the client to express feelings verbally or in other ways that are nondestructive and acceptable to the client (e.g., writing, drawing, or physical activity).	The client may need specific direction for the acceptable expression of feelings. He or she may never have learned to do so previously.
Give the client positive feedback when he or she is able to express anger verbally or in a nondestructive manner.	Positive feedback can give the client confidence and incentive to continue the positive behavior.
Describe and demonstrate specific social skills, such as eye contact, attentive listening, nodding. Discuss topics that are appropriate for casual conversation, such as the weather, local events.	The client may have little or no knowledge of social interaction skills. Modeling provides a concrete example of the desired skills.
Teach the client social skills, such as approaching another person for an interaction, appropriate conversation topics, and active listening. Encourage him or her to practice these skills with staff members and other clients, and give the client feedback regarding interactions.	The client may lack social skills and confidence in social interactions; this may contribute to the client's social isolation.

IMPLEMENTATION (continued)

Nursing Interventions *denotes collaborative interventions	Rationale
Introduce the client to other clients in the milieu and facilitate their interactions on a one client-to-one client basis. Gradually facilitate social interactions between the client and small groups, then larger groups.	Gradually increasing the scope of the client's social interactions will help the client build confidence in social skills.
Teach the client a step-by-step approach to solving problems: identifying problems, exploring alternatives, making a decision, and evaluating its success.	The client may be unaware of a logical process for examining and resolving problems.
Encourage the client to take direct action to meet personal needs (e.g., allow the client to obtain a newspaper to check want ads and identify possible jobs, make appointments, etc.) on his or her own as much as possible. Do not help the client unless it is necessary.	The client needs to learn independent living skills. This cannot happen if he or she does not do things without assistance even though it is uncomfortable initially.
Work with the client to help him or her anticipate future needs ("What will you do if…?"). It may help to write down specific strategies, people to contact, and so forth.	Because the client deals with change poorly (by history), anticipatory plans can help diffuse the emotional charge of change in the client's life and help the client develop planning skills.

Nursing Diagnosis

Powerlessness

The lived experience of lack of control over a situation, including a perception that one's actions do not significantly affect an outcome.

ASSESSMENT DATA

- Dependency on others to meet needs
- Feelings of inadequacy, dependency, worthlessness, failure, or hopelessness
- Apathy
- Doubt about role performance
- Perceived lack of control

EXPECTED OUTCOMES

Immediate

The client will

- Verbalize feelings openly, for example, talk with staff about present emotions at least once per day within 24 to 48 hours
- Identify present skills and level of functioning within 2 to 3 days

Stabilization

The client will

- Verbalize increased feelings of self-worth
- Identify people and resources in the community for support
- Terminate staff–client relationships

Community

The client will

- Use community support systems
- Tolerate discomfort associated with life stresses

IMPLEMENTATION

Nursing Interventions *denotes collaborative interventions	Rationale
Beginning with the initial interview, identify the goal of the client's discharge and independence from the hospital and reinforce this throughout the hospitalization.	It is essential to communicate the temporary nature of your relationship with a client who has excessive dependency.
*Rotate staff members who work with the client to avoid the client's developing dependence on particular staff members. It is not desirable to be the "only one" the client can talk to.	The client must learn self-reliance and avoid dependence on one or two people.
Remember: Do not give the client the addresses or personal telephone numbers of staff members. Do not allow the client to contact or socialize with staff members after discharge.	It is essential to separate professional and social relationships.
Encourage the client to express feelings, including anger, hostility, worthlessness, or hopelessness. Give the client support for expressing feelings openly and honestly.	The client can learn to ventilate feelings in a safe situation with you. Positive support encourages the client to continue to do so.
Encourage the client to share feelings with other clients, in small informal groups, then larger, more formal groups.	Including others as the client tolerates will minimize the client's dependence on one person or on hospital staff for communication.
*Encourage the client to build a support system that is as independent from the hospital as possible. If the client cannot achieve that level of independence, continued outpatient therapy or support groups may be indicated.	Use of an outside support system is a less dependent situation than hospitalization.
*Encourage the client to pursue relationships, personal interests, hobbies, or recreational activities that were positive in the past or that may appeal to the client. Consultation with a recreational therapist may be indicated.	The client may be reluctant to reach out to someone with whom he or she has had limited contact recently and may benefit from encouragement or facilitation. Recreational activities can serve as a structure for the client to build social interactions as well as to provide enjoyment.
*Encourage the client to identify resources in the community or on the Internet that he or she can use after discharge.	The client may be unfamiliar with existing resources (e.g., community centers, libraries, parks, recreational programs, volunteer opportunities). The Internet can be a source of social interaction, support, and recreation.
*Encourage the client to identify supportive people outside the hospital and to develop these relationships.	In addition to re-establishing past relationships or in their absence, increasing the client's support system by establishing new relationships may help decrease future depressive behavior and social isolation.
*When necessary, work with other agencies in the community to meet the client's needs, but do not undermine the client's progress by unnecessarily encouraging dependence on professional resources or institutions.	If other assistance is needed to maintain the client in the community, it should be used, but the client should do all he or she can independently. These clients may have all but exhausted community resources in the past, so work in this area may need special attention.

SECTION 12 REVIEW QUESTIONS

1. When working with a client with a paranoid personality disorder, the nurse would use which of the following approaches?

   a. Calm

   b. Cheerful

   c. Friendly

   d. Supportive

2. The client with an antisocial personality disorder approaches various staff with numerous requests. Which of the following interventions is the best response to this behavior?

   a. Give the client a written list of permissible requests.

   b. Have the client make requests only to the assigned staff person.

   c. Limit the client to the day room area.

   d. Tell the client to remain in his or her room until approached by staff.

3. The nurse assesses a client to be at risk for self-mutilation and implements a no self-harm contract. Which of the following would indicate that the safety contract was effective?

   a. The client withdraws to her room when feeling overwhelmed.

   b. The client notifies staff when anxiety is increasing.

   c. The client suppresses feelings of anger.

   d. The client talks to other clients about urges to harm herself.

4. A client with borderline personality disorder is admitted to the unit after attempting to cut her wrists with scissors. Her arms have multiple scars from previous episodes of self-injury. Another staff member says to the nurse, "She's not going to kill herself; she just wants attention."

Which of the following statements by the nurse would be most appropriate?

   a. "Any attempt at self-harm is serious and safety is a priority."

   b. "Don't let the nurse manager hear you talking like that; it's unprofessional."

   c. "She needs to be here until she learns to control her behavior."

   d. "She's here now and we'll have to try to do the best we can."

5. When planning care for a client with a schizoid personality disorder, which of the following outcomes would be most appropriate? The client will

   a. Communicate effectively with his or her landlord

   b. Express interest in a new hobby

   c. Join a community group for socialization

   d. Verbalize thoughts and feelings to peers

6. A 31-year-old client with dependent personality disorder has been living at home with very supportive parents. He is making plans for independent living in the community. The client tells the nurse, "I don't know if I can make it on my own without my parents." Which of the following responses by the nurse is most therapeutic?

   a. "You are a 31-year-old adult now, not a child who needs his parents to care for him."

   b. "You and your parents need a break from each other; it will be good for both of you."

   c. "Your parents have been supportive and can continue to be even if you live apart."

   d. "Your parents won't be around forever; you need to learn to take care of yourself."

SECTION 12 Recommended Readings

Black, D. W., Gunter, T., Loveless, P., Allen, J., & Sieleni, B. (2010). Antisocial personality disorder in incarcerated offenders: Psychiatric comorbidity and quality of life. *Annals of Clinical Psychiatry, 22*(2), 113–120.

Coid, J., & Ullrich, S. (2010). Antisocial personality on a continuum with psychopathology. *Comprehensive Psychiatry, 51*(4), 426–433.

Latalova, K., & Prasko, J. (2010). Aggression in borderline personality disorder. *The Psychiatric Quarterly, 81*(3), 239–251.

Lentz, V., Robinson, J., & Bolton, J. M. (2010). Childhood adversity, mental disorder comorbidity, and suicidal behavior in schizotypal personality disorder. *Journal of Nervous and Mental Diseases, 198*(11), 795–801.

Sadikaj, G., Russell, J. J., Moskowitz, D. S., & Paris, J. (2010). Affective dysregulation in individuals with borderline personality disorder: Persistence and interpersonal triggers. *Journal of Personality Assessment, 92*(6), 490–500.

Sansone, R. A., Chu, J. W., & Wieserman, M. W. (2010). Body image and borderline personality disorder among psychiatric inpatients. *Comprehensive Psychiatry, 51*(6), 579–584.

SECTION 12 Resources for Additional Information

Visit thePoint (http://thePoint.lww.com/Schultz9e) for a list of these and other helpful Internet resources.

Association for Research in Personality Disorders
Borderline Personality Disorder Central
Borderline Personality Disorder Family Support
International Society for the Study of Personality Disorders
MedlinePlus
National Education Alliance for Borderline Personality Disorder
National Institute of Mental Health
Personality Disorders Institute—Cornell University
S.A.F.E. Alternatives (Self Injury Treatment, Resources)
TARA Association for Personality Disorder

Behavioral and Problem-Based Care Plans

The behaviors and problems addressed in this section may occur in concert with other problems found in this *Manual*. Some of these problems may be manifested by a client who exhibits psychotic behavior, such as schizophrenia; others may be the primary problem in the client's current situation, such as hostile or aggressive behavior. These care plans are especially suited to choosing specific nursing diagnoses or elements of care to be incorporated into the client's individualized care plan.

CARE PLAN 45

Withdrawn Behavior

The term *withdrawn behavior* is used to describe a client's retreat from relating to the external world. The degree of the client's withdrawal can range from mild to severe and represents a disruption in his or her relating to the self, others, or the environment. Withdrawn behavior can occur in conjunction with a number of mental health problems, including schizophrenia, mood disorders, and suicidal behavior (see other care plans as appropriate).

Withdrawn behavior that is mild or transitory, such as a dazed period following trauma, is thought to be a self-protecting defense mechanism. This brief period of "emotional shock" allows the individual to rest and gather internal resources with which to cope with the trauma and is considered to be normal because it can be expected and does not extend beyond a brief period. However, withdrawn behavior that is protracted or severe can interfere with the client's ability to function in activities of daily living, relationships, work, or other aspects of life. Seemingly total withdrawal, such as *catatonic stupor*, involves autism, physical immobility, and no intake of food or fluid. Without treatment, it can lead to coma and death.

An especially important nursing goal with a client who is withdrawn is to establish initial contact by using a calm, nonthreatening, consistent approach. Using this type of approach repeatedly enables the client to recognize you as a safe contact with present reality to whom he or she can begin to respond, but does not demand a response from the client. As you build rapport with the client and provide a supportive environment, the client can begin to establish and maintain contact with you, the environment, and other people. Additional therapeutic goals include providing sensory stimulation, meeting the client's physiologic and hygienic needs, and promoting the client's physical activity and interactions with others.

NURSING DIAGNOSES ADDRESSED IN THIS CARE PLAN
Disturbed Thought Processes
Bathing Self-Care Deficit
Dressing Self-Care Deficit
Feeding Self-Care Deficit
Toileting Self-Care Deficit
Impaired Social Interaction

RELATED NURSING DIAGNOSES ADDRESSED IN THE MANUAL
Social Isolation
Imbalanced Nutrition: Less Than Body Requirements
Insomnia
Risk for Injury

Nursing Diagnosis

Disturbed Thought Processes

Disruption in cognitive operations and activities.

> *Note: This nursing diagnosis was retired in *NANDA-I Nursing Diagnoses: Definitions & Classification 2009–2011*, but the NANDA-I Diagnosis Development Committee encourages work to be done on retired diagnoses toward resubmission for inclusion in the taxonomy.

ASSESSMENT DATA

- Psychological immobility
- Hallucinations, delusions, or other psychotic symptoms
- Inability to attend
- Lack of spontaneity
- Apathy
- Decreased or absent verbal communication
- Lack of awareness of surroundings
- Decreased motor activity or physical immobility
- Fetal position, eyes closed, teeth clenched, muscles rigid
- Anergy (lack of energy)
- Changes in body posture, for example, slumping, curling up with knees to chin, holding arms around self
- Fear
- Anxiety, panic
- Depression
- Muteness

EXPECTED OUTCOMES

Immediate

The client will

- Begin to participate in the treatment program, e.g., tolerate sitting with a staff member for at least 15 minutes within 12 to 24 hours
- Demonstrate decreased hallucinations, delusions, or other psychotic symptoms within 24 to 48 hours
- Demonstrate adequate psychomotor activity to meet basic activities of daily living with staff assistance within 2 to 3 days
- Begin to interact with others, e.g., respond verbally to questions at least four times per day within 2 to 3 days

Stabilization

The client will

- Maintain contact with reality
- Demonstrate adequate psychomotor activity to meet basic activities of daily living independent of staff assistance
- Interact with others nonverbally and verbally, e.g., talk with staff or other clients for at least 10 minutes at least four times per day by a specified date
- Demonstrate improvement in associated problems (e.g., depression)

Community

The client will

- Be free of hallucinations, delusions, or other psychotic symptoms
- Function at his or her optimal level

IMPLEMENTATION

Nursing Interventions *denotes collaborative interventions	Rationale
Assess the client's current level of functioning and communication, and begin to work with the client at that level.	To make contact with the client, you must begin where he or she is now.
Sit with the client for regularly scheduled periods.	Your physical presence conveys caring and acceptance.
Tell the client your name and that you are there to be with him or her.	By telling the client you are there to be with him or her, you convey interest without making demands on the client.
Remain comfortable with periods of silence; do not overload the client with verbalization.	The client's ability to deal with verbal stimulation is impaired.
Use physical touch with the client (e.g., holding the client's hand) as tolerated. If the client responds to touch negatively, remove your hand at that time, but continue attempts to establish physical touch.	Your physical touch presents reality and conveys acceptance.
Talk with the client in a soft voice. If the client remains unresponsive, continue to do this with the positive expectation of a response from the client.	A soft voice can be comforting and nonthreatening, and expresses your caring and interest in the client. Expecting the client to respond increases the likelihood that he or she will do so.
Ask the client to open his or her eyes and look at you when you are speaking to him or her.	You will facilitate reality contact and the client's ability to attend by encouraging eye contact.
Be alert for subtle, nonverbal responses from the client.	The client's initial responses usually will not be verbal or dramatic but rather very gradual and subtle (hand movement, eyes opening).
Give the client positive feedback for any response to you or to the external environment. Encourage him or her to continue to respond and reach out to others.	Your encouragement can foster the client's attempts to re-establish contact with reality.
Use a radio, tape player, or television in the client's room to provide stimulation as tolerated.	Media can provide stimulation during times that staff are not available to be with the client.
Assess the client's tolerance of stimuli; do not force too much stimulation too fast.	Increasing stimuli too rapidly could result in the client's further withdrawal.
Avoid allowing the client to isolate himself or herself in a room alone for long periods.	Isolation will foster continued withdrawal.
Initially encourage the client to spend short periods with one other person, e.g., have the client sit with one person for 15 minutes of each hour during the day.	At first, the client will be more successful with minimal stimulation (e.g., interactions for short time periods) and minimal changes (e.g., interacting with the same staff member).
Interact with the client briefly on a one-to-one basis initially; gradually increase the amount of time and the number of people with whom the client interacts.	A gradual increase in the amount and variety of stimulation can foster the client's tolerance in a nonthreatening manner.
Talk with the client as though he or she will respond and avoid rapidly chattering at the client. Allow adequate time for the client to respond to you, either verbally or physically.	A positive expectation on your part increases the likelihood of the client's response. A client who is withdrawn may need more time to respond due to slowed thought processes.
Refer to other people and objects in the immediate environment as you interact with the client.	You will promote the client's contact with current reality by calling the client's attention to his or her environment.
Initially, encourage the client to express himself or herself nonverbally (e.g., by writing or drawing).	Nonverbal communication usually is less threatening to the client than verbalization.
Encourage the client to talk about these nonverbal communications and progress to more direct verbal communication as tolerated. Encourage the client to express feelings as much as possible.	By asking the client about writings or drawings rather than directly about himself or herself or emotional issues, you minimize the perception of threat by the client. Gradually, direct verbal communication becomes tolerable to the client.

IMPLEMENTATION (continued)

Nursing Interventions *denotes collaborative interventions	Rationale
At first, walk slowly with the client. Progress gradually from gross motor activity (walking, gestures with hands) to activities requiring fine motor skills (jigsaw puzzles, writing).	The client will be able to use gross motor skills first. Fine motor skills require more of the client's skill and attention.
See "Key Considerations in Mental Health Nursing: Nurse–Client Interactions" and other care plans as indicated.	Withdrawn behavior frequently is encountered with psychotic symptoms, depression, organic pathology, abuse, and post-traumatic stress disorder.
*Teach the client and family and significant others about withdrawn behavior, safe use of medications, and other disease process(es) if indicated.	The client and family and significant others may have little or no knowledge of the client's illness, care-giving responsibilities, or safe use of medications.

Nursing Diagnoses

Bathing Self-Care Deficit
Impaired ability to perform or complete bathing activities for self.

Dressing Self-Care Deficit
Impaired ability to perform or complete dressing activities for self.

Feeding Self-Care Deficit
Impaired ability to perform or complete self-feeding activities.

Toileting Self-Care Deficit
Impaired ability to perform or complete toileting activities for self.

ASSESSMENT DATA

- Inattention to grooming and personal hygiene
- Inadequate food or fluid intake; refusal to eat
- Retention of urine or feces
- Incontinence of urine or feces
- Decreased motor activity or physical immobility

EXPECTED OUTCOMES

Immediate   The client will

- Establish adequate nutrition and hydration, e.g., the client will eat 30% of meals within 2 to 3 days
- Establish adequate elimination within 2 to 3 days
- Begin to perform activities of daily living and personal hygiene with staff assistance within 24 to 48 hours
- Establish an adequate balance of rest, sleep, and activity

Stabilization   The client will

- Maintain adequate nutrition, hydration, and elimination
- Perform activities of daily living and personal hygiene without staff assistance
- Maintain an adequate balance of rest, sleep, and activity, e.g., the client will be awake and active during the day and evening until bedtime

Community   The client will

- Demonstrate independence in performing activities of daily living, personal hygiene, and meeting other self-care needs

IMPLEMENTATION

Nursing Interventions *denotes collaborative interventions	Rationale
Remain with the client during meals.	Your physical presence can stimulate the client and promote reality contact.
Feed the client if necessary.	The client needs to reestablish nutritional intake, without intravenous or tube feeding therapy if possible.
Try to find out what foods the client likes, including culturally based foods or foods from family members, and make them available at meals and for snacks (see Care Plan 52: The Client Who Will Not Eat).	The client may be more apt to eat foods he or she likes or has been accustomed to eating.
Assess and monitor the client's bowel elimination pattern.	Constipation may occur due to decreased food and fluid intake, decreased motor activity, or the client's inattention to elimination. Severe constipation and impaction can occur if the client has not had a bowel movement for an extended period before admission.
If the client is immobile or in the fetal position, provide passive range-of-motion exercises. Turn the client at least every 2 hours; provide skin care and observe for pressure areas and skin breakdown.	Range-of-motion exercises will maintain joint mobility and muscle tone. You must be alert to the prevention of physical complications due to immobility.
At first, walk slowly with the client. Progress gradually from slow walking to increasing levels of physical activity and from gross motor activity (walking, gestures with hands) to activities requiring fine motor skills or greater concentration.	The client will be able to use gross motor skills first, and walking will help reestablish flexibility. Physical movement facilitates digestion, elimination, and restful sleep.
Initially, assist the client as necessary to perform personal hygiene, such as brushing teeth, taking a shower, combing hair, and other activities of daily living.	The client may have little awareness of the need for hygiene or other activities of daily living or may have little or no interest in these.
Encourage the client to take gradually increasing levels of responsibility for hydration, nutrition, elimination, sleep, activity, and other self-care needs (see Care Plan 52: The Client Who Will Not Eat and Care Plan 38: Sleep Disorders).	Initially, the client may be totally passive regarding basic needs, and you may need to provide total care. Asking the client to perform self-care as his or her behavior improves will help the client assume more responsibility. Your positive expectations of the client will promote independence in these activities.

Nursing Diagnosis

Impaired Social Interaction

Insufficient or excessive quantity or ineffective quality of social exchange.

ASSESSMENT DATA

- Decreased or absent verbal communication
- Lack of energy or spontaneity
- Difficulty in interpersonal relationships
- Apathy
- Psychological immobility
- Fear
- Anxiety, panic
- Loneliness

EXPECTED OUTCOMES

Immediate	The client will
	• Demonstrate decreased withdrawn symptoms within 24 to 48 hours
	• Participate in the treatment program, e.g., interact with staff for at least 15 minutes at least four times per day within 2 to 3 days
Stabilization	The client will
	• Maintain contact with reality
	• Demonstrate increased interactions with others, e.g., interact verbally with other clients at least six times per day
Community	The client will
	• Participate in continued therapy or community support, if indicated
	• Communicate own needs effectively to others

IMPLEMENTATION

Nursing Interventions *denotes collaborative interventions	Rationale
Initially encourage the client to spend short periods with one other person, e.g., have the client sit with one person for 15 minutes of each hour during the day.	At first the client will deal more readily with minimal stimulation (e.g., interactions for short time periods) and minimal changes (e.g., interacting with the same staff member).
Initially encourage the client to express himself or herself nonverbally (e.g., by writing or drawing).	Nonverbal communication usually is less threatening than verbalization.
Encourage the client to talk about these nonverbal communications and progress to more direct verbal communication as tolerated. Encourage the client to express feelings as much as possible.	By asking the client about writings or drawings rather than directly about himself or herself or emotional issues, you minimize the client's perception of threat. Gradually, direct verbal communication becomes tolerable to the client.
Interact on a one-to-one basis initially, and then help the client progress to small groups, then larger groups as tolerated.	Gradual introduction of other people minimizes the threat perceived by the client.
Manage nursing assignments so that the client interacts with a variety of staff members, as the client tolerates.	Your social behavior provides a role model for the client. Interacting with different staff members allows the client to experience success in interactions within the safety of the staff–client relationship.
Teach the client social skills, such as approaching another person for an interaction, appropriate conversation topics, and active listening. Encourage him or her to practice these skills with staff members and other clients, and give the client feedback regarding interactions.	The client may lack social skills and confidence in social interactions; this may contribute to the client's depression and social isolation.
Encourage the client to identify relationships, social, or recreational situations that have been positive in the past.	The client may have been depressed and withdrawn for some time and have lost interest in people or activities that provided pleasure in the past.
*Encourage the client to pursue past relationships, personal interests, hobbies, or recreational activities that were positive in the past or that may appeal to the client. Consultation with a recreational therapist may be indicated.	The client may be reluctant to reach out to someone with whom he or she has had limited contact recently and may benefit from encouragement or facilitation. Recreational activities can serve as a structure for the client to build social interactions as well as provide enjoyment.
*Encourage the client to identify supportive people outside the hospital and to develop these relationships (see Care Plan 2: Discharge Planning and Section 2: Community-Based Care).	In addition to reestablishing past relationships or in their absence, increasing the client's support system by establishing new relationships may help decrease future withdrawn behavior and social isolation.

CARE PLAN 46

Hostile Behavior

Hostile behavior, or *hostility*, is characterized by verbal abuse, threatened aggressive behavior, uncooperativeness, and behaviors that have been defined as undesirable or in violation of established limits. Much hostility is the result of feelings that are unacceptable to the client, which the client then projects onto others, particularly authority figures (including staff members) or significant others. Often the client is afraid to express anger appropriately, fearing criticism or censure or a loss of control. Hostile behavior also can be related to the client's inability to express other feelings directly, such as shame, fear, or anxiety, or to other problems such as hallucinations, personality disorders (e.g., antisocial personality), conduct disorders, substance use, and post-traumatic stress disorder.

Although anger and hostility often may be seen as similar, hostility is characterized as purposely harmful. Anger is not necessarily hostility and may not be in need of control; it may be a healthy response to circumstances, feelings, or hospitalization (i.e., with the accompanying loss of personal control). When the client is not agitated, it is important to help the client examine his or her feelings and to support expressing anger in ways that are not injurious to the client or others and are acceptable to the client. Remember to be aware of the client's culture and how cultural values influence the client's perceptions and reactions.

Hostile behavior can lead to aggressive behavior. In assessing and planning care for these clients, it is important to be aware of past behavior: How has the client exhibited hostile behavior? What has the client threatened to do, and what was his or her actual behavior in these situations? What are the client's own limits for himself or herself? Remember that some medications (e.g., benzodiazepines) may agitate the client or precipitate outbursts of rage by suppressing inhibitions.

Nursing goals include preventing harm to the client and others and diminishing hostile or aggressive behavior, and assisting the client to develop skills in recognizing and managing feelings of anger safely and appropriately. Remember, the goal is not to control the client or to eliminate anger, but to protect the client and others from injury and to help the client develop and use healthy ways of controlling himself or herself and expressing feelings. It is extremely important in working with these clients to be aware of your own feelings. If you are angry with the client, you may tell the client that you are angry and explain the reason(s) for your anger, thereby modeling for the client an appropriate expression of anger. However, be sure that you do not act out your anger in a hostile or punitive way.

NURSING DIAGNOSES ADDRESSED IN THIS CARE PLAN
Risk for Other-Directed Violence
Noncompliance
Ineffective Coping

RELATED NURSING DIAGNOSES ADDRESSED IN THE MANUAL
Chronic Low Self-Esteem
Impaired Social Interaction

Nursing Diagnosis

Risk for Other-Directed Violence

At risk for behaviors in which an individual demonstrates that he or she can be physically, emotionally, and/or sexually harmful to others.

RISK FACTORS

- Feelings of anger or hostility
- Verbal aggression or abuse
- Agitation
- Restlessness (fidgeting, pacing)
- Inability to control voice volume (shouting)
- Outbursts of anger or hostility
- Uncooperative or belligerent behavior
- Physical combativeness, homicidal ideation, or destruction of property
- Lack of impulse control

EXPECTED OUTCOMES

Immediate   The client will

- Refrain from harming self or others throughout hospitalization
- Demonstrate decreased agitation, restlessness, or other risk factors within 24 to 48 hours

Stabilization   The client will

- Express angry feelings in a safe way, e.g., verbalize feelings to a staff member
- Be free of hostile behavior
- Verbalize knowledge of hostile behavior and alternatives to hostile behavior

Community   The client will

- Express emotions safely in stressful situations
- Continue with long-term therapy if appropriate

IMPLEMENTATION

Nursing Interventions *denotes collaborative interventions	Rationale
Withdraw your attention (ignore the client) when the client is verbally abusive. Tell the client that you are doing this and why (e.g., "I will not talk with you when you are being verbally abusive"), but you will give attention for appropriate behavior. If the client is physically abusive, provide for the safety of the client and others, and then withdraw your attention from the client.	Withdrawing attention can be more effective than negative reinforcement in decreasing unacceptable behaviors. The client may be seeking attention with this behavior. It is important to reinforce positive behaviors rather than unacceptable ones.
Be consistent and firm yet gentle and calm in your approach to the client.	As you provide limits, your behavior is a role model for the client.
Set and maintain firm limits.	Limits must be established by others when the client is unable to use internal controls effectively.
Remain calm. Control your own behavior, and communicate that control. If you are becoming upset, leave the situation in the hands of other staff members if possible.	Your behavior provides a role model for the client. If you behave in a hostile manner, it undermines limits and may exacerbate the client's hostile behavior.
Make it clear that you accept the client as a person, but that certain specified behaviors are unacceptable.	The client is acceptable as a person regardless of his or her behaviors, which may or may not be acceptable.

(continued on page 304)

IMPLEMENTATION (continued)

Nursing Interventions *denotes collaborative interventions	Rationale
Do not become insulted or defensive in response to the client's behavior.	Remember that your relationship with the client is professional. It is not a personal relationship, and it is not necessarily desirable for the client to like you. It may help to view verbal abuse as a loss of control or as projection on the client's part.
Do not argue with the client.	Arguing with the client can reinforce adversarial attitudes and undermine limits.
Be alert for a build-up of hostility in the client, such as increased verbal abuse or restless behavior.	Outbursts of hostility or aggression often are preceded by a period of increasing tension.
Be aware of and note situations and progression of events carefully, including precipitating factors, tension, level of stimuli, degree of structure, time, and staff members and others (clients, visitors) present.	Identifying patterns of behavior can be helpful in the anticipation of and early intervention in destructive behaviors.
Give support to those who are targets of the client's abuse (other clients, visitors, staff members) rather than giving the client attention for abusive behavior.	Others may not understand the client's behavior and may need support. If the client is seeking attention with hostile behavior, giving your attention to others may be effective in decreasing hostile behavior.
Do not attempt to discuss feelings when the client is agitated (see Care Plan 47: Aggressive Behavior).	Talking about feelings, especially anger, when the client is agitated may increase the agitation.
*Remain aware of your own feelings. It may be helpful if staff members express their feelings in a client care conference or informally to each other in private (away from the client and other clients).	A client who is hostile may be difficult to work with and engender feelings of anger, frustration, and resentment in staff members. These feelings need to be expressed so that they are not denied and subsequently acted out with the client. They should be discussed with other staff members; it is not therapeutic for the client to deal with the staff's feelings.
Encourage the client to seek a staff member when he or she is becoming upset or having strong feelings.	Seeking staff assistance allows intervention before the client can no longer control his or her behavior and encourages the client to recognize feelings and seek help.
Discuss with the client alternative ways of expressing emotions and releasing physical energy or tension.	The client needs to learn nondestructive ways to express feelings and release tension.
Encourage the client to increase his or her physical activity to release tension and plan to continue a regular exercise regimen after hospitalization. Encourage solitary or non-competitive activities to avoid placing the client in competitive sports situations.	Physical activity provides many health benefits, including decreasing physical tension. Competitive situations may trigger or exacerbate hostile behavior.
As early as possible, give the client the responsibility for recognizing and appropriately dealing with his or her feelings. Expect the client to take responsibility for his or her actions; make this clear to the client.	Assuming responsibility for his or her feelings and actions may help the client to develop or increase insight and internal controls. It may diminish the client's blaming others or feeling victimized.
Give the client positive feedback for controlling aggression, fulfilling responsibilities, and expressing feelings appropriately, especially angry feelings.	Positive feedback provides reinforcement for desired behaviors and can enhance self-esteem. It is essential that the client receive attention for positive behaviors, not only for unacceptable behaviors.

Nursing Diagnosis

Noncompliance

Behavior of a person and/or caregiver that fails to coincide with a health-promoting or therapeutic plan agreed on by the person (and/or family and/or community) and healthcare professional. In the presence of an agreed upon, health-promoting, or therapeutic plan, the person's or caregiver's behavior is fully or partially nonadherent and may lead to clinically ineffective or partially ineffective outcomes.

ASSESSMENT DATA

- Refusal to take medications
- Refusal to participate in treatment program
- Refusal to observe limits on behavior

EXPECTED OUTCOMES

Immediate

The client will

- Take medications as given within 24 to 48 hours
- Begin to participate in treatment plan, e.g., attend group activity at least once per day within 2 to 3 days

Stabilization

The client will

- Take medications without resistance
- Demonstrate full compliance with treatment plan, e.g., observe all behavioral limits, participate in all activities
- Verbalize plans to continue with long-term therapy if appropriate

Community

The client will

- Manage medication regimen independently
- Follow up with outpatient care

IMPLEMENTATION

Nursing Interventions *denotes collaborative interventions	Rationale
Involve the client in treatment planning and in decision making regarding his or her treatment as much as possible.	Participation in planning treatment can help reinforce the client's participation and help prevent the client from assuming a victim role or feeling that he or she has no choice (and no responsibility) in his or her treatment.
One staff member may verbally review limits, rationale, and other aspects of the treatment program with the client, but this should be done only once and should not be negotiated after limits have been set. You may provide a written plan to the client.	The client is entitled to an explanation of the treatment program, but justification, negotiation, or repeated discussions can undermine the program and reinforce the client's noncompliance.
Set and maintain firm limits. Do not argue with the client. Be specific and consistent regarding expectations; do not make exceptions.	Setting clear, specific limits lets the client know what is expected of him or her. Arguing with the client and making exceptions interject doubt and undermine limits.
It may be necessary to pay close attention to ensure the client ingests medication as ordered. Liquid medications, sprinkles, or dissolving tablets may be prescribed until the client accepts the need for medications.	The client may try to avoid taking prescribed medication. Using alternate forms of medications (when available) can prevent the client's hiding oral medications in his or her mouth and discarding them unobserved.
Withdraw your attention if possible (and safe) when the client refuses to participate or exceeds limits. Give positive support for the client's efforts to participate in treatment planning and treatment.	Withdrawing attention from unacceptable behavior can help diminish that behavior, but the client needs to receive attention for desired behaviors, not only for unacceptable behavior.

(continued on page 306)

IMPLEMENTATION (continued)

Nursing Interventions *denotes collaborative interventions	Rationale
It may be helpful to have one staff person per shift designated for decision making regarding the client and special circumstances (see "Key Considerations in Mental Health Nursing: Therapeutic Milieu").	Having one person designated as responsible for decisions minimizes the chance the client manipulating other staff members.
As the client's hostile behavior diminishes, talk with the client about underlying problems and feelings; continue to include the client in treatment planning.	When the client is less agitated, he or she will be better able to focus on feelings and other problems and more receptive to participation in treatment.
Help the client to identify factors involved in his or her noncompliance and other behaviors. Provide or encourage continued treatment for these underlying factors.	The client may have underlying personal, social, or psychiatric conditions that contribute to his or her behaviors. Developing insight into and addressing these issues will help prevent reoccurrence.

Nursing Diagnosis

Ineffective Coping

Inability to form a valid appraisal of the stressors, inadequate choices of practiced responses, and/or inability to use available resources.

ASSESSMENT DATA

- Inability to deal with feelings of anger or hostility
- Lack of insight
- Denial and projection of feelings that are unacceptable to the client
- Disordered thoughts
- Underlying feelings of anxiety, guilt, or shame
- Low self-esteem

EXPECTED OUTCOMES

Immediate   The client will

- Identify and verbalize feelings in a nonhostile manner within 3 to 4 days

Stabilization   The client will

- Express feelings to staff, other clients, or significant others, in a nonhostile manner
- Identify and demonstrate nonhostile ways to deal with feelings, stress, and problems, e.g., talking with others, writing in a journal, physical activity

Community   The client will

- Cope effectively with daily stress and life events in a nonhostile manner
- Seek assistance if hostile feelings return

IMPLEMENTATION

Nursing Interventions *denotes collaborative interventions	Rationale
Encourage the client to seek help from a staff member when he or she is becoming upset or having strong feelings.	Seeking staff assistance allows intervention before the client can no longer control his or her behavior and encourages the client to recognize feelings and seek help.
When the client is not agitated, discuss the client's feelings and ways to express them.	The client may need to learn how to identify feelings and ways to express them.
*Use role-playing and groups (formal and informal) to facilitate the client's expression of feelings.	The client can practice new behaviors in a nonthreatening, supportive environment.

IMPLEMENTATION (continued)

Nursing Interventions *denotes collaborative interventions	Rationale
Discuss the client's feelings about his or her hostile behavior, including past behaviors, their consequences, and so forth, in a nonjudgmental manner.	The client may be ashamed of his or her behavior, feel guilty, or lack insight into his or her behavior.
Discuss with the client alternative ways of expressing angry feelings and releasing physical energy or tension.	The client may need to learn other ways to express feelings and release tension.
Try to make physical activities available on a regular basis and when the client is becoming upset (e.g., running laps in a gymnasium). Encourage the client to use a regular exercise program to release tension.	Physical activity provides the client with a way to relieve tension in a healthy, nondestructive manner.
Provide opportunities for the client to succeed at activities, tasks, and interactions. Give positive feedback, and point out the client's demonstrated abilities and strengths.	Activities within the client's abilities will provide opportunities for success. Positive feedback provides reinforcement for the client's growth and can enhance self-esteem.
Help the client set goals for his or her behavior; give positive feedback when the client achieves these goals.	Setting goals promotes the client's sense of control and teaches goal-setting skills; achieving goals can foster self-confidence and self-esteem.
Be realistic in your feedback to the client; do not flatter the client or be otherwise dishonest.	Honesty promotes trust. Clients with low self-esteem do not benefit from flattery or undue praise.
*Teach the client and his or her family or significant others about hostile behavior, other psychiatric problems, and medication use if any.	Information about psychiatric problems and medications can promote understanding, compliance with treatment regimen, and safe use of medications.
*Encourage the client to follow through with continuing treatment for substance dependence or other psychiatric problems if appropriate.	Problems associated with hostile behavior may require long-term treatment.

CARE PLAN 47

Aggressive Behavior

Aggressive behavior is the acting out of aggressive or hostile impulses in a violent or destructive manner; it may be directed toward objects, other people, or the self. Aggressive behavior may be related to feelings of anger or hostility, homicidal ideation, fears, psychotic processes (e.g., delusions), substance use, personality disorders, or other factors (see other care plans as appropriate). Aggressive behavior may develop gradually or occur suddenly, especially in a client who is psychotic or intoxicated. Some signs that a client might become aggressive include restlessness, increasing tension, psychomotor agitation, making threats, verbal abuse, or increasing voice volume.

Safety is paramount with an aggressive client. The nursing staff needs to protect the client and others from harm and provide a safe, nonthreatening, and therapeutic environment. Preventing aggressive behavior, providing an outlet for the client's physical tension and agitation, and helping the client to express feelings in a nonaggressive manner are important goals. If the client acts out, nursing goals include dealing safely and effectively with physical aggression or weapons, providing safe transportation of the client from one area to another (e.g., into seclusion), providing for the client's safety and needs while the client is in restraints or seclusion, and providing for the safety and needs of other clients.

Important ethical and legal issues are involved in the care of clients who exhibit aggressive behavior. Because the client is not in control of his or her own behavior, it is the staff's responsibility to provide control to protect the client and others. This control is not provided to punish the client or for the staff's convenience. These clients may be difficult to work with and may invoke feelings of anger, fear, frustration, and so forth in staff members. It is essential to be aware of these feelings so that you do not act them out in nontherapeutic or dangerous ways. *Remember*: Clients who are aggressive continue to have feelings, dignity, and human and legal rights. The principle of treating the client safely with the least degree of restriction is important; do not overreact to a situation (e.g., if the client does not need to be restrained, do not restrain him or her). Because of legal considerations, accurate observation and documentation are essential.

Clients who exhibit aggressive behavior may pose real, sometimes life-threatening danger to others. Because of the possibility of sustaining injuries, nursing staff must be cautious when attempting to physically control or restrain a client. Appropriate precautions should be taken to avoid exposure to blood or other body substances, such as taking extreme care to avoid a needlestick injury when medicating an agitated client. If a situation progresses beyond the ability of nursing staff to control the client's behavior safely, the nurse in charge may seek outside assistance, such as security staff or police. When police are summoned, the nursing staff will completely relinquish the situation to them. The other clients then become the sole nursing responsibility until the situation is controlled.

NURSING DIAGNOSES ADDRESSED IN THIS CARE PLAN
Risk for Other-Directed Violence
Ineffective Coping
Risk for Injury

RELATED NURSING DIAGNOSES ADDRESSED IN THE MANUAL
Noncompliance
Impaired Social Interaction
Chronic Low Self-Esteem

Nursing Diagnosis

Risk for Other-Directed Violence

At risk for behaviors in which an individual demonstrates that he or she can be physically, emotionally, and/or sexually harmful to others.

RISK FACTORS

- Actual or potential physical acting out of violence
- Destruction of property
- Homicidal or suicidal ideation
- Physical danger to self or others
- History of assaultive behavior or arrests
- Neurologic illness
- Disordered thoughts
- Agitation or restlessness
- Lack of impulse control
- Delusions, hallucinations, or other psychotic symptoms
- Personality disorder or other psychiatric symptoms
- Manic behavior
- Conduct disorder
- Post-traumatic stress disorder
- Substance use

EXPECTED OUTCOMES

Immediate   The client will

- Refrain from harming others or destroying property throughout hospitalization
- Be free of self-inflicted harm throughout hospitalization
- Demonstrate decreased acting-out behavior within 12 to 24 hours
- Experience decreased restlessness or agitation within 24 to 48 hours
- Experience decreased fear, anxiety, or hostility within 2 to 3 days

Stabilization   The client will

- Demonstrate the ability to exercise internal control over his or her behavior
- Be free of psychotic behavior
- Identify ways to deal with tension and aggressive feelings in a nondestructive manner
- Express feelings of anxiety, fear, anger, or hostility verbally or in a nondestructive manner, e.g., talk with staff about these feelings at least once per day by a specified date
- Verbalize an understanding of aggressive behavior, associated disorder(s), and medications if any

Community   The client will

- Participate in therapy for underlying or associated psychiatric problems
- Demonstrate internal control of behavior when confronted with stress

IMPLEMENTATION

Nursing Interventions *denotes collaborative interventions	Rationale
Build a trust relationship with this client as soon as possible, ideally well in advance of aggressive episodes.	Familiarity with and trust in the staff members can decrease the client's fears and facilitate communication.
Be aware of factors that increase the likelihood of violent behavior or agitation. Use verbal communication or PRN medication to intervene before the client's behavior	A period of building tension often precedes acting out; however, a client who is intoxicated or psychotic may become violent without warning. Signs of increasing

(continued on page 310)

IMPLEMENTATION (continued)

Nursing Interventions *denotes collaborative interventions	Rationale
reaches a destructive point and physical restraint becomes necessary.	agitation include increased restlessness, motor activity (e.g., pacing), voice volume, verbal cues ("I'm afraid of losing control."), threats, decreased frustration tolerance, and frowning or clenching fists.
If the client tells you (verbally or nonverbally) that he or she feels hostile or destructive, try to help the client express these feelings in nondestructive ways (e.g., use communication techniques or take the client to the gym for physical exercise).	The client can try out new behaviors with you in a non-threatening environment and learn nondestructive ways to express feelings rather than acting out.
Anticipate the possible need for PRN medication and seclusion or restraint orders.	In an aggressive situation, you will need to make decisions and act quickly. If the client is severely agitated, medication may be necessary to decrease the agitation.
*Develop and practice consistent techniques of safe restraint as part of nursing orientation and continuing education.	Consistent techniques let each staff person know what is expected and will increase safety and effectiveness.
*Develop instructions in safe techniques for carrying clients.	Consistent techniques increase safety and effectiveness.
Be familiar with restraint, seclusion, and staff assistance procedures and legal requirements.	You must be prepared to act and direct other staff in the safe management of the client. You are legally accountable for your decisions and actions.
Always maintain control of yourself and the situation; remain calm. If you do not feel competent in dealing with a situation, obtain assistance as soon as possible.	Your behavior provides a role model for the client and communicates that you can and will provide control. Not all situations are within nursing's expertise or control; recognizing the need for outside assistance in a timely manner is essential.
Calmly and respectfully assure the client that you (the staff) will provide control if he or she cannot control himself or herself, but do not threaten the client.	The client may fear loss of control and may be afraid of what he or she may do if he or she begins to express anger or other feelings. Showing that you are in control without competing with the client can reassure the client without lowering his or her self-esteem.
*Notify the charge nurse and supervisor as soon as possible in a (potentially) aggressive situation; tell them your assessment of the situation and the need for help, the client's name, care plan, and orders for medication, seclusion, or restraint.	You may need assistance from staff members who are unfamiliar with this client. They will be able to help more effectively and safely if they are aware of this information.
*Follow the hospital staff assistance plan (e.g., use paging system to call for assistance to your location); then, if possible, have one staff member familiar with the situation meet the additional staff at the unit door to give them the client's name, situation, goal, plan, and so forth.	The need for help may be immediate in an emergency situation. Any information that can be given to arriving staff will be helpful in ensuring safety and effectiveness in dealing with this client.
If the client has a weapon:	
If you are not properly trained or skilled in dealing safely with a client who has a weapon, do not attempt to remove the weapon. Keep something (like a pillow, mattress, or a blanket wrapped around your arm) between you and the weapon.	*Avoiding personal injury, summoning help, leaving the area, or protecting other clients may be the only things you can realistically do. You may risk further danger by attempting to remove a weapon or subdue an armed client.*
If it is necessary to remove the weapon, try to kick it out of the client's hand. (Never reach for a knife or other weapon with your hand.)	*Reaching for a weapon increases your physical vulnerability.*
Distract the client momentarily to remove the weapon (e.g., throw water in the client's face, or yell suddenly).	*Distracting the client's attention may give you an opportunity to remove the weapon or subdue the client.*

IMPLEMENTATION (continued)

Nursing Interventions *denotes collaborative interventions	Rationale
*You may need to summon outside assistance (especially if the client has a gun). When this is done, total responsibility is delegated to the outside authorities.	Exceeding your abilities may place you in grave danger. It is not necessary to try to deal with a situation beyond your control or to assume personal risk.
Remain aware of the client's body space or territory; do not trap the client.	Potentially violent people have a body space zone up to four times larger than that of other people. That is, you need to stay farther away from them for them to not feel trapped or threatened.
Allow the client freedom to move around (within safe limits) unless you are trying to restrain him or her.	Interfering with the client's mobility without the intent of restraint may increase the client's frustration, fears, or perception of threat.
Decrease stimulation by turning television off or lowering the volume, lowering the lights, asking others to leave the area (or you can go with the client to another room).	If the client is feeling threatened, he or she can perceive any stimulus as a threat. The client is unable to deal with excess stimuli when agitated.
Talk with the client in a low, calm voice. Call the client by name, tell the client your name, where you are, and so forth.	Using a low voice may help prevent increasing agitation. The client may be disoriented or unaware of what is happening.
Tell the client what you are going to do and what you are doing as you actually do it. For example, "I will walk with you to another room to keep you safe" or "we are taking you to another room where you will be safe." Use simple, clear, direct speech; repeat if necessary. Do not threaten the client, but state limits and expectations.	The client's ability to understand the situation and to process information is impaired. Clear limits let the client know what is expected of him or her. Reassuring the client of his or her safety can lessen the client's perception of threat or harm, especially if he or she is experiencing psychotic symptoms.
Do not use physical restraints or techniques without sufficient reason.	The client has a right to the fewest restrictions possible within the limits of safety and prevention of destructive behavior.
*When a decision has been made to subdue or restrain the client, act quickly and cooperatively with other staff members. Tell the client in a matter-of-fact manner that he or she will be restrained, subdued, or secluded; allow no bargaining after the decision has been made. Reassure the client that he or she will not be hurt and that restraint or seclusion is to ensure safety.	Firm limits must be set and maintained. Bargaining interjects doubt and will undermine the limit. Reassuring the client of his or her safety can lessen the client's perception of threat or harm, especially if he or she is experiencing psychotic symptoms.
*While subduing or restraining the client, talk with other staff members to ensure coordination of effort (e.g., do not attempt to carry the client until everyone has verbally indicated they are ready).	Direct verbal communication will promote cooperation and safety.
Do not strike the client.	Physical safety of the client is a priority. The staff may subdue the client to prevent injury to the client or others but striking the client is not acceptable.
Do not help to restrain or subdue the client if you are angry (if enough other staff members are present). Do not restrain or subdue the client as a punishment.	Staff members must maintain self-control at all times and act in the client's best interest. There is no justification for being punitive to a client.
Do not recruit or allow other clients to help in restraining or subduing a client.	Physical safety of all clients is a priority. Other clients are not responsible for controlling the behavior of a client and should not assume a staff role.
If possible, do not allow other clients to watch staff subduing the client. Take them to a different area, and involve them in activities or discussion.	Other clients may be frightened, agitated, or endangered by a client with aggressive behavior. They need safety and reassurance at this time.
Obtain additional staff assistance when needed. Have someone clear furniture and so forth from the area through which you will be carrying the client.	Transporting a client who is agitated can be dangerous if attempted without sufficient help and sufficient space.

(continued on page 312)

IMPLEMENTATION (continued)

Nursing Interventions *denotes collaborative interventions	Rationale
When placing the client in restraints or seclusion, tell the client what you are doing and the reason (e.g., to regain control or protect the client from injuring himself, herself, or others). Use simple, concise language in a calm, non-judgmental, matter-of-fact manner (see Nursing Diagnosis: Risk for Injury).	The client's ability to understand what is happening to him or her may be impaired.
When the client is in restraints or seclusion, tell the client where he or she is, that he or she will be safe, and that staff members will continue to check on him or her. Tell the client how to summon the staff. Reorient the client or remind him or her of the reason for restraint as necessary.	Being placed in seclusion or restraints can be terrifying to a client. Your assurances may help alleviate the client's fears.
Reassess the client's need for continued seclusion or restraint according to the client's condition and facility policies. Release the client or decrease restraint as soon as it is safe and therapeutic. Base your decisions on the client's, not the staff's, needs.	The client has a right to the least restrictions possible within the limits of safety and prevention of destructive behavior. The client's safety and rights are priorities over staffing challenges or convenience.
Remain aware of the client's feelings (including fear), dignity, and rights.	The client is a worthwhile person regardless of his or her unacceptable behavior.
Carefully observe the client and promptly complete documentation in keeping with hospital policy. Bear in mind possible legal implications.	Accurate, complete documentation is essential, as restraint, seclusion, assault, and so forth are situations that may result in legal action.
Administer medications safely; take care to prepare correct dosage, identify correct sites for administration, withdraw plunger to aspirate for blood, and so forth.	When you are in a stressful situation and under pressure to move quickly, the possibility of errors in dosage or administration of medication is increased.
Take care to avoid needlestick injury and other injuries that may involve exposure to the client's blood or body fluids.	Hepatitis, HIV, and other diseases are transmitted by exposure to blood or body fluids.
Monitor the client for effects of medications, and intervene as appropriate.	Psychoactive drugs can have adverse effects, such as allergic reactions, hypotension, and pseudoparkinsonian symptoms.
Talk with other clients after the situation is resolved; allow them to express feelings about the situation.	Other clients have continued needs for therapeutic intervention in addition to their reactions to the acute situation. Be careful not to give attention only to the client who acts out or to withdraw to staff areas to discuss staff reactions and feelings.

Nursing Diagnosis

Ineffective Coping
Inability to form a valid appraisal of the stressors, inadequate choices of practiced responses, and/or inability to use available resources.

ASSESSMENT DATA

- Lack of problem-solving skills
- Destructive behavior
- Feelings of anger or hostility
- Feelings of anxiety, fear, or panic
- Feelings of worthlessness or guilt
- Inability to deal with feelings

EXPECTED OUTCOMES

Immediate	The client will

- Experience decreased fear, anxiety, or hostility within 24 to 48 hours
- Express feelings of anxiety, fear, anger, or hostility verbally or in a nondestructive manner within 3 to 4 days
- Verbalize feelings of self-worth, e.g., identify areas of strengths, abilities within 3 to 5 days

Stabilization	The client will

- Verbalize feelings of anxiety, fear, anger, hostility, worthlessness, and so forth
- Identify ways to deal with tension and aggressive feelings in a nondestructive manner, e.g., talking with others, physical activity
- Demonstrate or verbalize increased feelings of self-worth
- Verbalize plans to continue with long-term therapy if appropriate

Community	The client will

- Participate in therapy for underlying or associated psychiatric problems
- Deal with tension and aggressive feelings in a nondestructive manner in the community

IMPLEMENTATION

Nursing Interventions *denotes collaborative interventions	Rationale
Approach the client in a calm, matter-of-fact manner. Speak in a quiet, steady voice.	Your calm demeanor will communicate your confidence and sense of control to the client.
When the client is not agitated, encourage him or her to express feelings verbally, in writing, or in other nonaggressive ways.	The client will be most able to discuss emotional issues when he or she is not agitated. If the client is agitated, discussing emotional problems may increase agitation.
Teach the client about aggressive behavior, including how to identify feelings that may precede this behavior, such as increasing tension or restlessness. Help the client identify strategies that may help him or her avoid aggressive behavior.	The client may be unaware of the dynamics of aggressive behavior and feelings associated with it. Gaining this knowledge may help prevent aggressive behavior in the future.
Teach the client to use a problem-solving process: identifying the problem, evaluating possible solutions, implementing a solution, and evaluating the process.	The client may never have learned a systematic, effective approach to solving problems. Implementing a problem-solving process may help the client avoid frustration.
Encourage the client to identify and use nondestructive ways to express feelings or deal with physical tension.	The client may be able to avoid aggressive behavior using these techniques.
Talk with the client about coping strategies he or she has used in the past. Explore which strategies have been successful and which may have led to negative consequences.	The client may have had success using coping strategies in the past but may have lost confidence in himself or herself or in his or her ability to cope with stressors and feelings. Some coping strategies can be self-destructive (e.g., self-medication with drugs or alcohol).
Teach the client about positive coping strategies and stress management skills, such as increasing physical exercise, expressing feelings verbally or in a journal, or meditation techniques. Encourage the client to practice this type of technique while in the hospital.	The client may have limited or no knowledge of stress management techniques or may not have used positive techniques in the past. If the client tries to build skills in the treatment setting, he or she can experience success and receive positive feedback for his or her efforts.
*Teach the client and family or significant others about other disease process(es) and medication use if any.	The client's significant others may lack understanding of the client's behavior; they also can be supportive as the client attempts to change behavior.
Help the client set goals for his or her behavior; give positive feedback when the client achieves these goals.	Achieving goals can foster self-confidence and self-esteem. Allowing the client to set goals promotes the client's sense of control and teaches goal-setting skills.

(continued on page 314)

IMPLEMENTATION (continued)

Nursing Interventions *denotes collaborative interventions	Rationale
*Include the client's significant others in setting goals and planning strategies for change, as appropriate.	Including significant others can promote compliance with treatment and support for the client.
Provide opportunities for the client to succeed at activities, tasks, and interactions. Give positive feedback, and point out the client's demonstrated abilities and strengths.	Activities within the client's abilities will provide opportunities for success. Positive feedback provides reinforcement for the client's growth and can enhance self-esteem.
Be realistic in your feedback to the client; do not flatter the client or be otherwise dishonest.	Honesty promotes trust. Clients with low self-esteem do not benefit from flattery or undue praise.

Nursing Diagnosis

Risk for Injury
At risk for injury as a result of environmental conditions interacting with the individual's adaptive and defensive resources.

RISK FACTORS

- Actual or potential physical acting out of violence
- Destructive behavior toward objects or other people
- Agitation or restlessness
- Neurologic illness
- Delusions, hallucinations, or other psychotic symptoms
- Disordered thoughts
- Transportation of the client by staff under duress
- Confinement of the client in restraints or seclusion

EXPECTED OUTCOMES

Immediate   The client will

- Be free of self-inflicted harm throughout hospitalization
- Be free of accidental injury throughout hospitalization

Stabilization   The client will

- Remain free of injury
- Be free of psychotic behavior

Community   The client will

- Demonstrate internal control of behavior

IMPLEMENTATION

Nursing Interventions *denotes collaborative interventions	Rationale
*Develop and practice consistent techniques of restraint as part of nursing orientation and continuing education.	Consistent techniques let each staff person know what is expected and will increase safety and effectiveness.
*Obtain instructions in safe techniques for carrying clients as part of regular staff training.	Consistent techniques increase safety and effectiveness.
*Follow the hospital staff assistance plan (e.g., use paging system to call for assistance to your location); then, if possible, have one staff member familiar with the situation meet the additional staff at the unit door to give them the client's name, situation, goal, plan, and so forth.	The need for help may be immediate in an emergency situation. Any information that can be given to arriving staff will be helpful in ensuring safety and effectiveness in dealing with this client.

IMPLEMENTATION (continued)

Nursing Interventions *denotes collaborative interventions	Rationale
*While subduing or restraining the client, talk with other staff members to ensure coordination of effort. (For example, do not attempt to carry the client until everyone has verbally indicated they are ready.)	Direct verbal communication will promote cooperation and safety.
Obtain additional staff assistance when needed. Have someone clear furniture and so forth from the area through which you will be carrying the client.	Transporting a client who is agitated can be dangerous if attempted without sufficient help and sufficient space.
Apply mechanical restraints safely. Check extremities for color, temperature, and pulse distal to the restraints.	Mechanical restraints applied too tightly can impair circulation of blood.
Recheck extremities at least as often as specified in hospital policy (e.g., every 15 minutes) for color, temperature, and pulse distal to the restraints.	The client may increase the pressure of restraints against limbs when changing position.
If necessary, loosen and reapply restraints one at a time to exercise limbs or change the client's position.	The client may continue to be agitated; loosening one restraint and reapplying it before loosening another can minimize chances of injury to you and the client.
Administer medications safely; take care to prepare correct dosage, identify correct sites for administration, and so forth.	When you are in a stressful situation and under pressure to act quickly, the possibility of making an error in dosage or administration of medication is increased.
Monitor the client for effects of medications, and intervene as appropriate.	Psychoactive drugs can have adverse effects, such as allergic reactions, hypotension, and pseudoparkinsonian symptoms.
Check or observe the client at least as often as specified in hospital policy (e.g., every 15 minutes). Assess the client's safety, nutrition, hydration, and elimination. Offer fluids, food, and opportunities for hygiene and elimination; assist the client as necessary.	The client's safety is a priority. The client is in a helpless position and needs assistance with activities of daily living. The client's nutrition and hydration needs may be increased due to the physical exertion of his or her agitation.
Perform passive range of motion on restrained limbs, and reposition the client at least as often as specified in hospital policy (e.g., every 2 hours).	These actions minimize the deleterious effects of immobility.

CARE PLAN 48

Passive–Aggressive Behavior

Passive–aggressive personality disorder is characterized by the use of passive behavior to express hostility. This behavior includes obstructionism, pouting, procrastination, stubbornness, and intentional inefficiency. Clients with passive–aggressive personality disorder are resentful and negative and have difficulties in interpersonal relationships and work situations. These clients often also have another type of personality disorder, such as borderline, paranoid, dependent, or antisocial (APA, 2000).

Clients with this disorder manifest passive–aggressive and manipulative behaviors, but these behaviors also can be seen in clients with other problems. *Passive–aggressive behavior* is a type of indirect expression of feelings whereby a client does not express aggressive (angry, resentful) feelings verbally but denies them and reveals them instead through behavior. *Manipulative behavior* is characterized by the client's attempts to control his or her interactions and relationships with others, often to satisfy some immediate desire or to avoid discomfort or change.

Like other personality disorders, passive–aggressive personality disorder is persistent over time. Negativistic personality traits may be evident in childhood or adolescence, but the disorder per se is diagnosed only in adults (the diagnosis of *oppositional defiant disorder* is given to children with similar problems; APA, 2000).

It is especially important to remember your professional role when working with clients who have passive–aggressive personality disorder or who manifest passive–aggressive or manipulative behavior. Remember that it is neither necessary nor particularly desirable for the client to like you personally. It is not your purpose to be a friend to the client, nor is it the client's purpose to be a friend to you.

An important goal in working with these clients is to facilitate the client's accepting responsibility for his or her behavior. It may be beneficial to involve the client in care planning, but clients who manifest manipulative behavior may have little motivation to change their behavior or ways of relating to others. In seeking treatment, the client may want merely to get out of a crisis or stressful situation. Key nursing interventions include setting and maintaining consistent limits, encouraging direct expression of feelings, and promoting effective coping skills.

NURSING DIAGNOSIS ADDRESSED IN THIS CARE PLAN
Ineffective Coping

RELATED NURSING DIAGNOSES ADDRESSED IN THE MANUAL
Impaired Social Interaction
Chronic Low Self-Esteem
Noncompliance

Nursing Diagnosis

Ineffective Coping
Inability to form a valid appraisal of the stressors, inadequate choices of practiced responses, and/or inability to use available resources.

ASSESSMENT DATA

- Denial of problems or feelings
- Lack of insight
- Inability or refusal to express emotions directly (especially anger)
- Refusal to participate in activities
- Resistance to therapy
- Forgetfulness
- Dishonesty
- Anger or hostility
- Superficial relationships with others
- Somatic complaints
- Preoccupation with other clients' problems ("playing therapist") or with staff members to avoid dealing with his or her own problems
- Intellectualization or rationalization of problems
- Dependency
- Manipulation of staff or family
- Attempts to gain special treatment or privileges

EXPECTED OUTCOMES

Immediate

The client will

- Participate in the treatment program, activities, and so forth, e.g., participate in at least one activity per shift within 24 to 36 hours
- Verbalize fewer somatic complaints within 24 to 48 hours
- Demonstrate decreased manipulative, attention-seeking, or passive–aggressive behaviors within 3 to 4 days
- Express feelings directly, verbally and nonverbally, within 3 to 4 days

Stabilization

The client will

- Verbalize self-responsibility for behavior
- Communicate directly and honestly with staff and other clients about himself or herself
- Develop or increase feelings of self-worth
- Verbalize knowledge of problem behaviors, treatment plan, and other therapies
- Demonstrate independence from the hospital environment and staff
- Demonstrate increased responsibility for himself or herself

Community

The client will

- Express feelings, including anger, directly and in a nondestructive manner, e.g., by talking with a therapist or significant others
- Demonstrate increased feelings of self-worth
- Demonstrate appropriate interactions with others
- Demonstrate problem-solving skills when dealing with situations or others

IMPLEMENTATION

Nursing Interventions *denotes collaborative interventions	Rationale
*When the client voices a somatic complaint, immediately refer the client to a physician or treat according to the care plan. Then, tell the client that you will discuss other things, such as feelings. Do not engage in lengthy conversations about the client's physical complaints or condition.	Treating the somatic complaint in a matter-of-fact, consistent manner will minimize reinforcement of attention-seeking behavior. Emphasizing the client's feelings rather than physical complaints can help reinforce verbalization of feelings.
Note patterns in somatic complaints; e.g., does the client complain of having a headache when he or she is supposed to go to an activity?	The client may voice complaints because he or she finds a situation stressful, or the client may use complaints to avoid activities, and so forth.

(continued on page 318)

IMPLEMENTATION (continued)

Nursing Interventions *denotes collaborative interventions	Rationale
State the limits and the behavior you expect from the client. Do not debate, argue, rationalize, or bargain with the client.	Specific limits let the client know what is expected. Arguing, bargaining, or justifying interject doubt and undermine the limit.
Enforce all unit and hospital policies or regulations. Without apologizing, point out reasons for not bending the rules.	Institutional regulations provide a therapeutic structure. Apologizing for regulations undermines this structure and encourages manipulative behavior.
Be consistent, both with this client and all other clients; that is, do not insist that this client follow a rule while excusing another client from the same rule.	Consistency provides structure and reinforces limits. Making exceptions undermines limits and encourages manipulative behavior.
Be kind but firm with the client. Make it clear that limits and caring are not mutually exclusive, that you set and maintain limits because you care about the client, even though the client may feel hurt from experiencing a limit from someone who cares about him or her.	The client is acceptable as a person regardless of his or her behaviors, which may or may not be acceptable. Because you care about the client's well-being, you set and maintain limits to encourage the client's growth and health.
Be direct and use confrontation with the client if necessary; however, be sure to examine your own feelings. Do not react to the client punitively or in anger.	You are a role model of appropriate behavior and self-control. There is no justification for punishing a client. Remember, the client is acceptable as a person regardless of his or her behaviors, which may or may not be acceptable.
*Involve the client in care planning to assess motivation and establish goals, but do not allow the client to dictate the terms of therapy (e.g., which therapists, length and frequency of interactions). Involve the client in the full treatment program.	Including the client in planning of care can encourage the client's sense of responsibility for his or her health. Allowing the client to dictate his or her care may encourage manipulation by the client.
*Set limits on the frequency and length of interactions between the client and staff members, especially those significant to or preferred by the client. Set specific and limited appointment times with therapists (e.g., Thursday, 2:00 to 2:30 PM), and allow interactions only at those times.	Setting and maintaining limits can help decrease attention-seeking and manipulative behaviors and reinforce appropriate behaviors.
Do not discuss yourself, other staff members, or other clients with the client.	Your relationship with the client is professional. Sharing personal information about yourself or others is inappropriate and can be used in a manipulative way.
Do not attempt to be popular, liked, or the "favorite staff member" of this client.	It is not necessary or particularly desirable for the client to like you personally. A professional relationship is based on the client's therapeutic needs, not personal feelings.
Do not accept gifts from the client or encourage a personal dependency relationship.	Maintaining your professional role is therapeutic for the client. Your acceptance of gifts may foster manipulative behavior (e.g., the client may expect you to grant special favors).
Withdraw your attention from the client if he or she says "you are the only staff member I can talk to ..." or "the only one who understands" and so forth; tell the client that this is not desirable. Emphasize the importance of the milieu in his or her therapy.	It is important that the client establishes and maintains trust relationships with a variety of people, staff, and other clients. If you are "the only one" or the client's "favorite," the client may be too dependent or may be flattering you as a basis for manipulation.
Discuss the client's feelings (e.g., anger, feeling rejected) about being denied special privileges or experiencing limits. Encourage the client's expression of those feelings.	The client's ability to identify and express feelings impaired, especially feelings that are frustrating or otherwise uncomfortable for him or her. The client may not be used to accepting limits.
Discuss the client's problems in relation to his or her life at home, rather than in relation to the hospitalization. Do, however, point out how the client's behavior on the unit reflects behavior patterns in the client's life.	Focusing on unit activities may be a way for the client to avoid the problems he or she has in his or her life situation. Also, the goal is for the client to learn to manage his or her behavior effectively in the community, not to be a "good patient."

IMPLEMENTATION (continued)

Nursing Interventions *denotes collaborative interventions	Rationale
Discuss the client's behavior with him or her in a nonjudgmental manner, using examples in a nonthreatening way.	Providing nonjudgmental feedback can help the client to acknowledge problems and develop insight.
Help the client examine his or her behavior and relationships. You might say, "You seem to be …" or "What effect do you see …?"	Reflection and feedback can be effective in increasing the client's insight.
Encourage the client to express feelings directly in verbal and nonverbal ways (such as writing in a journal).	Appropriate expression of feelings is a healthy behavior. The client's ability to identify and express feelings is impaired.
In your interactions with the client, emphasize expression of feelings rather than intellectualization.	The client may use intellectualization as a way of avoiding dealing with emotions.
Withdraw your attention when the client refuses to be involved in activities or other therapies or when the client's behavior is otherwise inappropriate.	Minimizing or withdrawing attention can be more effective than negative reinforcement in decreasing unacceptable behaviors.
Give attention and support when the client's behavior is appropriate (e.g., attends activities, expresses feelings).	Positive feedback provides reinforcement and can enhance self-esteem. It is essential that the client is given attention for appropriate behavior, not only for unacceptable behaviors.
Teach the client the problem-solving process: identifying the problem, exploring alternatives, making a decision, and evaluating its success.	The client may be unaware of a logical process for examining and resolving problems.
Describe and demonstrate social skills, such as eye contact, attentive listening, nodding, and so forth. Discuss topics that are appropriate for social conversation, such as the weather, local events, and so forth.	The client may have little or no knowledge of social interaction skills. Modeling provides a concrete example of the desired skills.
Encourage the client to practice these skills with staff members and other clients, and give the client feedback regarding interactions.	Practicing skills and receiving feedback within the therapeutic milieu provides an opportunity to learn and build skills in a nonthreatening environment.
Talk with the client about his or her interactions and observations of interpersonal dynamics.	Awareness of interpersonal and group dynamics is an important part of building social skills. Sharing observations provides an opportunity for the client to express his or her feelings and receive feedback about his or her progress.
Encourage the client to identify relationships that have been positive in the past and to identify other supportive people outside the hospital.	The client may have had supportive relationships in the past that can be reestablished or strengthened. The client may need to identify other people to form positive relationships using new skills for interactions and seeking support.

CARE PLAN 49

Sexual, Emotional, or Physical Abuse

Abusive behavior, also known as *family violence*, *battering*, or *abuse*, is the physical, sexual, or psychological maltreatment of one person by another (or others). This behavior can include the infliction of minor to life-threatening injuries; homicide; sexual abuse (including *incest*, *date rape*, and *marital rape*); or refusal to provide needed care, emotional nurturing, or economic assistance to a dependent person. Emotional abuse may be perceived by the victim as more devastating than even severe physical abuse, and the emotional consequences of any kind of abuse may be lifelong.

Cultural values and beliefs may be related to abusive behaviors or seem conducive to or consistent with them, such as ideas of personal ownership (e.g., that a child is the property of the parents), masculinity, discipline, marriage roles, and so forth. For example, a battered woman may not recognize an abusive marital relationship because she feels that *she* has failed at making a successful marriage, which she sees as her responsibility and which is central to her self-concept. Cultural factors also can influence the identification and treatment of an abusive situation; for example, a client's culture may have strong prohibitions against revealing information about family behavior to others, especially strangers or people in authority positions. It is imperative for the nurse to be aware of these factors and to help the client reconcile his or her needs with his or her cultural values.

Certain myths also contribute to the difficulty of recognizing abuse. Two examples of these myths are as follows: abuse happens only in low-income or alcoholic families; and the victim enjoys or provokes the abuse. *Remember*: There is *never* any justification for abuse.

Behavior related to abuse often resembles post-traumatic behavior (see Care Plan 31: Post-Traumatic Stress Disorder). Both abusers and adult victims of abuse may have witnessed or been the victims of abuse as children, but some may not recall the abuse until well into their adult lives, if at all. The behavior of victims of abuse has been described as "learned helplessness," in that they come to see themselves as powerless (because their actions have no effect on the abuser's behavior), and they become extremely passive. The abuser and the adult victim of abuse often share certain characteristics, such as low self-esteem, dependency needs, social isolation, lack of trust, and dysfunctional personal relationships. Domestic abuse may be seen as a dysfunctional family behavior, and family therapy may be indicated as a part of intervention.

Abusive behavior may be a factor in a number of other psychiatric problems, such as depression, suicidal behavior, aggressive behavior, withdrawn behavior, conduct disorders, eating disorders, substance abuse, and personality disorders. Abusive behavior can occur in any relationship, but it often takes place in intimate, family, or care-giving relationships, such as between parent and minor child, spouses or partners, or adult child and elderly parent. Abuse is extremely common and should be considered when you assess any client, especially those who present with any of the previous problems. In the United States, spouse or intimate partner abuse accounts for significant injury, death, and psychological and economic cost: approximately 4.8 million women and 2.9 million men experience intimate partner assaults each year (CDC, 2010d). In 2008, there were 3.3 million cases of child abuse or neglect reported to Child Protective Services (CDC, 2010b); however, these data include only confirmed cases and are considered to underestimate the situation. Elder abuse and neglect are also common and often not reported by the victim, who may feel completely dependent upon the perpetrator(s) of the abuse (CDC, 2010c).

Abusive behavior is characterized by a pattern of abusive episodes over time; without intervention, abuse is likely to continue, with episodes increasing in severity. An abusive episode has been identified as a cycle with three stages:

1. a buildup of tension;
2. an outburst of physical or emotional assault; and
3. a period of contrition, when the abuser demonstrates remorse and loving behavior toward the victim.

People involved in abusive behavior often deny that abuse is occurring and may be quite resistant to change. The abuser also may deny the abuse to himself or herself and justify the behavior or blame it on others, especially the victim. Adult victims of abuse often seek help in crisis situations but return to the abusive relationship when the crisis is past. Reasons for this return include economic dependence, fear of retribution, and love for the abusive person. Child, elder, and dependent adult abuse often must be reported by health care workers to appropriate authorities by law, but reporting abuse of other adult victims of abuse often requires the victim to agree to reporting and intervention.

Initial nursing goals include protecting the client from harm and decreasing withdrawn, depressive, aggressive, or suicidal behavior. Other therapeutic goals include promoting the client's recognition of the abuse, facilitating the client's participation in treatment, and promoting the client's self-esteem. As treatment progresses, it is important to help the client learn coping skills, to identify ways in which he or she can make changes, to make concrete plans to implement those changes, and to identify community resources for long-term support.

NURSING DIAGNOSES ADDRESSED IN THIS CARE PLAN
Post-Trauma Syndrome
Ineffective Coping
Chronic Low Self-Esteem

RELATED NURSING DIAGNOSES ADDRESSED IN THE MANUAL
Powerlessness
Risk for Other-Directed Violence
Risk for Suicide
Ineffective Denial
Risk for Self-Mutilation
Anxiety
Fear
Hopelessness
Impaired Social Interaction
Risk for Loneliness
Deficient Knowledge (Specify)

Nursing Diagnosis

Post-Trauma Syndrome
Sustained maladaptive response to a traumatic, overwhelming event.

ASSESSMENT DATA

Note: These parameters may be appropriate in the assessment of a victim of abuse or a perpetrator of abuse.

- Reexperience of abuse through dreams, intrusive thoughts, and so on
- Feelings of helplessness or powerlessness
- Denial of abuse
- Fatigue
- Apathy
- Poor grooming
- Excessive or inadequate body weight

- Sleep disturbances (nightmares, insomnia)
- Stress-related physiologic problems, such as headaches and gastrointestinal (GI) disturbances
- History of repeated hospitalizations or emergency room visits
- Substance abuse
- Fear, anxiety
- Feelings of shame or humiliation
- Feelings of guilt or remorse
- Depressive behavior
- Anger or rage (may not be overt)
- Difficulty in interpersonal relationships, such as lack of trust, excessive dependence, manipulative behavior, social isolation
- Poor impulse control
- History of assaultive behavior
- Anhedonia (inability to experience pleasure)
- Sexual problems
- Suicidal behavior
- Low self-esteem

EXPECTED OUTCOMES

Immediate

The client will

- Be free of self-inflicted harm throughout hospitalization
- Demonstrate decreased abusive behavior within 12 to 24 hours
- Identify the abusive behavior within 24 to 48 hours
- Participate in self-care for basic needs (e.g., personal hygiene, nutrition, and so forth) within 24 to 48 hours
- Demonstrate decreased withdrawn, depressive, or anxious behaviors within 2 to 3 days
- Demonstrate a decrease in stress-related or psychosomatic symptoms within 2 to 3 days
- Express feelings of helplessness, fear, anger, guilt, anxiety, and so forth, e.g., talk with staff about these feelings for at least 30 minutes at least twice per day within 2 to 4 days

Stabilization

The client will

- Verbalize acceptance of losses related to the abusive relationship(s)
- Remain free of abusive behavior
- Identify support systems outside the hospital, e.g., support groups or significant others
- Identify choices available for future plans, e.g., housing, employment

Community

The client will

- Make future plans based on awareness of abusive patterns
- Complete self-care for basic needs and activities of daily living independently
- Verbalize knowledge of abusive behavior and recovery process
- Participate in treatment for associated problems

IMPLEMENTATION

Nursing Interventions *denotes collaborative interventions	Rationale
Remain aware of the client's potential for self-destructive or aggressive behavior, and intervene as necessary (see Care Plan 26: Suicidal Behavior and Care Plan 47: Aggressive Behavior).	Clients who are in abusive situations are at increased risk for aggressive or self-destructive behavior, including homicide and suicide.
Be aware of state laws regarding reporting abuse and report to authorities required by law (e.g., child abuse). If not required by law, remember that adult victims of abuse must decide whether or not to report abuse.	State laws require that specific types of abuse (e.g., child, dependent adult abuse) be reported. An adult victim of abuse may be in greater danger by reporting abuse if he or she has continued contact with the abuser.

IMPLEMENTATION (continued)

Nursing Interventions *denotes collaborative interventions	Rationale
If the client is an independent adult, assure the client of confidentiality and that any decisions made will be his or hers to make, unless the abuse involves a child, elder, or other situation requiring reporting by law.	The client may feel pressured to make a change he or she does not feel ready to make and may fear that the abuser will find out that he or she has identified abuse.
Allow the client to give his or her perceptions of the situation. Initially, you may ask if the client feels he or she is the victim of abuse (e.g., you might ask the client if he or she "feels safe at home") or point out your observations that may indicate an abusive situation, but do not pressure the client to identify abuse, per se, at this time.	Denial often occurs in abusive situations and can be seen as a part of grieving, in that the client is experiencing and grieving for multiple losses.
With the client's consent, you may want to limit the client's visitors, or have a staff member present during visits.	The client may not feel safe if the abuser is present. Your presence decreases the likelihood of abusive behavior.
Be nonjudgmental with the client, whether he or she is an abuser or a victim of abuse. Be aware of your own feelings (e.g., anger, blaming) and attitudes about abuse.	The abuser may be in denial or defensive about abusive behavior and needs to receive help. The victim may feel powerless, even if you disagree. You may have feelings from your own experiences and cultural values.
Encourage the client to tell you the extent of the abuse and his or her perception of the need for protection.	The client may need to be referred to a shelter or other sanctuary after hospitalization for his or her safety.
Document information accurately, carefully, and objectively. Do not put your opinions in the client's record.	Legal proceedings may develop, perhaps at a much later time, for which documentation will be required.
Encourage the client to take care of himself or herself by meeting basic needs and performing activities of daily living. Give the client positive support for doing so. See Care Plan 25: Major Depressive Disorder and Care Plan 52: The Client Who Will Not Eat.	The client may have neglected his or her own needs and self-care due to distress or low self-esteem or may have suffered abuse for meeting his or her own needs in the past.
Spend time with the client, and encourage him or her to express feelings through talking, writing, crying, and so forth. Be accepting of the client's feelings, including guilt, anger, fear, and caring for the abuser.	Abusive situations engender feelings that the client needs to express, including grieving losses (such as a healthy relationship, trust, security, and home). Victims of abuse often feel that they deserved abuse, or it would not have happened. Finally, abuse does not preclude feelings of caring toward an abuser.
*If the client has been abused, encourage him or her to talk about experiences of abuse, but do not push the client to recall experiences. Maintain a nonjudgmental attitude. Refer the client to long-term therapy if needed.	Retelling traumatic experiences is part of the grieving process and recovery. However, these feelings may create extreme anxiety, and the client may not be ready to face these feelings. Long-term supportive therapy may be indicated.
*Involve the client in or refer the client to a group therapy situation that includes other victims of abuse, abusers, or both, as appropriate to the client's situation.	Therapeutic groups led by a professional can help decrease a sense of isolation and shame, increase self-respect, examine behaviors, and give support for change.
*Teach the client and his or her significant others about abusive behavior.	Learning about abuse can help the client to identify and express feelings and face the abusive situation.
Teach the client about the stress of being in an abusive situation, the relationship between stress and physical health, and stress management techniques.	The client may need to learn to recognize stress and develop skills that deal effectively with stress. The client may have neglected his or her own health and may need encouragement to take positive steps to improved physical health, such as good nutrition and physical activity.
Encourage the client to identify and list options for the future, including positive and negative aspects of these options. Encourage the client to discover what he or she would like and to explore choices.	Clients in abusive relationships often see themselves as powerless, with no options, desires, or choices.

(continued on page 324)

IMPLEMENTATION (continued)

Nursing Interventions *denotes collaborative interventions	Rationale
*Help the client identify and contact community resources, such as crisis centers and shelters. Provide written information (such as telephone numbers for these resources), especially if he or she returns to an abusive situation.	Clients in abusive relationships often are isolated and unaware of available resources. Contacting resources before discharge can help ensure continued contact.
*Help the client arrange follow-up care or therapy. Make referrals to therapists, support groups, or other community or Internet resources as appropriate. When referring a client to Internet resources, provide guidance on how to evaluate the quality of the resource and disclosing personal identity.	Family, marital, or individual therapy may be indicated. Support or therapy groups are available in many communities and on the Internet, including groups for battered women, survivors of child abuse or incest, child abusers (e.g., Parents Anonymous groups), men who are abusive, and lesbians or gay men in abusive situations. Internet resources vary widely in quality, credibility and value and carry risks for inappropriate disclosure of personal identity (see Using the Internet that appears in Part 1).
*Provide the client with information regarding legal issues and options. Make referrals as appropriate.	The client may wish to obtain legal protection, pursue prosecution, or retain information for future consideration.
Remember that an adult client needs to make his or her own decisions about changes in his or her life situation. Be aware of your own feelings, such as frustration and fear for the client's safety, and remain nonjudgmental.	Realizing and grieving for the losses involved in abuse can be a long process. The client may not feel ready to make changes at the present time. The nonjudgmental support and information you give may help motivate the client to seek help or make changes in the future.

Nursing Diagnosis

Ineffective Coping

Inability to form a valid appraisal of the stressors, inadequate choices of practiced responses, and/or inability to use available resources.

ASSESSMENT DATA

- Verbalization of inability to cope
- Inability to solve problems
- Difficulty in interpersonal relationships
- Lack of trust
- Self-destructive behavior
- Denial of abuse
- Guilt
- Fear
- Anxious, withdrawn, or depressive behavior
- Manipulative behavior
- Social isolation

EXPECTED OUTCOMES

Immediate

The client will

- Demonstrate decreased withdrawn, depressive, or anxious behaviors within 2 to 3 days
- Demonstrate a decrease in stress-related symptoms within 2 to 3 days
- Express feelings of helplessness, fear, anger, guilt, and so forth, e.g., talk with staff about these feelings for at least 30 minutes at least twice per day within 2 to 4 days

Stabilization   The client will

- Identify support systems outside the hospital, e.g., support groups or significant others
- Verbalize knowledge of positive coping strategies, such as using the problem-solving process
- Continue to express feelings directly
- Verbalize plans for continued therapy if indicated

Community   The client will

- Cope effectively with stress and stressful life events
- Participate in treatment for associated problems
- Use community support systems effectively

IMPLEMENTATION

Nursing Interventions *denotes collaborative interventions	Rationale
Spend time with the client, and encourage him or her to express feelings through talking, writing, crying, and so forth. Be accepting of the client's feelings, which may include guilt, anger, fear, and caring for the abuser.	Abusive situations engender feelings that the client needs to express, including grieving losses (e.g., trust, health, security, and home). Victims of abuse often feel that they deserved abuse, or it would not have happened. Abuse does not preclude feelings of caring toward the abuser.
When interacting with the client, point out and give support for his or her efforts in decision making, seeking assistance, expressing strengths, problem solving, interactions, and successes.	The client may not see his or her strengths and may have suffered abuse when displaying strengths in the past. Positive support may help reinforce the client's efforts and promote self-esteem.
Give the client choices as much as possible. Structure some activities at the client's present level of accomplishment to provide successful experiences.	Offering choices to the client conveys that the client can and has the right to make choices. Achievement at any level is an opportunity for the client to receive positive feedback.
Teach the client problem solving and coping skills. Support his or her efforts at decision making; do not make decisions for the client or give advice.	The client needs to learn effective skills in making his or her own decisions. When the client makes a decision, he or she can enjoy a successful outcome or learn that he or she can survive a mistake and identify alternatives.
Talk with the client about coping strategies he or she has used in the past. Explore which strategies have been successful and which may have led to negative consequences.	The client may have had success using coping strategies in the past but may have lost confidence in himself or herself or in his or her ability to cope with stressors and feelings.
Teach the client about positive coping strategies and stress management skills, such as increasing physical exercise, expressing feelings verbally or in a journal, or meditation techniques. Encourage the client to practice this type of technique while in the hospital.	The client may have limited or no knowledge of stress management techniques or may not have used positive techniques in the past. If the client tries to build skills in the treatment setting, he or she can experience success and receive positive feedback for his or her efforts.
Teach the client to use a structured problem-solving process: identifying the problem, evaluating possible solutions, implementing a solution, and evaluating the process.	The client may feel overwhelmed by changes and problems and may never have learned a systematic, effective approach to solving problems. Using a structured process may help the client address one problem at a time and build confidence in his or her ability to cope.
*Use role-playing and group therapy to explore and reinforce effective behaviors.	The client can try out new or unfamiliar behaviors in a non-threatening, supportive environment.
*Encourage the client to pursue educational, vocational, or professional avenues as desired. Refer the client to a vocational rehabilitation or educational counselor, social worker, or other professional as appropriate.	Development of the client's abilities can increase self-confidence and enable the client to work toward independence from the abusive relationship.
*Encourage the client to interact with other clients and develop relationships with others outside the hospital. Facilitate interactions as necessary.	Clients in abusive relationships often are socially isolated and lack social skills or confidence.

(continued on page 326)

IMPLEMENTATION (continued)

Nursing Interventions *denotes collaborative interventions	Rationale
*Refer the client to appropriate resources to obtain child care, economic assistance, and other services.	Abusive behavior often occurs when economic or other stressors are present or increased.
*Help the client identify and contact community resources, such as crisis centers, hot lines, shelters, and Internet resources. Provide written information (e.g., telephone numbers for these resources), especially if he or she returns to an abusive situation.	Clients in abusive relationships often are isolated and unaware of available resources. Contacting resources before discharge can help ensure continued contact.

Nursing Diagnosis

Chronic Low Self-Esteem
Longstanding negative self-evaluating/feelings about self or self-capabilities.

ASSESSMENT DATA

- Verbalization of low self-esteem, negative self-characteristics, or low opinion of self
- Verbalization of guilt or shame
- Feelings of worthlessness, hopelessness, or rejection
- Feelings of helplessness, powerlessness, or despair

EXPECTED OUTCOMES

Immediate   The client will

- Express feelings related to self-esteem and self-worth issues within 24 to 48 hours
- Assess own strengths and weaknesses realistically, e.g., make a written list of abilities and areas needing support or development within 2 to 4 days

Stabilization   The client will

- Recognize own accomplishments or progress
- Demonstrate increased self-esteem and self-confidence

Community   The client will

- Make decisions and solve problems independently
- Continue therapy regarding self-esteem issues or follow-up care

IMPLEMENTATION

Nursing Interventions *denotes collaborative interventions	Rationale
Convey that you care about the client and that the client is a worthwhile human being.	Often, feedback received by clients in abusive situations is consistently negative and demeaning; the client may not have experienced acceptance of himself or herself.
Encourage the client to express feelings; convey your acceptance of the client's feelings.	Expressing feelings can help the client to identify, accept, and work through them, even if they are painful or uncomfortable. Feelings are not inherently bad or good.
Acknowledge and support the client for efforts to interact with others, participate in treatment, and express emotions.	Regardless of the level of accomplishment, the client can benefit from acknowledgment of his or her efforts.
In interacting with the client, point out and give support for his or her efforts in decision making, seeking assistance, expressing strengths, solving problems, interactions, and achieving successes.	The client may not see his or her strengths and may have suffered abuse when displaying strengths in the past. Positive support may help reinforce the client's efforts and promote self-esteem.

IMPLEMENTATION (continued)

Nursing Interventions *denotes collaborative interventions	Rationale
Initially, provide activities at the client's present level of accomplishment to provide successful experiences. Give the client positive feedback for even small accomplishments.	Positive feedback provides reinforcement and can enhance self-esteem. The client's abilities to concentrate and interact with others may be impaired.
Encourage the client to take on progressively more challenging activities. Give the client positive support for efforts to participate in activities or interactions.	As the client's abilities increase, he or she may be able to feel increasing self-regard related to accomplishments. Your direct feedback can help the client take credit for accomplishments.
If the client is reluctant to make something for himself or herself in an activity initially, you may encourage him or her to make it as a gift for someone else, e.g., a friend or family member. Gradually help the client to make or do something for himself or herself.	The client's self-esteem may be so low that he or she may feel undeserving of anything, even something he or she has made. Making and giving a gift may foster positive feelings of self-regard and can be a step toward doing something for himself or herself.
Help the client identify positive aspects about himself or herself and his or her behavior. You may point out positive aspects as observations without arguing with the client about his or her feelings.	The client may see only his or her negative self-evaluation; his or her ability to recognize the positive may be impaired. The client's feelings of low self-esteem are very real to him or her, but your positive observations present a different viewpoint that he or she can begin to integrate.
Do not flatter the client or be otherwise dishonest. Give honest, genuine, positive feedback to the client whenever possible.	The client will not benefit from insincerity; dishonesty undermines trust and the therapeutic relationship.
Teach the client problem solving and coping skills. Support the client's efforts at decision making; do not make decisions for the client or give advice.	The client needs to learn effective skills in making his or her own decisions. When the client makes a decision, he or she can enjoy a successful outcome or learn that he or she can survive a mistake and identify alternatives.
Encourage the client to identify relationships that have been positive in the past.	The client may have been socially isolated for some time and have not maintained relationships that provided support in the past. The client may be reluctant to reach out to someone with whom he or she has had limited contact recently or feel ashamed of the abusive situation and may benefit from encouragement or facilitation.
*Encourage the client to identify other supportive people outside the hospital and to develop these relationships.	In addition to reestablishing past relationships or in their absence, increasing the client's support system by establishing new relationships may help decrease future social isolation.
*Encourage the client to identify and pursue personal interests, hobbies, or recreational activities that were positive in the past or that may appeal to the client. Consultation with a recreational therapist may be indicated.	Recreational activities can serve as a structure for the client to build social interactions as well as provide enjoyment.
*Referral to a clergy member or spiritual advisor of the client's faith may be indicated.	Feelings of shame, guilt, or inadequacy may be related to the client's religious beliefs.
*Encourage the client to pursue long-term therapy for self-esteem issues if indicated.	Self-esteem problems can be deeply rooted and require long-term therapy.

CARE PLAN 50

Grief

Grief, or grieving, is a subjective state that occurs in response to a loss. Grieving may be called *grief work* because the client must work through the phases and tasks, expressing and accepting the feelings involved. If the client does not do this work, *dysfunctional grieving* (also called *unresolved grief* or a *morbid grief reaction*) may result, in which conscious grieving may be absent, delayed, distorted, exaggerated, or prolonged (chronic). In dysfunctional grieving, the client may deny the loss; deny feelings related to the loss; experience impaired social relationships and functioning; exhibit depressed, withdrawn, or self-destructive behavior; develop symptoms of a physical or psychiatric illness; or continue to experience intense grief long after the acute mourning period.

A client's experience of the grief process is influenced by many factors, including spiritual beliefs, culture, previous experiences of loss and grief, and social support. The client's religion and customs can form a framework that provides solace, support, and a means of expressing feelings. If the client lacks this support, however, his or her grief can be compounded and prolonged. *Disenfranchised grief* is a term used to describe the experience of individuals whose grief is not acknowledged or supported by their social network or who are excluded from participating in grief-related rituals (such as funerals). Examples of *disenfranchised grief* situations include a client whose relationship with someone who has died was not known or respected by others (e.g., a gay or lesbian relationship or an extramarital affair); a child or impaired adult whom others feel is incapable or is inappropriate to include in grieving discussion or events; or a loss that is significant to the client but not recognized by others (e.g., the loss of a beloved pet or a job). It is especially important for the nurse to be aware of this kind of situation and to help validate and support the client's grief in a nonjudgmental way.

A number of factors can contribute to dysfunctional or unresolved grieving. Traumatic losses earlier in life, inability to share grief with others, and a lack of interpersonal support make unresolved grief more likely. Factors that increase the likelihood of *complicated grief* include social learning (such as denying or repressing the pain of grief), a lack of knowledge of the grief process, and a lack of participation in rituals of grief that could help facilitate social support and the expression of feelings (Zisook & Shear, 2009).

Grief can occur in response to the loss of anything that is significant to the client, such as health (e.g., injury, disability, or chronic illness), a job or status, a loved one (through death, separation, or termination of a relationship), a pet, a role (e.g., the mother role when the last child leaves the parental home), or the future (e.g., when diagnosed with a terminal illness). Losses are described as *actual*, when the loss has already occurred or is occurring, or *anticipated*, when the client is aware that a loss will occur. An anticipated loss, such as when a client has a terminal illness, involves *anticipatory grieving,* or working through the grief process in anticipation of the loss. A loss may be *observable* to others or may be *perceived* only by the client (as with the loss of an ideal the client has held). Grief may be in response to any *change* because change involves loss.

Grief can be experienced on many levels in response to different types of losses. In addition to the loss of an individual person, object, life change, and so forth, a loss on the community level can trigger deep and lasting grief. *Community grieving* refers to grief shared by members of a community in response to a significant loss or change, such as a natural disaster, accident, or crime in which many people are killed or injured, a key individual is killed or dies, or when there is severe or widespread destruction of property. This type of grief can occur on a national level (sometimes called *national grief*), as occurred in response to the assassinations of Dr. Martin Luther King, Jr., Robert Kennedy, and John F. Kennedy. Widespread grief shared among people in many countries also can occur, for example, in response to terrorist attacks or the death of an internationally known individual (see "Key Considerations in Mental Health Nursing: Community Grief and Disaster Response").

Grief has been described by various authors as a process that includes a number of stages, characteristic feelings, experiences, and tasks. These include shock, denial, numbness, being stopped or seriously impaired in one's daily functioning, developing awareness of the loss, and preoccupation with the loss; feelings such as yearning, anger, ambivalence, depression, despair, and guilt; disorganization; and tasks such as managing feelings, accepting the loss, reorganizing relationships, and integrating the loss into one's life. Progression through these stages or processes does not necessarily occur in a certain order, and it is characterized by stress, emotional pain, and an impairment of daily life functioning (Bowlby, 1980; Kübler-Ross, 1969; Zisook & Shear, 2009). Moreover, the grief process is not linear, feelings vary in intensity, and the time spent in the grieving process varies considerably (from weeks to years).

Chronic sorrow refers to recurrent grief that occurs in response to an ongoing loss or to a series of losses, such as the losses resulting from a chronic, debilitating, or terminal disease or from the birth of a child who has a serious condition that is disabling or terminal. In chronic sorrow, an individual sustains loss after loss, and grieving for these losses is complicated by the awareness that losses will continue to occur, that the situation will not improve, and that the individual will never have a "normal" life. Chronic sorrow, like grieving for any loss, can have a variable course, with the intensity of emotional responses waxing and waning over time. Intense grief episodes may be triggered by an event, such as a medical crisis; a normative or developmental milestone that is reached by others in a cohort or peer group but not achieved in the individual's situation (e.g., when others in a peer group graduate or get married, but the individual's situation precludes such an event); anniversary dates (e.g., a birthday or the anniversary of the loss); holidays; or sensory triggers that recall the loss (e.g., songs, smells, or foods).

Many clients are unfamiliar with grief and may be overwhelmed by their emotions, fearful, depressed, or even suicidal. Important nursing goals are to provide information about grieving and help the client understand that the goal in grief work is not to avoid or eliminate painful feelings but to experience, express, and work through the emotions involved, toward successful integration of the loss. Nursing therapeutic goals with the grieving client include the following:

- Validate the client's loss (especially with disenfranchised grief and chronic sorrow).
- Facilitate the client's movement through the feelings and tasks of grieving.
- Decrease depressive, withdrawn, self-destructive, or aggressive symptoms.
- Diminish secondary gain from depressive symptoms.
- Help alleviate the client's fears of having feelings that are undesirable or of being overwhelmed by feelings.
- Ensure that the client's physiologic and hygienic needs are met.
- Promote the client's independence in meeting physiologic and hygienic needs, expressing feelings, and accomplishing grief work.

Discharge planning is extremely important in working with the grieving client. Alternative methods of managing life tasks and dealing with stress must be developed if the lost person or object was integral to previous coping strategies, and the client's lifestyle must be adapted to the loss and new life situation. In the case of anticipatory grieving, it is important to help the terminally ill client identify a support structure or other resources (e.g., hospice services) to assist the client after discharge. Loss and grief work involve significant physical stress as well as emotional stress, and they can increase the client's vulnerability to illness and even death. Rest, exercise, nutrition, hydration, and elimination should be monitored during hospitalization and addressed in discharge plans.

NURSING DIAGNOSES ADDRESSED IN THIS CARE PLAN
Complicated Grieving
Grieving
Hopelessness

RELATED NURSING DIAGNOSES ADDRESSED IN THE MANUAL
Risk for Other-Directed Violence
Risk for Suicide
Disturbed Body Image
Social Isolation
Ineffective Health Maintenance
Insomnia

Note: The nursing process for the Nursing Diagnoses of both Complicated Grieving and Grieving are addressed in the Assessment implementation sections below, and included grieving related to actual, perceived, and anticipated losses (e.g., terminal illness).

Nursing Diagnosis

Complicated Grieving

A disorder that occurs after the death of a significant other, in which the experience of distress accompanying bereavement fails to follow normative expectations and manifests in functional impairment.

Grieving

A normal complex process that includes emotional, physical, spiritual, social, and intellectual responses and behaviors by which individuals, families, and communities incorporate an actual, anticipated, or perceived loss into their daily lives.

ASSESSMENT DATA

* Actual or potential loss of health, abilities, or life
* Denial of loss
* Difficulty in accepting significant loss
* Denial of feelings
* Difficulty in expressing feelings
* Fear of intensity of feelings
* Suicidal ideas or feelings, self-destructive behavior, accident proneness
* Anger, hostility, rage, or aggressive behavior
* Depressive behavior
* Withdrawn behavior
* Expression of distress regarding potential loss
* Sorrow
* Rumination
* Feelings of despair, hopelessness, disillusionment
* Feelings of helplessness, powerlessness
* Loss of interest in activities of daily living
* Anhedonia (inability to experience pleasure)
* Ambivalent feelings toward the lost person or object
* Guilt feelings
* Crying
* Anxiety or fear
* Agitation
* Fatigue
* Sleep disturbance
* Changes in eating habits
* Resentment

EXPECTED OUTCOMES

Immediate

The client will

- Be free of self-inflicted harm throughout hospitalization
- Verbally identify the loss, potential loss, or illness within 12 to 24 hours
- Verbalize or demonstrate decreased suicidal, aggressive, depressive, or withdrawn behaviors within 24 to 48 hours
- Express feelings, verbally and nonverbally, e.g., talk with staff about the grief situation for at least 30 minutes at least twice a day within 2 to 4 days
- Establish or maintain adequate nutrition, hydration, and elimination, e.g., eat at least 30% of all meals with staff assistance within 2 to 4 days

Stabilization

The client will

- Verbalize acceptance of the loss or illness
- Verbalize knowledge of the grief process
- Establish or maintain an adequate balance of rest, sleep, and activity
- Discuss loss or illness with significant others
- Verbalize changes in lifestyle and coping mechanisms incorporating the fact of the loss
- Demonstrate initial integration of the loss into his or her life, e.g., verbalize realistic future plans integrating the loss

Community

The client will

- Demonstrate physical recuperation from the stress of loss and grieving
- Progress through the grieving process
- Participate in continued therapy, if indicated, e.g., identify a therapist and make an initial appointment prior to discharge
- Demonstrate reestablished relationships or social support in the community

IMPLEMENTATION

Nursing Interventions *denotes collaborative interventions	Rationale
Be alert to risk of suicidal behavior. Institute suicide precautions as needed (see Care Plan 26: Suicidal Behavior).	Clients experiencing significant loss or facing loss of health and functioning may be at increased risk for suicide.
Initially, assign the same staff members to the client, and then gradually vary the staff people (see Care Plan 1: Building a Trust Relationship).	The client may be overwhelmed by and fear facing the loss. The client's ability to respond to others may be impaired. Limiting the number of new contacts provides consistency and facilitates familiarity. However, the number of people should increase as tolerated to minimize dependency.
Approach the client and initiate interactions; use silence and active listening to facilitate communication.	The client may fear rejection from others if he or she talks about the loss or illness. Your presence indicates caring and acceptance.
After establishing rapport with the client, bring up the loss in a supportive manner; if the client refuses to discuss it, withdraw and state your intention to return. ("I can understand that you may not want to talk with me about this now. I will come to talk with you again at 11:00, maybe we can discuss it then.") Return at the stated time, then continue to be supportive.	Your presence and telling the client you will return demonstrate caring and support. The client may need emotional support to face and express painful feelings. Confronting the client or pushing him or her to express feelings may increase anxiety and lead to further denial or avoidance.
Approach the client in a nonjudgmental way. Be sure to deal with your own feelings of discomfort, if any, related to the client's situation or grief.	The client may fear others' reactions to the loss or terminal illness. Being aware of and dealing with your own feelings will help prevent them from interfering in your work with the client.

(continued on page 332)

IMPLEMENTATION (continued)

Nursing Interventions *denotes collaborative interventions	Rationale
*As the client tolerates, encourage discussion of the client's loss or illness, first with staff members, then with the client's significant others and other clients. Be gentle in your approach to the client; talk about the situation in simple, matter-of-fact terms.	Acknowledging the loss or illness is necessary to the grief process. Gentleness demonstrates regard for the client's feelings. Being matter-of-fact about an illness can help separate the illness itself from emotional issues.
Talk with the client in realistic terms concerning the loss; discuss concrete changes that have occurred or that the client must now make as a result of the loss.	Discussing the loss on this level may help to make it more real for the client.
With the client, identify his or her strengths; resources; and sources of hope, pleasure, and support.	The client may feel so overwhelmed that he or she is unable to see anything positive.
Give the client honest praise for the things that he or she is able to do; acknowledge the client's efforts in the context of the loss, illness, impaired abilities, or dying.	The client will not benefit from dishonesty or flattery, but small accomplishments may indeed merit praise in the context of a major illness.
Assure the client that a loss or illness is not a form of punishment and that he or she does not deserve to experience the loss or illness.	The client or others may feel that illness is a punishment or that the client is to blame.
Encourage the client to express feelings in ways with which he or she is comfortable (e.g., talking, writing, drawing, crying). Convey your acceptance and give support for attempts to express feelings.	Expressing feelings can help the client to identify, accept, and work through feelings, even if these are difficult for the client.
Encourage the client to recall experiences and talk about the relationship with the lost person and so forth. Discuss changes in the client's feelings toward self, others, and the lost person.	Discussing the lost object or person can help the client identify and express what the loss means to him or her, and his or her feelings.
Encourage appropriate (i.e., safe) expression of all types of feelings toward the lost person or object. Provide assurance to the client that "negative" feelings like anger and resentment are normal and healthy in grieving and that feeling relieved that someone has died after a difficult illness or stressful emotional situation is also normal and acceptable.	Feelings are not inherently bad or good. Giving the client support for expressing feelings may help the client accept uncomfortable feelings. Feelings are not inherently bad or good, and expressing feelings that one is experiencing can help the client progress through grief.
Note: If you feel uncomfortable with the client's expression of feelings or with your role in bringing up painful feelings, then withdraw temporarily. Examine your feelings and have the client speak with someone who is more comfortable (see "Key Considerations in Mental Health Nursing: Nurse–Client Interactions").	Your comfort with the client's feelings conveys support and acceptance. If you are uncomfortable, you may inadvertently convey disinterest or disapproval or may reinforce the client's avoidance of feelings.
Convey to the client that although feelings may be uncomfortable, they are natural and necessary and they will not harm him or her.	The client may fear the intensity of his or her feelings.
Discourage the client's using activities to avoid grieving ("to get my mind off it"). Convey that although the client does not have to think about feelings at all times, a part of each day should be spent dealing with them. At least once per shift, invite the client to talk about the loss, feelings, plans, and so forth.	It is important to reinforce the client's grief work as necessary and healthy. Avoiding feelings may delay the client's progress through grieving.
Discourage the client from ruminating on guilt or worthlessness. After listening to the client's feelings, tell him or her you will discuss other aspects of the loss or grief that may underlie these feelings.	The client needs to identify and express the feelings that underlie the rumination and to proceed through the grief process. It may help the client to write down regrets or other factors underlying feelings of guilt or worthlessness, then address other aspects of the loss verbally with others.

IMPLEMENTATION (continued)

Nursing Interventions *denotes collaborative interventions	Rationale
Limit the amount of therapeutic interactions with the client. Encourage independent expression of feelings (e.g., writing, interacting with others, physical activity). Plan staff interactions at times that allow the client to fulfill responsibilities and maintain personal care.	The client needs to develop independent skills of communicating feelings and to integrate the loss into his or her daily life, while meeting his or her own basic needs.
Expect the client to fulfill responsibilities, and give support for doing so. Withdraw your attention if the client does not fulfill responsibilities (e.g., do not have a therapeutic interaction if the client refuses to participate in an activity).	It is important to minimize secondary gain and to convey that the client can fulfill responsibilities while grieving.
Encourage the client to talk with others about the loss, his or her feelings, and changes resulting from the loss.	The client needs to develop independent skills of communicating feelings and expressing grief to others.
*Facilitate sharing, ventilating feelings, and support among clients. Use larger groups for a general discussion of loss and grief. However, help the client understand that there are limits to sharing grief in a social context.	Sharing grief with others can help the client identify and express feelings and feel normal. Dwelling on grief in social interactions can result in other people's discomfort with their own feelings and avoiding the client.
*Referral to the facility chaplain, clergy, or other spiritual resource person may be indicated.	The client may be more comfortable discussing spiritual issues with an advisor who shares his or her belief system.
Provide opportunities for the client to release tension, anger, and so forth through physical activity and promote this as a healthy means of dealing with stress.	Physical activity provides a way to relieve tension in a healthy, nondestructive manner.
*Point out to the client and his or her significant others that experiencing a loss or chronic or terminal illness and grieving are difficult tasks and give the client positive feedback for his or her efforts.	The client may not realize the difficulty of the work that he or she is doing to face and live with the loss or illness.
Point out to the client that a major aspect of loss is a real physical stress. Encourage good nutrition, hydration, rest, and daily physical exercise (such as walking, swimming, or cycling).	The client may be unaware of the physical stress of the loss or may lack interest in basic needs. Physical exercise can relieve tension in a healthy manner.
*Teach the client and significant others about the grief process.	The client and significant others may have little or no knowledge of grief or the process involved in recovery.
Point out to the client that grieving can be a time of learning from which to gather the strength to go forward.	The grief process allows the client to adjust to a change and to begin to move toward the future.
Urge the client to identify and pursue his or her own strengths; facilitate activities that promote their development.	The client's strengths are a major factor in his or her ability to deal with continuing grief work.
*In each interaction with the client, try to include some discussion of goals, the future, and discharge plans. Help the client identify resources that can provide continuing support, such as church or support groups in the community or on the Internet.	The client needs to integrate the loss into his or her life. The grief process may continue for months or years to some extent. Supportive groups can help the client meet needs for expressing feelings and adjusting to the loss.
*Encourage the client to identify and maintain supportive relationships outside the hospital.	The client may fear rejection from others in his or her life and may need encouragement to contact others.
*Encourage the client to pursue past relationships, personal interests, hobbies, or recreational activities that he or she may enjoy. Consultation with a recreational therapist may be indicated.	The client may need to reestablish relationships with others with whom he or she has had limited contact, especially if the client was in a caretaker role during a protracted illness or if the loss was of a partner who was key to mutual relationships. Recreational activities can serve as a structure for the client to build social interactions as well as provide enjoyment.

(continued on page 334)

IMPLEMENTATION (continued)

Nursing Interventions *denotes collaborative interventions	Rationale
*Help the client to identify resources for assistance in the community or Internet. Referral to a social worker may be indicated.	The client may need continued support after discharge. Social workers can help the client to identify and contact resources. Many communities and organizations provide information, services, and support groups for clients experiencing grief or terminal illnesses.
*Help the client plan for the future regarding any changes resulting from the loss (e.g., living arrangements, finances, social activities) or illness (e.g., advance directives, powers of attorney, wills).	Planning the future with regard to the loss or illness will help the client integrate the loss and effectively plan for the future.

Nursing Diagnosis

Hopelessness

Subjective state in which an individual sees limited or no alternatives or personal choices available and is unable to mobilize energy on own behalf.

ASSESSMENT DATA

* Anger, hostility, or rage
* Anhedonia (inability to experience pleasure)
* Suicidal ideas or feelings
* Depression
* Sorrow, despair
* Passivity
* Decreased communication
* Lack of initiative, anergy
* Impaired social interaction
* Withdrawn behavior
* Sleep disturbances
* Changes in eating habits

EXPECTED OUTCOMES

Immediate

The client will

* Be safe and free of self-inflicted harm throughout hospitalization
* Demonstrate decreased suicidal, withdrawn, or depressive symptoms within 2 to 4 days

Stabilization

The client will

* Demonstrate a maximum level of decision making in planning his or her own care
* Be free of suicidal, withdrawn, and depressive symptoms
* Demonstrate the ability to identify choices or alternatives, e.g., list alternatives with pros and cons of each and review with staff or significant others
* Demonstrate active participation in self-care and plans for life after discharge

Community

The client will

* Meet self-care needs independently
* Make decisions and solve problems independently

IMPLEMENTATION

Nursing Interventions *denotes collaborative interventions	Rationale
Assess the client's suicide potential, and institute suicide precautions if indicated (see Care Plan 26: Suicidal Behavior).	Clients with a chronic or terminal illness or who are grieving are at increased risk for suicide. The client's safety is a priority.
Encourage the client to express his or her feelings verbally and nonverbally, in nondestructive ways.	Ventilation of feelings can help lessen feelings of despair and so forth and helps the client to progress through the grief process.
See Care Plan 25: Major Depressive Disorder.	
Teach the client the problem-solving process: describe the problem, list and evaluate alternatives, implement an alternative, and evaluate the effectiveness of the action.	The client may feel overwhelmed by the situation and may not know how to implement a systematic approach to solving problems.
*Referral to the facility chaplain, clergy, or other spiritual resource person may be indicated.	The client may be more comfortable discussing spiritual issues with an advisor who shares his or her belief system.
Encourage the client to identify relationships, social, or recreational situations that have been positive in the past.	The client may feel isolated from others and lost interest in people or activities that provided pleasure in the past.
Encourage the client to contact supportive individuals or resources; facilitate these contacts if necessary.	The client may be lack the motivation or energy to make the first contact with individuals or resources that can be helpful to him or her.
*Encourage the client to continue therapy after discharge if indicated. Encourage the client to identify resources for therapy and to make an initial appointment before discharge.	Grieving and chronic or terminal illness may require long-term therapy.

CARE PLAN 51

Disturbed Body Image

Body image is a person's perception of his or her physical self. This perception includes conscious and unconscious perceptions of physical attributes and functioning, emotions, and sensations. It extends beyond the body to include objects such as clothing or items used in work. A person's body image forms and changes as he or she develops, and is closely tied to self-esteem and identity, both of which are threatened by a change in body image. Body image also is influenced by cultural beliefs and values and messages one receives from others. Feelings of body image and the sense of self include those related to sexuality, femininity, masculinity, parenthood, youthfulness, maturity, health, strength, and ability (Black & Andreasen, 2011).

Disturbed body image is a change in a person's perception of and attitudes about his or her physical self. Often, this alteration is a response to a change or loss related to physical appearance or functioning and involves grieving. Grieving in response to a change in body image can include shock, denial or disbelief, fear, anger, depression, and acceptance or reorganization; it can be a functional adaptation, or it may be dysfunctional or unresolved (see Care Plan 50: Grief). However, grief related to a change in one's own body image differs from the grief that results from the loss of a person or thing outside oneself because a permanent change in body image or loss of physical function remains present and cannot be replaced. Thus, the resolution of the grief becomes adaptation to a change that does not get better or disappear or, in the case of terminal illness, may continue to worsen over time. Remember that progression through the various stages of grieving is not necessarily orderly; these phases may overlap, and the client may vacillate among them. A change in body image is more traumatic when it is external and visible to the person and others; involves the face, genitals, or breasts; or is unforeseen, uncontrolled, or unwanted (Zisook & Shear, 2009). The client's perception of and feelings about his or her changed body image are not necessarily proportional to the observable change, and the removal of an internal body part or a change in health status may be as traumatic to the client as the loss of a visible extremity.

A disturbance in body image affects the client's need to feel normal, and it often involves social stigma. The client's reaction to the disturbed body image may be strongly influenced by his or her cultural background, so it is important to be aware of the client's cultural values related to a change in physical appearance, health status, and so forth. The client's significant others are also affected by the change, and the client faces their responses and the responses of each new person he or she encounters. It is essential to remember that this client is still a person, whatever the alteration in his or her body.

Note: Disturbed body image differs from body image *distortion*, such as occurs in anorexia nervosa, when a client perceives his or her body to be larger than it actually is. Such a distortion may be of delusional proportions and may occur in clients with neurologic or psychiatric illness. (See other care plans as appropriate.)

The change or loss that precipitates a disturbance in body image may be the result of a burn or trauma; a chronic, debilitating, disfiguring, or terminal illness; surgery (especially radical or mutilating), stoma, or amputation; or stroke. The loss also may be the result of changes in appearance, fitness, or abilities related to growth, maturation, or aging (see Care Plan 11: Adjustment Disorders of Adolescence, Care Plan 39: Adjustment Disorders of Adults, and

"Key Considerations in Mental Health Nursing: The Aging Client"). It also may be related to a procedure the client has chosen, such as gender change or breast augmentation or reduction.

Health care personnel sometimes tend to minimize the change in a client's body and communicate to the client, directly or indirectly, that the loss is not as bad as the client feels it is. Nurses must be aware of this possibility because they may have become accustomed to seeing illness, surgery, and so forth and no longer experience strong feelings in response to these events. Medical and nursing staff also may insulate themselves emotionally from such traumatic events as a defense mechanism; they may view these medical situations in a matter-of-fact, "clinical" way; or they may see them as positive events (such as having a stoma or an amputation versus dying), without recognizing or appreciating the emotional implications for the client. It is also important to remain aware of cultural factors, including beliefs about self-worth and value to others (e.g., spouse or family) regarding a loss of health or abilities.

Therapeutic goals with clients experiencing a disturbance in body image include preventing suicidal or other self-destructive behavior, helping the client acknowledge the loss and progress through grief work, and facilitating the client's integration of the change into daily living and relationships with others. Effective discharge planning includes working with the interdisciplinary care team to identify community resources for longer-term support, especially with clients who have a terminal illness.

NURSING DIAGNOSES ADDRESSED IN THIS CARE PLAN
Disturbed Body Image
Situational Low Self-Esteem
Ineffective Role Performance

RELATED NURSING DIAGNOSES ADDRESSED IN THE MANUAL
Complicated Grieving
Risk for Suicide
Risk for Loneliness
Anxiety
Deficient Knowledge (Specify)

Nursing Diagnosis

Disturbed Body Image
Confusion in mental picture of one's physical self.

ASSESSMENT DATA

- Actual or perceived physical change or illness
- Verbal or nonverbal response to change in body structure or function
- Denial of physical change or illness
- Anger, hostility, or rage
- Guilt
- Resentment
- Confusion
- Anxiety or fear
- Feelings of hopelessness or worthlessness
- Depressive behavior
- Despair
- Withdrawn behavior
- Dissociation or depersonalization
- Grief
- Self-destructive behavior
- Regression
- Dependency
- Refusal to perform self-care activities (when physically capable)
- Identity concerns (sexual role, role as wage earner, parental role, and so forth)

EXPECTED OUTCOMES

Immediate   The client will

- Be safe and free of injury throughout hospitalization
- Verbalize the physical change, loss, or disability within 24 to 48 hours
- Discuss disturbed body image with staff members and significant others within 2 to 3 days
- Express feelings, verbally and nonverbally, e.g., talk with staff about feelings related to the physical change for at least 15 minutes at least twice per day within 2 to 3 days
- Establish or maintain adequate nutrition, hydration, and elimination within 3 to 4 days
- Establish or maintain an adequate balance of rest, sleep, and activity within 3 to 4 days

Stabilization   The client will

- Participate in treatment program and activities
- Participate in self-care related to surgery, injury, or illness
- Verbalize knowledge of his or her physical condition, treatment, and safe use of medication, if any
- Demonstrate skills in activities of daily living and self-care
- Verbalize knowledge of the grief process and recovery

Community   The client will

- Identify and use sources of support outside the hospital
- Participate in social activities or groups
- Verbalize changes in lifestyle and coping mechanisms incorporating the loss or change
- Verbalize realistic future plans integrating the loss or change
- Progress through the grief process

IMPLEMENTATION

Nursing Interventions *denotes collaborative interventions	Rationale
Be alert to the risk of suicidal behavior and institute suicide precautions as needed (see Care Plan 26: Suicidal Behavior).	Clients with disturbed body image may be at increased risk for suicide.
Initially, assign the same staff members to work with the client. Gradually increase the number of people interacting with the client (see Care Plan 1: Building a Trust Relationship).	The client's ability to respond to others may be impaired; he or she may expect rejection from others due to the physical change. Initially limiting new contacts will facilitate familiarity and trust. Increasing the number of people interacting with the client will promote the client's ability to communicate with a variety of people.
Approach the client and initiate interaction; use silence and active listening to facilitate communication.	The client's ability to initiate interactions may be impaired due to low self-esteem, anger, and so on. Your presence will demonstrate interest, caring, and acceptance.
*Be aware of your own feelings and behavior regarding the client's physical change, such as not looking at or not touching the client. Talk with other staff members about feelings of discomfort, repulsion, disapproval, and so forth.	Extreme physical changes or disfigurement can be disturbing, especially initially. Identifying and exploring your own feelings will allow you to be more comfortable and less likely to inadvertently communicate feelings of discomfort to the client.
View the client as a whole person, not only as a person with a disability; however, do not ignore the disability.	The client needs to know that others can see him or her as a person, and that the physical change is not all that others see. Ignoring the disability may reinforce the client's denial or fears of others' intolerance.
As the client tolerates, encourage discussion of the physical change in simple, matter-of-fact terms. Ask for the client's perceptions, and begin teaching the client about the change or illness.	Acknowledgment of the change is necessary to the grief process. Frank but sensitive discussion will convey your acceptance and promote feelings of normalcy. Eliciting the client's perceptions may facilitate expression of feelings and help you identify areas in which information is needed.

IMPLEMENTATION (continued)

Nursing Interventions *denotes collaborative interventions	Rationale
Encourage expression of feelings, including anger, resentment, guilt, self-blame, envy of healthy people, fears of rejection and inadequacy, and feelings about the change itself (repulsion, fear, and so forth).	Expressing these feelings is a part of grieving and can help the client work through the feelings, even if they are painful or uncomfortable. The client needs to know that these feelings are normal and acceptable, not bad.
Encourage discussion of the client's perception of what the change means, changes in his or her abilities, feelings of helplessness, guilt, and so forth.	The client may be experiencing overwhelming feelings of fear, worthlessness, and powerlessness or may feel that he or she is being punished with the disability. The client may feel unable to survive having to depend on others for needs that were formerly met independently.
Allow the client quiet time alone to think and express feelings through writing, crying, and other outlets.	The client may need privacy to express certain feelings and needs to develop independence in expressing feelings.
See "Key Considerations in Mental Health Nursing: The Aging Client, Nurse–Client Interactions," Care Plan 50: Grief, and Care Plan 25: Major Depressive Disorder.	
Help the client identify strengths and abilities that are not affected by this physical change or that are changed in some way but not lost.	Body image includes feelings about abilities and is linked to self-esteem. The client may feel that the change has destroyed all of his or her strengths.
Communicate realistic expectations of the client; do not expect *less* than the client is capable of doing.	Expecting less than the client is capable of will undermine the client, but if the client perceives inability, he or she may indeed not be capable at this time.
Encourage the client to express feelings of isolation, fears of rejection, and the reactions of others.	The client may project his or her own negative feelings about the change onto others and expect rejection.
*Talk with the client's significant others about impact of the client's change, their feelings, and responses to the change; show acceptance of these feelings. Family therapy may be indicated.	The client's significant others are affected by this change and may have feelings of fear, repulsion, inadequacy, guilt, and so forth. Expressing these feelings may help work through them.
Use role-playing and rehearsal to help the client prepare for the reactions of others, learn to ask for help, and teach others about his or her condition and care.	Anticipatory guidance can increase the client's abilities and confidence in facing others. The client may have been independent and may not be comfortable asking for help.
*Teach the client and significant others about the physical change and needed skills, including self-care, caregiving, and safe use of medications if any. Ask for the client's perceptions, return demonstration, of skills and so forth. Encourage the client to practice skills and share them with others. Refer the client to a nurse practitioner; occupational, physical, recreational, or vocational therapists; and a support group as appropriate (local or Internet).	The client needs information and skills to promote self-care and confidence and to help develop and accept a new body image, integrating the change, prostheses, and so forth. Support groups of people who have experienced the same or a similar change can help the client adapt to the loss.
*Referral to the facility chaplain, clergy, or other spiritual resource person may be indicated.	The client may be more comfortable discussing spiritual issues with an advisor who shares his or her belief system.
*Teach the client and family and significant others about the grief process.	The client and family or significant others may have little or no knowledge of the grief process.
*Discuss sexual concerns and information with the client as appropriate. Remain nonjudgmental and aware of the client's feelings and cultural values in this area. Refer the client to a support group (e.g., sexual assertiveness group for the disabled) or a therapist if appropriate.	Sexuality is a basic need for both female and male clients. The client may be afraid to discuss sexuality, may not know how, or may fear disapproval. The client may need to learn new ways to perceive sexuality and to give and receive sexual pleasure. If you are unaware of your own feelings, you may inadvertently express disapproval to the client (see "Key Considerations in Mental Health Nursing: Sexuality").

(continued on page 340)

IMPLEMENTATION (continued)

Nursing Interventions *denotes collaborative interventions	Rationale
Explore with the client ways of adapting his or her lifestyle and activities. Identify alternatives, resources, new or changed roles, goals, plans, and so forth.	The client needs to develop and integrate new or altered behaviors, perceptions of self, and goals to adapt to the change.
Help the client prepare to achieve and sustain his or her optimal level of functioning in the future.	It is important not to undermine or underestimate the client's abilities simply because he or she has a disability.
*Help the client identify and use support systems outside the hospital.

See Care Plan 2: Discharge Planning. | Long-term therapy may be indicated. Social support (family, friends, community, or Internet support groups) can help the client feel normal and integrate the new body image into his or her life. |

Nursing Diagnosis

Situational Low Self-Esteem

Development of a negative perception of self-worth in response to a current situation (specify).

ASSESSMENT DATA

- Feelings of hopelessness or worthlessness
- Self-deprecatory verbalization
- Lack of self-confidence
- Anxiety or fear
- Depressive behavior
- Despair
- Withdrawn behavior
- Self-destructive behavior
- Regression
- Dependency

EXPECTED OUTCOMES

Immediate   The client will

- Demonstrate decreased depressive symptoms within 2 to 4 days
- Verbalize increased feelings of self-worth within 3 to 5 days

Stabilization   The client will

- Be free of depressive symptoms
- Demonstrate increased feelings of self-worth
- Assess own strengths and weaknesses realistically, e.g., list capabilities and areas needing support or development, and discuss with staff

Community   The client will

- Demonstrate confidence in coping skills
- Make decisions and solve problems independently

IMPLEMENTATION

Nursing Interventions *denotes collaborative interventions	Rationale
Review with the client his or her strengths and abilities that are not affected by the physical change and those that are changed in some way but not lost.	Body image includes feelings about abilities and is linked to self-esteem. The client may feel that the physical change has destroyed all of his or her strengths.

IMPLEMENTATION (continued)

Nursing Interventions *denotes collaborative interventions	Rationale
Provide opportunities for the client to succeed at activities, tasks, and interactions. Give positive feedback, and point out the client's demonstrated abilities and strengths.	The client may feel incapable of succeeding at anything and may need encouragement to attempt activities. Activities within the client's abilities provide opportunities for success. Positive feedback can enhance self-esteem.
Be realistic in your feedback to the client; do not flatter or be otherwise dishonest.	Clients with low self-esteem do not benefit from flattery or undue praise.
*Encourage the client to make contact with friends and family or to continue personal interests, hobbies, or recreational activities, as he or she is able.	The client may be reluctant to reach out to others due to the difficulty of his or her situation or fears of others' reactions. Interest or recreational activities the client is able to do can provide enjoyment and continue a sense of self-regard.
*Encourage the client to identify supportive people and resources outside the hospital and to develop these relationships.	The client may need additional support to rebuild self-esteem and confidence in his or her new situation.
See "Key Considerations in Mental Health Nursing: Building Self-Esteem."	

Nursing Diagnosis

Ineffective Role Performance

Patterns of behavior and self-expression that do not match the environmental context, norms, and expectations.

ASSESSMENT DATA

- Apathy
- Inability to continue preillness role
- Loss of independence (current or anticipated)
- Attention deficits
- Low self-esteem
- Fear of unknown
- Inability to concentrate

EXPECTED OUTCOMES

Immediate

The client will

- Identify life areas that require alterations due to the loss, illness, or physical change within 2 to 4 days
- Verbalize abilities and limitations realistically within 3 to 5 days

Stabilization

The client will

- Maintain independence within his or her limitations
- Verbalize increased feelings of self-worth
- Discuss current or anticipated changes in family with significant others

Community

The client will

- Demonstrate effective performance in new or changed roles within limits of the illness or change
- Verbalize needs effectively to others

IMPLEMENTATION

Nursing Interventions *denotes collaborative interventions	Rationale
Allow the client to complete any tasks that are within his or her physical capabilities.	Completion of self-care and other tasks without assistance allows the client to retain independence and enhances self-esteem.
Provide ample time for task completion to avoid rushing the client.	The client's psychomotor skills may be slower. Rushing the client will increase frustration and impair task completion.
Provide rest periods at regular intervals. Do not wait until the client is too exhausted to continue.	Rest periods prevent overtiring. Once fatigue is present, the client's ability to recover is impaired.
Break complex tasks into small steps.	Small tasks will be easier for the client to complete and provide an increased number of opportunities for success.
Allow the client to continue decision making about tasks, even if he or she is unable to perform the task.	Decision making allows the client to retain some control, even when he or she is dependent on others for physical care. The client may retain cognitive abilities longer than psychomotor skills.
Approach the client on an adult level, using a matter-of-fact approach regarding personal care.	A matter-of-fact attitude lessens the possibility that the client will feel awkward.
If the client becomes frustrated, have him or her stop the task and try again later. Avoid doing the task for the client at these times.	Allowing the client to stop a frustrating situation, relax, and try again decreases frustration and teaches the client to do this in the future. Performing the task for the client may convey that the client is unable to do the task.
When possible involve the client in discussions about how care is given, who will give care, and so forth.	This allows the client to remain included and, when possible, retain personal control.
*If the client's energy is diminished, allow him or her to choose which tasks he or she would like to perform and which to delegate to a caregiver.	Allowing the client choices within his or her ability enhances a sense of personal control.
*Provide information to the client, significant others, and caregivers about realistic expectations for the client's abilities.	The client and his or her significant others may lack knowledge of how the client's situation affects his or her abilities.
Discuss with the client ways in which he or she might deal with future changes when they do occur.	Anticipatory planning can alleviate the client's anxiety.

CARE PLAN 52

The Client Who Will Not Eat

Nurses in mental health treatment settings often encounter clients who will not eat. Because nutrition and hydration are such basic physiologic needs, it is important for nurses to be able to help these clients, regardless of the etiology of the problem. Emotional problems related to eating can include guilt, depression, associating food or not eating with punishment, manipulating others, or receiving secondary gain from not eating. In working with these clients, the nurse needs to remember that food and eating may have emotional, religious, or cultural meanings that can be quite powerful.

Clients may not eat for physiologic or psychological reasons. A client may refuse to eat, be uninterested in eating, or be unaware of the need or desire to eat. Psychiatric problems that may underlie a client's not eating include (see related care plans as indicated) the following:

- Eating disorders
- Depression
- Withdrawal
- Grief
- Self-destructive behavior
- Confusion
- Agitation
- Anger and hostility
- Manic behavior
- Delusions or other psychotic symptoms
- Stress, anxiety, or phobias
- Guilt
- Low self-esteem
- Manipulative behavior
- Personality disorders

A client may be experiencing physical problems that interfere with appetite or that make it difficult to eat. Physical problems that may contribute to a client's not eating include the following:

- Effects of medications, such as altered taste sensation
- Effects of acute or chronic physical illness, such as nausea or decreased appetite
- Poor dentition or gum disease
- Poorly fitting dentures
- Difficulty swallowing or chewing
- Difficulty feeding self
- Physical disability, such as hemiplegia

Nursing care is focused on meeting the client's basic needs and treating the client's underlying problem(s). Nursing goals include an accurate assessment of the client's present physical and nutritional state, recent and usual eating habits, and current intake and output. Treatment goals include promoting homeostasis, increasing the client's intake of food and liquids, and assisting the client to establish independent, nutritionally adequate eating habits.

NURSING DIAGNOSES ADDRESSED IN THIS CARE PLAN
Imbalanced Nutrition: Less Than Body Requirements
Ineffective Coping

RELATED NURSING DIAGNOSES ADDRESSED IN THE MANUAL
Bathing Self-Care Deficit
Dressing Self-Care Deficit
Feeding Self-Care Deficit
Toileting Self-Care Deficit
Noncompliance

Nursing Diagnosis

Imbalanced Nutrition: Less Than Body Requirements
Intake of nutrients insufficient to meet metabolic needs.

ASSESSMENT DATA

- Lack of appetite
- Lack of interest in eating
- Aversion to eating
- Weight loss
- Body weight 20% or more under ideal body weight
- Refusal to eat
- Difficulty eating
- Malnutrition
- Inadequate hydration
- Electrolyte imbalance
- Starvation
- Disturbance in elimination
- Difficulty swallowing
- Lack of awareness of need for food and fluids
- Delusions, other psychotic symptoms, or other psychiatric problems

EXPECTED OUTCOMES

Immediate   The client will

- Establish adequate nutrition, hydration, and elimination, e.g., eat at least 30% of all food offered within 1 to 3 days
- Demonstrate adequate fluid and electrolyte balance, i.e., electrolyte levels will be within normal limits within 2 to 4 days
- Be free of signs and symptoms of malnutrition within 4 to 5 days

Stabilization   The client will

- Demonstrate weight gain if appropriate
- Demonstrate independence in food and fluid intake, e.g., eat 80% of all meals without staff assistance

Community   The client will

- Maintain regular, adequate, nutritional eating habits
- Maintain adequate or normal body weight

IMPLEMENTATION

Nursing Interventions *denotes collaborative interventions	Rationale
*Do a thorough assessment using physical assessment and interviews with the client and significant others. Obtain detailed information regarding the client's eating patterns before the illness; familiar or liked foods; special diets (e.g., religious or vegetarian); recent changes in eating	Accurate baseline information is essential in planning and providing nursing care.

IMPLEMENTATION (continued)

Nursing Interventions *denotes collaborative interventions	Rationale
habits; GI or other physical complaints and disorders; circumstances that affect the client's appetite; and any other problems that may affect eating.	
Strictly monitor intake and output in an unobtrusive way. Record the type and amount of food, and the times and circumstances of eating. For example, was the client alone? Was eating encouraged? What was the level of stimuli?	Information on intake and output is necessary to assess the client's nutritional state. Unobtrusive observations minimize the client's secondary gain.
It may be necessary for you to feed the client, offer food to the client, accompany the client to get food, or sit with the client through mealtime. Nasogastric tube feedings or intravenous therapy also may be necessary.	The client's physical health is a priority.
Keep a record of the client's elimination. Record the color, amount, consistency, and frequency of stools.	If the client is consuming little or no food, stools may be less frequent or loose. The client may have been using laxatives, enemas, or suppositories to promote elimination.
Weigh the client regularly, at the same time of day and in a matter-of-fact manner. The client should consistently wear only a hospital gown or pajamas when being weighed.	Being matter-of-fact about weight measurement will help to separate issues of weight and eating from emotional issues. The client may conceal weights under his or her clothing to appear to have gained weight.
*Provide nursing care (and facilitate medical treatment) for physical problems related to the client's not eating.	The client's physical health is a priority. Many physical problems can contribute to or result from the client's not eating.
Provide fruit, juices, and foods high in fiber.	Fruit, juices, and foods high in fiber content promote adequate elimination.
Have some food and liquids available for the client at all times.	The client may be interested in eating at times other than mealtimes.
Offer food, nutritious liquids, and water to the client frequently in small amounts.	The client may be overwhelmed by or may not tolerate large amount of foods.
Discourage the intake of nonnutritional or diuretic substances (e.g., coffee, tea, or diet soda) except water. Encourage the use of milk or sugar (rather than artificial sweetener) in coffee or tea.	It is important to maximize nutrition when the client can or will eat or drink.
Encourage the intake of liquids highest in nutritional value and calories, such as fruit juice, chocolate milk, and whole milk.	If the client will not eat solid foods, liquids can provide many calories and nutrients.
Offer the client fortified shakes, made by blending ice cream, milk, and powdered milk (stir just before giving to the client), or dietary supplements.	Fortified liquids can be effective in providing maximal nutrition to a client who will not eat solid foods.
Offer foods that require little effort to eat (i.e., are easily chewed and swallowed) and are visually and aromatically pleasant.	The client may feel that he or she does not have much energy to eat. Foods that are appealing can stimulate the client's interest and appetite.
If the client has GI complaints (e.g., nausea), offer light, bland foods; clear soups; and clear carbonated beverages. Avoid fried foods, gravy, or spicy foods.	Light, bland foods or clear liquids may be more easily tolerated by (and more appealing to) the client with GI complaints.
If the client initially will take only liquids, gradually attempt to introduce solid foods, such as cream soups, crackers, cooked cereal, pudding, and light foods.	Gradual introduction of solid foods may be effective in overcoming the client's resistance.
Try to accommodate the client's normal or previous eating habits as much as possible.	Reinforcing previous normal eating habits increases the likelihood that the client will eat.

(continued on page 346)

IMPLEMENTATION (continued)

Nursing Interventions *denotes collaborative interventions	Rationale
*Make culturally or ethnically appropriate foods available; the client's significant others may be able to provide guidance or food acceptable to the client.	The client may be more apt to eat foods that are culturally acceptable or provided by family members or significant others.
When offering foods, *tell* the client you have something for him or her to eat; do not *ask* if he or she wants to eat or feels like eating. However, do not order the client to eat.	The client's ability to make decisions may be impaired, or the client may refuse to eat if asked. However, he or she may eat in response to your suggestion or expectation that he or she will eat.
Gradually progress from feeding the client to offering food to asking the client to get his or her food. Record changes in the frequency of eating and the amount eaten.	The client needs to develop independent eating habits.
Gradually decrease the frequency of suggestions, and allow the client to take responsibility for eating; again, record changes.	The transition from feeding the client to independent eating is more likely to be successful if it is gradual.

Nursing Diagnosis

Ineffective Coping

Inability to form a valid appraisal of the stressors, inadequate choices of practiced responses, and/or inability to use available resources.

ASSESSMENT DATA

- Inability to meet basic needs for nutrition
- Inability to ask for help
- Inability to solve problems
- Self-destructive behavior (refusal to eat)
- Difficulty identifying and expressing feelings
- Ineffective expression of emotional needs and conflicts
- Delusions, other psychotic symptoms, or other psychiatric problems

EXPECTED OUTCOMES

Immediate

The client will

- Demonstrate beginning ability to meet basic needs or ask for help within 24 to 48 hours
- Demonstrate decreased delusions, phobias, guilt, or other related psychiatric problems within 2 to 4 days

Stabilization

The client will

- Demonstrate non–food-related coping mechanisms, such as verbalizing feelings to staff or significant others, physical activity, and stress management
- Demonstrate improvement in related psychiatric problems

Community

The client will

- Participate in continued therapy after discharge if indicated
- Cope with stress and stressful life events independently

IMPLEMENTATION

Nursing Interventions *denotes collaborative interventions	Rationale
Do not tell the client that he or she will get sick, weak, or may die from not eating.	The client may hope to become ill or die from not eating or drinking or may believe this is true.
Do not threaten the client (e.g., "If you don't eat, you'll have to have an intravenous line."). However, use limits, consequences, consistency, and the giving and withdrawing of attention as appropriate (see Care Plan 36: Anorexia Nervosa).	Threatening the client will undermine trust and is not therapeutic. The effective use of limits is helpful in reinforcing positive behaviors and minimizing secondary gain. *Remember*: Intravenous and tube feeding therapy are medical treatments, not punishments.
Give positive support and attention when the client eats; withdraw your attention when he or she refuses to eat.	Positive feedback provides reinforcement. It is essential to support the client in positive ways and to minimize attention for unacceptable behaviors.
*Talk with the client's significant others about the concept of secondary gain; explain the treatment program and enlist their cooperation.	Significant others may be unaware of the dynamics of secondary gain and unwittingly reinforce the client's not eating.
If necessary, ask other clients to minimize attention given to the client for not eating.	Other clients may be unaware of the dynamics of secondary gain and may unwittingly reinforce the client's not eating.
Set up structured times and limits regarding eating (e.g., try to feed the client for 10 minutes, then withdraw for half an hour). Be consistent in your approach and behavior.	Consistency and limits minimize the possibility of manipulation. Limiting mealtimes decreases the amount of time the client is dealing with issues of food and eating and receiving attention for not eating.
Assess or explore the client's history, particularly his or her attitudes and feelings regarding food and eating.	The client may associate food or eating with stress, pleasure, reward, guilt, resentment, religion, or morality. The client's family may emphasize food or use eating (or not eating) as a means of manipulation, control, and so forth.
Encourage the client to eat at appropriate meal and snack times; allow food only at those times.	This can prevent the client from eating when he or she feels anxious or stressed and will help to decrease these associations.
Encourage the client to express his or her feelings at times other than mealtimes.	Focusing on feelings without food present can help decrease associations between emotions and food.
Discourage (withdraw your attention from) rituals or other emotional associations with meals, food, and so forth.	Withdrawing attention from undesired behaviors will minimize reinforcement and may help decrease or eliminate these behaviors.
*Teach the client and significant others about disorders related to the client's not eating and stress management techniques. Record the client's perceptions of and responses to stress; encourage the client to approach a staff member when experiencing stress.	The client and his or her family or significant others may have little or no knowledge of the client's behavior, underlying disorder(s), or stress management. The client may need to learn to recognize stress and his or her responses to it, as well as techniques for stress management.
*Encourage the client to identify others in his or her environment with whom the client can talk and to identify activities that might decrease stress (e.g., hobbies, physical activities).	The client can learn to ask for help, express feelings, and learn other ways to deal directly with emotions and stress rather than using food.
*Work with the client regarding psychiatric problems that may be related to eating behaviors.	Psychiatric problems related to the client's not eating must be resolved to ensure independence in healthful eating patterns.

SECTION 13 REVIEW QUESTIONS

1. The nurse is working with a client who has a potential for violence and aggressive behavior. Which of the following immediate outcomes would be most appropriate for the nurse to include in the plan of care? The client will

   a. Ask the nurse for medication when upset

   b. Discuss feelings of anger with staff

   c. Participate in therapy to resolve underlying issues

   d. Use indirect behaviors to express anger

2. A client is preparing for discharge from a substance dependence treatment program. Which of the following would be the priority in the discharge plan?

   a. A list of goals

   b. Family forgiveness

   c. Follow-up care

   d. Supportive friends

3. A client who was raped has difficulty expressing her feelings of anger and outrage. Which of the following activities would the nurse suggest to assist the client in expressing her feelings?

   a. Meditating

   b. Listening to music

   c. Using a punching bag

   d. Writing in a journal

4. A client who is newly widowed tells the nurse that she wishes she could "join her husband in heaven." After assessing the client for suicidal ideation, which of the following would be the best response by the nurse?

   a. "Do you have children that can help you at this time?"

   b. "Things will get better with time."

   c. "Tell me what feelings you've been experiencing."

   d. "What was the cause of your husband's death?"

SECTION 13 Recommended Readings

Boelen, P. A., van de Schoot, R., van den Hout, M. A., de Keijser, J., & van den Bout, J. (2010). Prolonged grief disorder, depression, and posttraumatic stress disorder are distinguishable syndromes. *Journal of Affective Disorders, 125*(1–3), 374–378.

Bonner, G., & Wellman, N. (2010). Postincident review of aggression and violence in mental health settings. *Journal of Psychosocial Nursing and Mental Health Services, 48*(7), 35–40.

Daignault, I. V., & Hebert, M. (2009). Profiles of school adaptation: Social, behavioral, and academic functioning in sexually abused school girls. *Child Abuse & Neglect, 33*(2), 102–115.

Fujisawa, D., Miyashita, M., Nakajima, S., Ito, M., Kato, M., & Kim, Y. (2010). Prevalence and determinants of complicated grief in the general population. *Journal of Affective Disorders, 127*(1–3), 352–358.

Walker, D. C., Anderson, D. A., & Hildebrandt, T. (2009). Body checking behaviors in men. *Body Image, 6*(3), 164–170.

SECTION 13 Resources for Additional Information

Visit thePoint (http://thePoint.lww.com/Schultz9e) for a list of these and other helpful Internet resources.

Academy of Psychosomatic Medicine
Alzheimer's Association
Alzheimer's Disease Education and Referral (ADEAR) Center
American Hospice Foundation
Brain Injury Association of America
CDC (violence information)
Child Welfare Information Gateway
Hospice Foundation of America
Institute on Domestic Violence in the African American Community
National Center on Elder Abuse
National Coalition Against Domestic Violence
National Institute of Justice—Elder Abuse
National Latino Alliance for the Elimination of Domestic Violence
Partnership Against Domestic Violence
Sena Foundation (grief and loss)

REFERENCES

Aguilera, D. C. (1998). *Crisis intervention: Theory and methodology* (8th ed.). St. Louis, MO: Mosby.

Alcoholism Information. (2010). Alcoholism statistics. Retrieved from http://www.alcoholism-information.com/Alcoholism_Statistics.html

Alcoholism-Statistics.com. (2010). Alcoholism in the population. Retrieved from http://alcoholism-statistics.com/facts.php

American Academy of Child and Adolescent Psychiatry. (2007). Practice parameter for the assessment and treatment of children and adolescents with attention-deficit/hyperactivity disorder. *Journal of the American Academy of Child and Adolescent Psychiatry, 46*(7), 894–921.

American Academy of Child and Adolescent Psychiatry and American Psychiatric Association. (2010). ADHD: Parents medication guide. Retrieved from http://www.psych.org/Share/Parents-Med-Guide.aspx

American Diabetes Association. (2011). *Diabetes Care, 34*(Supp. 1).

American Psychiatric Association. (2000). *DSM-IV-TR: Diagnostic and statistical manual of mental disorders* (4th ed., Text Rev.). Washington, DC: Author.

American Psychiatric Association. (2010a). American psychiatric association practice guidelines for the treatment of psychiatric disorders: Compendium 2006. Retrieved from http://psychiatryonline.org/guidelines.aspx

American Psychiatric Association. (2010b). Homeless statistics. Retrieved from http://pn.psychiatryonline.org/content/45/3/7.2full

American Psychiatric Nurses Association. (2010). Standards of practice. Retrieved from http://www.apna.org/i4a/pages/index.cfm?pageid=3335

Bartels, S. J., & Pratt, S. I. (2009). Psychosocial rehabilitation and quality of life for older adults with serious mental illness: Recent findings and future research directions. *Current Opinion in Psychiatry, 22*(4), 381–385.

Black, D. W., & Andreasen, N. C. (2011). *Introductory textbook of psychiatry* (5th ed.). Arlington, VA: American Psychiatric Publishing.

Bowlby, J. (1980). *Attachment and loss, Vol. 3: Loss, sadness and depression*. New York, NY: Basic Books.

Caplan, G. (1964). *Principles of preventive psychiatry*. New York, NY: Basic Books.

Carbray, M. J., & McGuinness, T. (2009). Pediatric bipolar disorder. *Journal of Psychosocial Nursing and Mental Health Nursing, 47*(12), 22–26.

Centers for Disease Control. (2010a). Attention-deficit/hyperactivity disorder. Retrieved from http://www.cdc.gov/ncbddd/adhd/facts.html

Centers for Disease Control. (2010b). Child abuse statistics. Retrieved from http://www.cdc.gov/violenceprevention/pdf/CM-datasheet-a.pdf

Centers for Disease Control. (2010c). Elder abuse statistics. Retrieved from http://www.cdc.gov/violenceprevention/pdf/EM-FactSheet-a.pdf

Centers for Disease Control. (2010d). Violence statistics. Retrieved from http://www.cdc.gov/violenceprevention/pdf/IPV-factsheet-a.pdf

Day, J., Ternouth, A., & Collier, D. A. (2009). Eating disorders and obesity: Two sides of the same coin? *Epidemiologia e Psichiatria Siciale, 18*(2), 96–100.

Eisenman, D. P., Glik, D., Ong, M., Zhou, Q., Tseng, C.-H., Long, A., … Asch, S. (2009). Terrorism-related fear and avoidance behavior in a multiethnic urban population. *American Journal of Public Health, 99*(1), 168–174.

Giger, J. N., & Davidhizar, R. E. (2008). *Transcultural nursing*. St. Louis, MO: Mosby.

Gilmer, T. P., Stefancic, S., Ettner, S. L., Manning, W. G., & Tsemberis, S. (2010). Effect of full-service partnerships on homelessness, use and cost of mental health services, and quality of life among adults with serious mental illness. *Archives of General Psychiatry, 67*(6), 645–652.

Goldman, M. B. (2009). The mechanism of life-threatening water imbalance in schizophrenia and its relationship to the underlying psychiatric illness. *Brain Research Review, 61*(2), 210–220.

Gorman, J. M. (2006). Gender differences in depression and response to psychotropic medication. *Gender Medicine, 3*(2), 93–109.

Gwynne, K., Blick, B. A., & Duffy, G. M. (2009). Pilot evaluation of an early intervention programme for children at risk. *Journal of Paediatrics and Child Health, 45*(3), 118–124.

Horsfall, J., Cleary, M., Hunt, G. E., & Walter, G. (2009). Psychosocial treatments for people with co-occurring severe mental illnesses and substance use disorders (dual diagnoses): A review of empirical evidence. *Harvard Review of Psychiatry, 17*(1), 24–34.

Hudson, J. I., Hiripi, E., Pope, H. G., & Kessler, R. C. (2006). The prevalence and correlates of eating disorders in the National Comorbidity Survey Replication. *Biological Psychiatry, 61*(3), 348–358.

Kneisl, C. R., & Trigoboff, E. (2009). *Contemporary psychiatric-mental health nursing* (2nd ed.). Upper Saddle River, NJ: Prentice Hall.

Kübler-Ross, E. (1969). *On death and dying.* New York, NY: McGraw-Hill.

Logan, J. E. (2009). Prevention factors for suicide ideation among abused pre-early adolescent youths. *Journal of the International Society for Child and Adolescent Injury Prevention, 15*(4), 278–280.

Mohamed, S., Neale, M. S., & Rosenheck, R. (2009). Veteran's affairs intensive case management for older veterans. *American Journal for Geriatric Psychiatry, 17*(8), 671–681.

NANDA International. (2009). *Nursing diagnoses: Definitions and classification 2009–2011.* Somerset, NJ: Wiley-Blackwell.

National Center for Complementary and Alternative Medicine. (2007). Statistics. Retrieved from http://nccam.nih.gov/news/camstats/2007/camsurvey_fs1.htm

National Coalition for the Homeless. (2009). Mental illness and homelessness. Retrieved from http://www.nationalhomeless.org

National Institute of Mental Health. (2010). Schizophrenia statistics. Retrieved from http://www.nimh.nih.gov/statistics/index.shtml

Peplau, H. (1963). A working definition of anxiety. In S. E. Bird & M. A. Marshall (Eds.), *Some clinical approaches to psychiatric nursing.* New York, NY: Macmillan.

Ross, C. A. (2009). Psychodynamics of eating disorder behavior in sexual abuse survivors. *American Journal of Psychotherapy, 63*(3), 211–226.

Sadock, B. J., & Sadock, V. A. (2008). *Kaplan & Sadock's concise textbook of clinical psychiatry* (3rd ed.). Philadelphia, PA: Wolters Kluwer Lippincott Williams & Wilkins.

Stanford School of Medicine. (2010). Pediatric bipolar disorders program. Retrieved from http://pediatricbipolar.Stanford.edu

University of Iowa College of Nursing. (2010). Acute confusion and delirium. Retrieved from http://www.nursing.uiowa.edu/sites/default/files/documents/hartford/EBP_Catalog2012.pdf

Videbeck, S. L. (2011). *Psychiatric mental health* nursing (5th ed.). Philadelphia, PA: Wolters Kluwer Lippincott Williams & Wilkins.

Zisook, S., & Shear, K. (2009). Grief and bereavement: What psychiatrists need to know. *World Psychiatry, 8*(2), 67–74.

ANSWERS TO SECTION REVIEW QUESTIONS

Section 1

1. **C** The nurse encourages the client to discuss the medication noncompliance in a nonthreatening, nonjudgmental, and neutral manner.
2. **B** When the client is actively involved in the process, he or she is more likely to follow through with discharge plans.
3. **A** Giving feedback about negative behavior can assist the client to identify problem areas and increase self-awareness.
4. **B** If the caregiver has assumed the entire caregiving burden and isn't willing to ask for or accept assistance, the risk for caregiver role strain is increased.

Section 2

1. **A** Going to day treatment would give the client a meaningful place to go and provide opportunities to meet people and socialize.
2. **D** Developing a daily routine that includes activities will encourage the client to be more engaged in his or her environment.
3. **B** Psychosocial rehabilitation focuses on improving the quality of life by promoting independent functioning in the community rather than focusing on abstract concepts such as insight.
4. **A** Accepting and validating the client's feelings will acknowledge the client's concerns and promote further therapeutic interaction.

Section 3

1. **B** Limit setting provides the client with clear expectations for acceptable behavior as well as consequences for exceeding limits.
2. **C** A child with ADHD is generally overstimulated and active, rarely demonstrating sullen, withdrawn, or pouting behavior.
3. **D** Lack of self-worth and perceived low regard from others are major components of low self-esteem.
4. **D** The 16-year-old has multiple, acute psychosocial stressors in her life—parental divorce, a new and unfamiliar school, and separation from friends—which increases her risk for adjustment disorder.

Section 4

1. **A** In early dementia, the client may retain many ADL skills, but is slower or more awkward in completing self-care, thus requiring more time.
2. **B** The client is experiencing a sensory (tactile) misperception, which is an hallucination.
3. **A** When the nurse states her name, function, and location, she reorients the client without sounding critical or challenging the client.
4. **A** Delirium is usually an acute condition, which is resolved as soon as the causative condition is identified and successfully treated.
5. **A** The client needs to be oriented in order to accomplish other, more complex goals.
6. **B** The client is better able to focus on the nurse when the surrounding environment is quiet and nonstimulating.

Section 5

1. **B** The onset of alcohol withdrawal includes tremulousness, sweating, and elevated blood pressure.
2. **C** Alcohol is metabolized in the body at a consistent rate, so only time will lead to sobriety—it is unaffected by exercise, caffeine, or cold water.
3. **A** Ambulation is contraindicated for a client in severe withdrawal since he or she is confused, frightened, unsteady, and doesn't perceive the environment correctly.
4. **D** Caffeine will further increase anxiety and tremors and has no nutritive value.
5. **C** Safety is a priority. The nurse's presence may reassure the client, whereas using restraints or touching the client may be threatening or increase confusion.
6. **D** One of the most significant safety risks for PCP is the increased incidence of violent behavior.

Section 6

1. **B** The client is expressing a delusional idea, which is addressed in NANDA nursing diagnosis Disturbed Thought Processes.
2. **B** It is important that the nurse doesn't respond to the client's paranoid delusion as though it was reality based.

3. **C** The client is reporting an auditory hallucination, which is addressed by NANDA nursing diagnosis Disturbed Sensory Perceptions.

4. **A** The nurse can validate what the client is experiencing while using the technique of Presenting Reality to let the client know the nurse doesn't share the experience.

5. **B** Trying to meet the client's need for safety and security is a priority.

Section 7

1. **D** The nurse would respond to the client's second statement (I want you to remember me), which may indicate the client's suicidal ideas or intent.

2. **A** It is essential for the nurse to maintain the client's dignity and privacy when she is unable to do so for herself.

3. **D** The nurse can nonverbally convey genuine interest by spending time with the client even when he or she is not responding verbally.

4. **A** The nurse focuses on the client's current feelings about the loss.

5. **C** Walking with the client provides a large muscle activity to channel the client's energy constructively.

6. **B** The client's safety is always a priority.

Section 8

1. **D** The client's ability to understand complex or abstract ideas is often impaired by anxiety.

2. **B** Relaxation techniques help the client to reduce anxiety to a manageable level.

3. **B** Factual feedback is one of the best behavioral reinforcers.

4. **D** Initially the nurse can assist the client to complete the ritual and be on time for breakfast to help minimize the client's anxiety.

Section 9

1. **C** This statement indicates the client's understanding of the relationship between coping with stress and somatic symptoms.

2. **B** La belle indifference, or seeming unconcerned about the physical impairment, is a classic sign of conversion disorder.

3. **B** This approach minimizes potential secondary gain and indicates the nurse's belief that the client can go to the dining room.

4. **A** The nurse initially helps the client express feelings about his current condition as a first step in therapeutic communication.

Section 10

1. **A** The client may be purging to compensate for the increased nutritional intake.

2. **B** Coping mechanisms for clients with bulimia have been primarily food related, so non—food-related coping is a sign of progress.

3. **D** The client has described the binging and purging as her way of responding when she is upset—this represents an ineffective food-related attempt to cope.

4. **C** All three of the findings are symptoms of anorexia nervosa.

Section 11

1. **D** The client with difficulty sleeping needs to establish a regular bedtime with little stimulation before retiring. Relaxation can facilitate falling asleep.

2. **A** When a client is feeling overwhelmed, identifying and expressing feelings is necessary before the client is ready for problem solving.

3. **C** It is important to determine the client's perception of the change, which will have both positive and negative effects on the client's life.

4. **B** Alcohol intake often causes early wakening and doesn't produce restful sleep.

Section 12

1. **A** Being calm is a neutral approach—being cheerful or friendly may heighten the client's suspicion.

2. **B** When one assigned staff person makes decisions, the potential for staff splitting and manipulation is decreased.

3. **B** Safety contracts usually specify clients' ability to be safe or to notify staff if they feel they cannot be safe—the client is following the contract.

4. **A** It is important to view any self-harm as a serious problem and safety issue.

5. **A** Effective community functioning is a primary goal for clients with schizoid personality disorder—they do not value or desire social interests.

6. **C** The nurse can help the client see that living independently does not mean the loss of a positive, supportive, parental relationship.

Section 13

1. **B** Direct, open discussion of angry feelings may facilitate coping. Internalizing angry feelings is often a precursor to aggression.

2. **C** Without follow-up care, the client is not likely to maintain his or her sobriety. Recovery in substance

abuse disorders requires ongoing effort and involvement.

3. **D** Writing feelings may be less difficult than verbalizing the feelings to someone else. Music, meditation, and exercise are relief behaviors, but do not address the client's problems.

4. **C** It is important for the nurse to encourage the client to express her feelings and actively listen to the client, rather than changing the subject or trying to "cheer her up."

GLOSSARY

A

Acquired immunodeficiency syndrome (AIDS) A condition caused by infection with human immunodeficiency virus (HIV) that results in severe, life-threatening impairment of the immune system.

Acting out Behavior that occurs as a means of expressing feelings. It may be acceptable (crying when sad) or unacceptable, even destructive (throwing chairs or hitting another person when angry).

Adaptation The adjustment that occurs in response to a change in the environment, in a static sense. Dynamically, the process by which the adjustment is made. An adjustment that occurs but does not meet the individual's needs constructively is called maladaptation.

AD/HD See Attention deficit/hyperactivity disorder.

Adjustment disorder A disorder in which a client has an excessive reaction to an identified psychosocial stressor.

Adult child of an alcoholic An adult who was raised in an environment in which at least one parent was an alcoholic.

Affect The behavioral expression of an individual's mood.

Aggressive behavior Behavior that is violent or destructive, ranging from threatening verbalizations to striking other persons or throwing objects. This behavior is often associated with anger, hostility, or intense fear.

Agitation A state of restlessness characterized by hyperactivity, increased response to stimuli, and an inability to relax or become calm.

Agnosia Inability to recognize objects in spite of intact sensory function.

Agoraphobia The fear of being in a place or situation from which one may not be able to escape or obtain help for overwhelming anxiety or panic if needed.

AIDS See Acquired immunodeficiency syndrome.

Alogia Decreased, or poverty of, speech.

Alzheimer's disease An organic mental disorder characterized by cerebral atrophy, plaque deposits in the brain, and enlargement of the third and fourth ventricles. It results in loss of speech and motor function, profound changes in behavior and personality, and death.

Anergy The lack of normal levels of energy, ambition, or drive.

Anhedonia The inability to experience pleasure.

Anorexia nervosa An eating disorder characterized by refusal to eat or eating only minimal amounts of food.

Anticipatory grieving Grief that occurs prior to an actual loss, such as in anticipation of death from a terminal illness.

Anticipatory guidance A process used to assist people to cope with an impending event or situation before its occurrence. The process includes identification of the future event and identification and evaluation of possible responses to the event.

Antisocial behavior Behavior frequently in conflict with society's social, moral, and/or legal mores.

Antisocial personality disorder A personality disorder characterized by a disregard for and violation of the rights of others and behaviors that are in conflict with societal norms.

Anxiety Feelings of apprehension cued by a threat to a person's self-esteem, values, or beliefs.

Apathy A seeming lack of feelings or emotional response; apparent indifference to surroundings, circumstances, or situation.

Aphasia Impaired language function.

Appropriate Fitting the circumstances, situation, or environment at a given time.

Apraxia Impairment in the ability to do motor tasks, despite having the ability to comprehend the task and having intact sensory function and motor ability.

Attention deficit/hyperactivity disorder (AD/HD) A pattern of hyperactivity, impulsivity, and inattention that is greater than expected at a client's developmental level.

Attention-seeking behavior Actions that occur for the primary purpose of gaining another's attention. It is frequently a type of behavior (such as throwing dishes when upset) that attempts to force another person to become engaged or to intervene (see also Manipulative behavior).

Avolition The inability to engage in self-initiated, goal-directed activity.

B

Best practices Documents written by an individual, group, or organization to guide care for clients with a specific diagnosis or situation.

Bipolar disorder A mood disorder characterized by periods of manic behavior and periods of depressive behavior, formerly called "manic depressive illness" or "bipolar affective disorder."

Blocking The inability to verbalize thoughts.

Body image The individual's perception of his or her physical self, although it also may include nonphysical attributes.

Borderline personality disorder A personality disorder characterized by unstable behavior, mood, self-esteem, and relationships.

Bulimia nervosa, bulimia An eating disorder characterized by food consumption binges usually followed by purging or vomiting.

C

Caregiver An individual providing care for a client, usually in a home setting.

Caregiver's syndrome The situation in which a caregiver feels overwhelmed by the negative effects of providing care to a client, for example, stress, lack of sleep, and lack of attention to the caregiver's needs.

Case manager A health care professional who acts to coordinate the client's care.

Catatonic A state of disrupted relatedness and withdrawal that is characterized by physical and psychological immobility.

Chemical dependence See Substance abuse.

Chronic sorrow Recurrent grief that occurs in response to an ongoing loss or a series of losses (e.g., losses resulting from a debilitating or terminal disease).

Clanging Rhyming speech.

Collaborative care The concept of working together with health care professionals from other disciplines to provide care that includes the expertise, clinical perspective, and resources from a variety of disciplines (see also Interdisciplinary team).

Commitment The legal detainment of a person without his or her consent in a facility for mental health treatment. Usually, the person must meet one of the following criteria to be committed: (1) dangerous to self, (2) dangerous to others, and (3) incapable of caring for self in a reasonable manner. (Specific laws vary from state to state.)

Community grieving Grief shared by members of a community in response to a significant loss or change.

Comorbid disorder Two or more diagnoses existing together.

Complementary and alternative medicine A term that denotes a range of treatments, treatment disciplines, dietary supplements, vitamins, and health practices considered to be alternatives and supplements to conventional medical treatments and medications.

Complicated grieving A state that occurs when a person fails to progress through normal or expected phases of the grief process when mourning a significant loss; emotional distress may be excessive or minimal; the person's ability to function in daily life is impaired.

Compulsive behaviors Ritualistic acts, usually repetitive and purposeless in nature, used in an effort to deal with anxiety or unacceptable thoughts.

Conduct disorder A pattern of behavior in which a client who is a minor consistently violates rules, societal norms, or the rights of others.

Confrontation The technique of presenting a person with one's perception of that person's behavior or with conflicts one sees between what the person says and what he or she does. The goal of confrontation is for the client to gain insight or to progress in the problem-solving process.

Conversion disorder The expression of an emotional conflict through a physical symptom, which is usually sensorimotor in nature; also called *conversion reaction*.

Co-occurring disorder See Comorbid disorder.

Coping strategy The means used by an individual in an effort to achieve adaptation to events or situations in one's life.

Creutzfeldt–Jakob disease A CNS disorder, caused by a "slow virus" or prion, typically seen in adults between 40 and 60 years of age. This encephalopathy includes altered vision, loss of coordination or abnormal movements, and a dementia that progresses rapidly in a few months.

Critical care unit psychosis A psychotic state related to the constant stimuli (lights, sounds), disruptions of diurnal patterns, frequent interruption of sleep, and so on, experienced in critical care units.

Critical incident stress Feelings of profound grief, anxiety, vulnerability, and loss of control in response to terrorism, large-scale violence, natural disasters, or major accidents.

D

Date rape Sexual assault by an individual with whom the victim agreed to have a social engagement or date. The victim declines sexual activity, but is assaulted regardless of his or her wishes.

Defense mechanism An unconscious process that functions to protect the self or ego from anxiety; a coping mechanism.

Delirium A change in cognition and disturbance in consciousness that develops over a short period.

Delirium tremens The most severe result of alcohol withdrawal, characterized by disorientation, hallucinations, combative behavior and/or suicidal behavior, or life-threatening physical sequelae.

Delusion A false belief that has no base in reality.

Delusion, bizarre A false belief that is not related to a plausible or possible situation.

Delusion, fixed A false belief that persists over time and does not respond to psychotropic medications or treatment.

Delusion, grandiose A false belief that one has talents, abilities, experiences, relationships, or fame that one does not actually have.

Delusion, jealous A false belief that one's partner or spouse is unfaithful when that is not true.

Delusion, nonbizarre A belief that is false in the present situation, but could possibly be true in other circumstances.

Delusion, persecutory A false belief that one is being spied on, judged, pursued, or harassed.

Delusion, somatic A false belief that one's body or body part(s) is contaminated, infested, deformed, or ugly and unacceptable.

Delusion, transient A false belief that diminishes in response to psychotropic medications, treatment, or time.

Dementia A deteriorating condition characterized by losses in memory and other cognitive deficits.

Denial The unconscious process of putting aside ideas, conflicts, problems, or any source of emotional discomfort. This is sometimes a healthy response (e.g., as a stage in the grief process) to give the person a chance to organize thoughts and align resources to deal with the current crisis. However, if this is a person's only response, or if it is prolonged, it becomes an unhealthy response and a means of avoiding problems and conflicts. These may then be acted out in other nonproductive ways.

Depression An affective state characterized by feelings of sadness, guilt, and low self-esteem, often related to a loss.

Depressive disorder, major A diagnosis of depression that includes one or more major depressive episodes and occurs without a history of manic (or hypomanic) episodes.

Disaster nursing Direct involvement in crisis intervention, community response, and education designed to help communities deal with traumatic events.

Disaster response See Critical incident stress.

Disenfranchised grief The grief experience of individuals whose grief is not acknowledged or supported by their social network or who are excluded from participating in grief-related rituals.

Disordered water balance Excessive intake of water or other fluids; also called *psychogenic polydipsia*.

Disorientation A state in which the individual has lost the ability to recognize or determine his or her position with respect to time, place, and/or identity.

Dissociation A disruption in the usually integrated functions of consciousness, memory, identity, or perception of the environment.

Dual diagnosis Coexisting diagnoses of a major mental illness and chemical dependence. (*Note:* Some authors define dual diagnosis as mental illness and mental retardation or any two coexisting primary diagnoses.)

E

Ego boundary In the differentiation of the self from the not-self or environment, the point or boundary of the self.

Erotomania A type of delusion in which an individual falsely believes he or she is loved by another person, usually someone famous.

Evidence-based practice Care planning and treatment decisions based on research or expert opinion that supports the efficacy of the intervention.

Executive functioning The ability to engage in abstract thinking, including planning, initiating, executing, and stopping complex behaviors.

Extrapyramidal symptoms (EPS) A group of neurological symptoms that can be caused by side effects of certain medications, such as antipsychotic drugs. Types of EPS include dystonia, parkinsonism, and akathisia.

F

Feedback Information provided to a person to increase insight, facilitate the problem-solving process, or give an external interpretation of behavior.

G

Gratification The meeting of one's needs in a satisfactory or pleasing manner.

Grief, grieving, grief work Behavior associated with mourning a loss, whether observable or perceived. It can be viewed as tasks necessary for adaptation to the loss (identification of loss, expression of related feelings, and making lifestyle changes that incorporate the loss).

H

Hallucination A sensory experience that is not the result of external stimuli. It may be visual, auditory, kinesthetic, tactile, olfactory, or gustatory in nature.

Histrionic, hysterical The appearance of physical (sensory or motor) symptoms in the absence of organic pathology, or behavior that is dramatic, not appropriate to place or situation.

HIV See Human immunodeficiency virus.

Homeostasis A tendency toward stability and balance among the individual's bodily processes.

Homicidal ideation Thoughts about killing other people.

Hostility Feelings of animosity and resentment that are expressed by verbal abuse or threatened aggressive or violent behavior, intended to be harmful to others.

Human immunodeficiency virus (HIV) The virus that causes AIDS.

Hypochondriacal Exhibiting physical symptoms that have no organic pathology; caused by or influenced by psychological stress.

I

Ideas of reference The belief of an individual that statements made by others or events are caused by or specifically meant for him or her (e.g., that a television program was produced in order to send him or her a message).

Illusion The misinterpretation of sensory stimulation.

Incest Sexual contact or activity between family members.

Insight Understanding or self-awareness that occurs when connections between conscious behavior and feelings, desires, or conflicts are recognized.

Intellectualization A defense mechanism that separates and denies or ignores the emotions associated with an event from ideas and opinions about the event. The rational discussion of facts devoid of the feelings aroused by the person, event, or situation.

Interdisciplinary team In mental health care, a group of health care professionals from different disciplines working together to provide collaborative care. Disciplines represented on the team can include psychiatric nursing, psychiatry, psychology, psychiatric social work, occupational therapy, recreational therapy, and vocational rehabilitation.

Interpersonal Involving a dynamic interchange between two or more people.

Intrapersonal Occurring as an internal process; occurring within oneself.

K

Knowledge deficit Lack of information or understanding; may be related to a lack of prior education, impaired ability to understand or retain information, resistance to learning, or other problems.

Korsakoff's syndrome A type of dementia characterized by severe mental impairment, including memory loss and disorientation, resulting from chronic alcoholism and the associated vitamin B_1 (thiamine) deficiency, usually occurring after a minimum of 5 to 10 years of heavy drinking.

L

La belle indifference A phrase used to describe an individual's lack of concern about a symptom related to a conversion reaction, such as paralysis.

Labile Unstable; quickly and easily changed, frequently from one extreme to another.

Loose associations A symptom of disordered thought processes in which successive ideas are expressed in an unrelated or only slightly related manner.

M

Major depressive disorder See Depressive disorder, major.

Manic behavior Hyperactive behavior characterized by excessive response to stimuli, push of speech, short attention span, lack of impulse control, low frustration tolerance, inability to impose internal controls, and possibly aggressive and/or self-destructive actions.

Manipulative behavior Actions designed to indirectly influence another person's response. It frequently helps the person avoid the logical consequences of his or her negative actions.

Marital rape Sexual assault by a legal spouse.

Milieu Any specific environment, including a group of persons.

Milieu therapy A group of persons interacting in a given environment, usually with a mental health orientation, with specific goals of problem solving, improved mental health, and resolution of difficulties achieved by the interaction within the milieu.

N

Negativism A pervasive mood resulting in perceptions and responses that are pessimistic in nature.

Neologisms Invented words.

Noncompliance Failure to accurately adhere to therapeutic recommendations.

Nursing diagnosis A statement of an actual or potential problem, human response, or situation amenable to nursing intervention.

O

Obsessive thoughts Ideas that occupy the individual's time and energy to the point of interfering with daily life. The thoughts are often ruminative, deprecatory, or persecutory in nature.

Obsessive-compulsive disorder A disorder characterized by the presence of obsessions or compulsions that cause significant stress or impairment.

One-to-one Involving one client and one nurse (staff member). This may be for the purpose of interaction or for observation, as with suicide precautions.

Optimal level of functioning The highest level of mental and physical wellness attained by a given individual. This is influenced by the person's inherent capabilities, the environment, coping mechanisms, and internal and external stressors.

P

Panic An extreme, disabling state of acute anxiety.

Paranoia Behavior characterized by mistrust and suspicion. It may involve delusions of grandiosity or persecution.

Parkinson's disease A progressive neurological disease characterized by tremor, muscle rigidity, and loss of postural reflexes.

Passive–aggressive behavior A type of manipulative behavior in which a client does not express hostile (angry, resentful) feelings directly, but denies them and reveals them indirectly through behavior.

Perseveration Repetitive speech or thoughts.

Persistent and severe mental illness See Serious and persistent mental illness (SPMI).

Personality disorder Maladaptive traits or characteristics that involve behaviors manifested as a result of maladaptive coping mechanisms. These mechanisms are used as a method of dealing with stress or problems and are often disturbing to others in terms of relationships, impulse control, and a sense of responsibility for one's behaviors.

Phobia The persistent fear of an object or situation that presents no real threat or in which the threat is magnified out of proportion to its actual severity.

Pick's disease An organic mental disorder characterized by frontal and temporal lobe atrophy, resulting in loss of speech, poor motor function, profound behavioral and personality changes, and death within 2 to 5 years.

Post-traumatic stress disorder A disorder characterized by behaviors that occur as a response to experiencing an unusually traumatic event or situation, such as a violent crime, combat experience, or incest.

Poverty of content Speech that contains much verbalization but little or no substance.

Poverty of speech See Alogia.

Precipitating factor A factor or situation of importance to the client that is related to the development of an unhealthy response. It may be a major event (death in the family, loss of a job) or something that may seem minor to others (an argument with a friend). The client's perception of the magnitude of the event is the most significant factor to assess.

Presenile dementia A general category of organic mental disorders involving progressive behavioral and personality changes due to primary degeneration and loss of brain neurons in people under age 65.

Problem-solving process A logical, step-by-step approach to problem resolution that includes identifying the problem, identifying and evaluating possible solutions, choosing and implementing a possible solution, and evaluating its effectiveness.

Projection A defense mechanism that uses unconscious transfer of blame or responsibility for unacceptable thoughts, feelings, or actions to someone else.

Psychogenic polydipsia Excessive intake of water and/or other fluids seen in clients with chronic mental illness; also called *disordered water balance*.

Psychotic Refers to a dysfunctional state in which the individual is unable to recognize reality or communicate effectively with others, and/or the individual exhibits regressive or bizarre behavior; characterized by delusions, hallucinations, and grossly disordered thinking, affect, and behavior.

Psychotic depression A mood disorder involving extreme sadness, withdrawal, and a disruption in relatedness, characterized by delusions, hallucinations, and loss of reality contact.

Push of speech Rapid verbalization that sounds forced from the person. Words are run together and spoken so rapidly that speech may be unintelligible.

R

Rape trauma syndrome A specific type of post-traumatic behavior following a rape.

Rationalization A justification for an unreasonable, illogical, or destructive act or idea to make it appear reasonable or justified.

Reactive depression, depressive neurosis A mood disorder, usually milder than major depression, often precipitated by an identifiable event, situation, or stressor.

Reinforcement A response to behavior that may encourage or discourage that behavior. Reinforcement can be planned to be positive (giving a reward that has value to the client and designed to perpetuate certain behavior) or negative (a consequence that the client perceives as negative that is designed to eliminate or decrease certain behavior).

Relaxation techniques Specific techniques to promote physical and mental relaxation, which can be taught by a nurse to a client. These may include breathing exercises (slow, deep, regular conscious breathing) and skeletal muscle tensing/relaxing exercises as well as suggestions for prebedtime measures, such as a warm bath or warm milk.

Respite A temporary relief from one's customary situation, usually lasting 1 to 3 days. For example, a client may stay somewhere other than his or her current living situation, or a caregiver may take a break from caregiving responsibilities.

Ritualistic Behavior that is automatic and repetitive in nature, frequently without reason or purpose; often elaborate and/or rigid.

Role modeling The demonstration of a behavior as a teaching technique.

Rumination Persistent meditation or pondering of thoughts. Carried to excess, rumination over past or present feelings (e.g., worthlessness or guilt) can replace constructive problem solving.

S

Schizoid personality disorder A personality disorder characterized by restricted emotions in interpersonal relationships and detachment from other people.

Schizotypal personality disorder A personality disorder characterized by peculiarity of ideas, appearance, and behavior as well as deficits in interpersonal relationships.

Seclusion A safe, controlled environment that has markedly decreased stimulation (no other people, no noise, minimal furnishings). It can be beneficial for individuals who are unable to tolerate stimulation or are exhibiting aggressive or self-destructive behavior to be confined in a seclusion room.

Secondary gains Benefits that a client derives from exhibiting certain behaviors, or from illness or hospitalization, that are not the most direct logical consequences of those behaviors. For example, the client may be successfully avoiding certain responsibilities, receiving attention, or manipulating others as a result of destructive behaviors or illness.

Seizure precautions Measures taken to ensure the client's safety when and if seizure activity occurs. They generally include padding the side rails of the client's bed, placing an airway at bedside, and alerting staff members to the potential for seizures.

Self-esteem The degree to which a person feels valued and worthwhile.

Self-medicating behavior Behavior in which a client attempts to alter moods, alleviate symptoms or distress, or manage his or her disease by using alcohol or illicit drugs, making changes in a prescribed medication regimen, or obtaining prescription medications from others.

Senile dementia A general category of organic mental disorders involving progressive behavioral and personality changes due to primary degeneration and loss of brain neurons in people over age 65.

Separation anxiety Apprehension or dread in response to future separation from a significant person or others or future uncertainty or change.

Serious and persistent mental illness (SPMI) A term used to describe chronic mental illness, in which a client manifests "positive" symptoms, such as delusions and hallucinations, and "negative" symptoms, such as social withdrawal, anhedonia, anergy, and apathy, that often persist over time and do not necessarily respond to medications.

Shaping A procedure that rewards successive approximations of a behavior toward the successful performance of a target behavior.

Sheltered setting An environment in which certain limits exist, some factors are controlled, and supportive elements are in place for the specific purpose of protecting clients who are unable to protect themselves adequately at a given time (e.g., a hospital, a rehabilitation work environment, a group home, supervised apartments).

Significant other A person who is important or valuable to another. This person may be a spouse or relative but could also be a partner, a friend, an employer, or a roommate, and so forth.

Somatic Physiologic in nature; pertaining to the body.

Somatization disorder A disorder in which the client has a number of physical symptoms, usually including pain, gastrointestinal, sexual, and neurological symptoms; historically called hysteria.

Somatoform disorder A disorder in which the client has physical symptoms that are suggestive of a medical problem, but there is no physical problem that fully accounts for the symptoms.

SPMI See Serious and persistent mental illness.

Stressor Any stimulus that requires a response from the individual.

Substance abuse The taking of any element into the body to produce a specific effect to the extent that, in time, achieving this effect gains priority over any or all major life concerns. Substances such as alcohol, glue, medication, and drugs are frequently the elements used. The substance is desired and used even when overall effects to physical or emotional health are deleterious.

Substance use The ingestion of chemicals to alter mood, behavior, or feelings.

Suicidal gesture A behavior that is self-destructive in nature but not lethal (e.g., writing a suicide note, then taking 10 aspirin tablets). It is usually considered to be manipulative behavior, but its nonlethality may be a result of the client's ignorance of the nonlethal nature of his or her behavior, and it may be a true suicide attempt.

Suicidal ideation Thoughts of committing suicide or thoughts of methods to commit suicide.

Suicide attempt A self-destructive behavior that is potentially lethal.

Suicide precautions Specific actions taken by the nursing staff to protect a client from suicidal gestures and attempts and to ensure close observation of the client.

Support systems or groups Persons, organizations, or institutions that provide help and assistance to a person in coping or dealing with problems or life situations (e.g., family, friends, Alcoholics Anonymous, Weight Watchers, an outpatient program).

Systematic desensitization A behavioral procedure using conscious relaxation to decrease the anxiety response to an identified phobic trigger.

T

Tangentiality A pattern of thinking expressed by the individual's verbalization straying away from the central topic on to vaguely related details. The individual is unable to discuss a central idea due to thoughts evoked by a word or phrase in the idea.

Therapeutic milieu See Milieu and Milieu therapy.

Thought blocking A sudden interruption in train of thought, which cannot be immediately retrieved.

Thought broadcasting The belief that one's thoughts are broadcast to the external world, so others can hear them.

Thought control The belief that others are in control of one's thoughts.

Thought insertion The belief that thoughts are placed into one's mind by others.

Thought withdrawal The belief that thoughts are being removed from one's mind by others.

Time out Retreat to a neutral environment to provide the opportunity to regain internal control.

Tolerance (drug) The need to increase the dose of a drug to achieve the same effect achieved in the past.

V

Volition A conscious choice or decision.

W

Waxy flexibility A condition in which the client's extremities are easily moved by another person but remain rigidly in the position in which they are placed, no matter how awkward or uncomfortable the position.

Withdraw attention Ignoring a client or physically leaving a client alone for the purpose of reducing or eliminating an undesirable behavior or topic of interaction. This is effective only if attention is valuable to that client and if attention is given to the client for desired behaviors.

Withdrawal syndrome Symptoms or behaviors that occur when use of a chemical substance is terminated abruptly.

Withdrawn behavior Behavior manifested by emotional and physical distancing from the external world, resulting from a disruption in relatedness between the self and others and/or the environment.

Word salad Speech that is composed of random, incoherent words and phrases that does not convey meaning.

Sample Psychosocial Assessment Tool

Date: _____ Client initials: _____ Advance directive signed? Y/N

Admission date: _____ Admission status: _____

Age: _____ Gender: _____ Primary language (written, spoken): _____

Allergies: _____

Diagnoses: Axis I: _____

Axis II: _____

Axis III: _____

Axis IV: _____

Axis V: _____

Reason for admission, primary problem

• Client's perception (i.e., what the client states as reason for admission):
• Perception of others (i.e., information from concerned others, health care providers about reason for client's admission):

Precipitating factors (e.g., recent stressors, medication noncompliance, life events):

Predisposing (risk) factors, family history:

Treatment history (inpatient and/or outpatient treatment):

Current medications (include dosage, frequency):

• **Prescription medications** (include compliance, e.g., "Do you take your medication as prescribed?" "Do you ever skip doses or take additional doses?" "Do you ever take another person's medications?"):
• **Over-the-counter (OTC) medications:**
• **Vitamins, herbal, and other supplements:**

Substance use, dependence (include type, quantity, frequency, compliance, e.g., "How often do you drink alcohol?" "On average, how many drinks do you have?"

"How often do you drink to the point of intoxication?" "Do you drink alone or with others?"):

Physiologic and self-care concerns

• **Medical problems:**
• **Physical impairments, disabilities, prostheses:**
• **Self-care abilities, deficits, personal hygiene:**
• **Review of systems** (include weight gain or loss, note if intentional or unintentional):
• **Sleep** (include pattern, amount, and quality):
• **Nutrition** (include appetite, food intake, food preferences, or dietary requirements):

Ethnicity/culture

• Cultural and spiritual beliefs and practices:
• Health beliefs and practices:

• **Appearance** (dress, facial expression, posture, eye contact; dressed appropriately for weather and occasion):

• **Motor behavior** (e.g., agitated, fidgety, unable to sit, pacing, no movement):

• **Speech** (include quantity, e.g., poverty of speech or minimal verbalization, one-word answers, hyperverbal, incessant talking; quality, e.g., poverty of content, latent responses, circumstantial, tangential, nonsensical, clanging or rhyming, perseveration, echolalia):

Mental status

- **Mood and affect** (mood, e.g., labile or stable, depressed, anxious, serious, paranoid, giddy, scared, angry; affect, e.g., broad range or restricted, flat, blunted, silly, inappropriate):
- **Thought process, cognition** (i.e., how the client thinks; e.g., logical, organized, rational or fragmented, loose associations, flight of ideas, thought blocking):
- **Thought content** (i.e., what the client thinks about; e.g., suicidal or homicidal thoughts, delusions—paranoid, somatic, religious, grandiose, ideas of reference):
- **Sensorium and intellectual processes** (include orientation to person, place, and time; confusion; recent and remote memory; concentration and attention spans; auditory, visual, olfactory, gustatory, tactile, or command hallucinations; fund of general knowledge; and concrete or abstract thinking abilities, e.g., interpretation of proverbs):
- **Suicidal or homicidal ideation** (include suicidal ideas, active, i.e., thinking of ways to kill self; or passive, wishing to be dead or never wake up; plan for suicide; whom the client wishes to harm and why):
- **Judgment and insight—limited, poor, good, fair** (e.g., ability to solve problems or make sound decisions; can the client see the relationship between own behavior and situation?):

Self-concept (how client perceives self; "How would you describe yourself as a person?"):

Client strengths (as identified by client and as identified by nurse):

Living situation (include other persons living with client; house, apartment, and group home):

Educational and work history (e.g., college, trade school, GED; current and past employment, when; type of job or career; volunteer work; income):

Roles and relationships (Is the client fulfilling current roles? Are roles satisfying? Whom does the client have relationships with? Are relationships supportive, satisfying, close, estranged, antagonistic, troubled? Does the client lack relationships?):

Coping skills and defense mechanisms (effective and ineffective, e.g., relief behaviors, "What do you do to relax when you are upset or stressed?" "How do you solve a problem—think about it, spend time alone, talk it over with a friend?"):

Interests and hobbies (include what the client currently does and what the client has done in the past, when stopped and why):

How the client spends a typical day (outside the hospital, when the client is feeling good/well and when having problems or stressed):

Teaching needs:

Barriers to learning (e.g., language or literacy barrier, lack of motivation/available energy, inability to concentrate/pay attention, lack of insight, defense mechanisms such as denial):

Client's expectations for care (e.g., "How can we help you?" "What would you like to accomplish while in the hospital?"):

Priorities for nursing care:

Discharge planning (include what client needs to be successful in community living, e.g., placement, case manager, financial or legal help, transportation, socialization; what client needs to manage illness; what the client needs to improve quality of life):

Signature: _____

Psychiatric-Mental Health Nursing: Scope and Standards of Practice

STANDARDS OF CARE

Standard I. Assessment

The psychiatric-mental health nurse collects client health data.

Standard II. Diagnosis

The psychiatric-mental health nurse analyzes the data in determining diagnoses.

Standard III. Outcome Identification

The psychiatric-mental health nurse identifies expected outcomes individualized to the client.

Standard IV. Planning

The psychiatric-mental health nurse develops a plan of care that prescribes interventions to attain expected outcomes.

Standard V. Implementation

The psychiatric-mental health nurse implements the interventions identified in the plan of care.

Standard Va. Counseling

The psychiatric-mental health nurse uses counseling interventions to assist clients in improving or regaining their previous coping abilities, fostering mental health, and preventing mental illness and disability.

Standard Vb. Milieu Therapy

The psychiatric-mental health nurse provides, structures, and maintains a therapeutic environment in collaboration with the client and other health care providers.

Standard Vc. Self-Care Activities

The psychiatric-mental health nurse structures interventions around the client's activities of daily living to foster self-care and mental and physical well-being.

Standard Vd. Psychobiologic Interventions

The psychiatric-mental health nurse uses knowledge of psychobiologic interventions and applies clinical skills to restore the client's health and prevent further disability.

Standard Ve. Health Teaching

The psychiatric-mental health nurse, through health teaching, assists clients in achieving satisfying, productive, and healthy patterns of living.

Standard Vf. Case Management

The psychiatric-mental health nurse provides case management to coordinate comprehensive health services and ensure continuity of care.

Standard Vg. Health Promotion and Maintenance

The psychiatric-mental health nurse employs strategies and interventions to promote and maintain mental health and prevent mental illness.

(Interventions Vh–Vj are advanced practice interventions and may be performed only by the certified specialist in psychiatric-mental health nursing.)

Standard VI. Evaluation

The psychiatric-mental health nurse evaluates the client's progress in attaining expected outcomes.

STANDARDS OF PROFESSIONAL PERFORMANCE

Standard I. Quality of Care

The psychiatric-mental health nurse systematically evaluates the quality of care and effectiveness of psychiatric-mental health nursing practice.

Standard II. Performance Appraisal

The psychiatric-mental health nurse evaluates his or her own psychiatric-mental health nursing practice in relation to professional practice standards and relevant statutes and regulations.

Standard III. Education

The psychiatric-mental health nurse acquires and maintains current knowledge in nursing practice.

Standard IV. Collegiality

The psychiatric-mental health nurse contributes to the professional development of peers, colleagues, and others.

Standard V. Ethics

The psychiatric-mental health nurse's decisions and actions on behalf of others are determined in an ethical manner.

Standard VI. Collaboration

The psychiatric-mental health nurse collaborates with the client, significant others, and health care providers in providing care.

Standard VII. Research

The psychiatric-mental health nurse contributes to nursing and mental health through the use of research.

Standard VIII. Resource Utilization

The psychiatric-mental health nurse considers factors related to safety, effectiveness, and cost in planning and delivering client care.

Reprinted with permission from American Nurses Association, American Psychiatric-Mental Health Nurses Association, and the International Society of Psychiatric-Mental Health Nurses. (2007). *Psychiatric-mental health nursing: Scope and standards of practice.* Silver Springs, MD: Nursebooks.org.

Canadian Standards of Psychiatric and Mental Health Nursing Practice

BELIEFS ABOUT PSYCHIATRIC AND MENTAL HEALTH NURSING

Psychiatric and mental health nursing (PMHN) is a specialized area of nursing that has as its focus the promotion of mental health, the prevention of mental illness, and the care of clients experiencing mental health problems and mental disorders.

The psychiatric and mental health nurse works with clients in a variety of settings, including institutional facility and community settings. Clients may be unique in their vulnerability, in this area of nursing practice, as they can be involved involuntarily and can be committed to an institution under the law. Further, clients may receive treatment against their will. This fact affects the nature of the nurse–client relationship and often raises complex ethical dilemmas.

The centrality of PMHN practice is the therapeutic use of self; nurse–client interactions are purposeful and goal directed. The psychiatric and mental health nurse understands how the psychiatric disease process, the illness experience, the recuperative powers, and the perceived degree of mental health are affected by contextual factors. Advances in knowledge (for instance, the current increase in understanding the biological basis of mental disorders and the sociological determinants of behavior) require that psychiatric and mental health nurses continually incorporate new research-based findings into their practice. PMH nurses acknowledge a responsibility to promote evidence-based, outcomes-oriented practice to enhance knowledge and skill development within the specialty. PMH nurses also acknowledge a responsibility to personal mental health promotion and maintenance.

PMHN knowledge is based on nursing theory, which is integrated with physical science theory, social science theory, and human science theory. PMHN shares with other mental health disciplines a body of knowledge based on theories of human behavior. In addition, "reflection on practice" continues to develop the nurses' habitual practices and skills of being truly present to the client situation at hand (Benner, Tanner, & Chesla, 1996, p. 325). In some settings, there may be an overlapping of professional roles and/or a sharing of competencies. PMH nurses recognize their accountability to society for both the discrete and shared functions of practice.

STANDARD I: PROVIDES COMPETENT PROFESSIONAL CARE THROUGH THE HELPING ROLE

The helping role is fundamental to all nursing practice. PMH nurses "enter into partnerships with clients, and through the use of the human sciences, and the art of caring, develop helping relationships" (CNA, 1997, p. 43) and therapeutic alliances with clients. A primary goal of PMHN is the promotion of mental health and the prevention or diminution of mental disorder.

The Nurse

1. Assesses and clarifies the influences of personal beliefs, values, and life experiences on the therapeutic relationship.
2. Establishes and maintains a caring goal-directed environment.
3. Uses a range of therapeutic communication skills, both verbal and nonverbal, including core communication skills (e.g., empathy, listening, observing).
4. Makes distinctions between social and professional relationships.
5. Recognizes the influence of culture and ethnicity on the therapeutic process and negotiates care that is culturally sensitive.
6. Mobilizes resources that increase clients' access to mental health services.
7. Understands and responds to human responses to distress such as anger, anxiety, fear, grief, helplessness, hopelessness, and humor.
8. Guides the client through behavioral, developmental, emotional, or spiritual change while acknowledging and supporting the client's participation, responsibility, and choices in own care.
9. Supports the client's sense of resiliency, for example, self-esteem, power, and hope.
10. Offers supportive and therapeutic care to the client's significant others.
11. Reflectively critiques therapeutic effectiveness of nurse–client relationships by evaluating client responses

Standard Committee of the Canadian Federation of Mental Health Nurses. (1998). *Canadian standards of psychiatric mental health nursing practice* (2nd ed.). Ottawa, ON: Canadian Nurses Association.

to therapeutic processes and by evaluating personal responses to client. The nurse seeks clinical supervision with ongoing therapeutic skill development.

STANDARD II: PERFORMS/REFINES CLIENT ASSESSMENTS THROUGH THE DIAGNOSTIC AND MONITORING FUNCTION

Effective diagnosis and monitoring is central to the nurse's role and is dependent upon theory, as well as upon understanding the meaning of the health or illness experience from the perspective of the client. This knowledge, integrated with the nurse's conceptual model of nursing practice, provides a framework for processing client data and for developing client-focused plans of care. The nurse makes professional judgments regarding the relevance and importance of these data, and acknowledges the client as a valued and respected partner throughout the decision-making process.

The Nurse

1. Collaborates with clients to gather holistic assessments through observation, examination, interview, and consultation, while being attentive to issues of confidentiality and pertinent legal statutes.
2. Documents and analyzes baseline data to identify health status, potential for wellness, health care deficits, potential for danger to self and others; alterations in thinking, perceiving, communicating, and decision-making abilities; substance abuse and dependency; and history of abuse (emotional, physical, sexual, or verbal).
3. Formulates and documents a plan of care in collaboration with the client and with the mental health team, recognizing variability in the client's ability to participate in the process.
4. Refines and extends client assessment information by assessing and documenting significant change in the client's status, and by comparing new data with the baseline assessment and intermediate client goals.
5. Anticipates problems in the future course of the client's functional status, for example, shifts in mood indicative of change in potential for self-harm: effects of "flashbacks."
6. Determines the most appropriate and available therapeutic modality that will potentially best meet client's needs, and assists the client to access these resources.

STANDARD III: ADMINISTERS AND MONITORS THERAPEUTIC INTERVENTIONS

Due to the nature of mental health problems and mental disorders, there are unique practice issues confronting the psychiatric and mental health nurse in administering and monitoring therapeutic interventions. Safety in PMHN has unique meaning since many clients are at risk for self-harm and/or self-neglect. Clients may not be mentally competent to participate in decision making. The PMH nurse needs to be alert to adverse reactions as client's ability to self-report may be impaired. The PMH nurse uses evidence-based and experiential knowledge from nursing, health sciences, and related mental health disciplines to both select and tailor nursing interventions. This is accomplished in collaboration with the client to the greatest possible extent.

The Nurse

1. Assists and educates clients to select choices, which will support positive changes in their affect, cognition, behavior, and/or relationships (CNA, 1997, p. 68).
2. Supports clients to draw on own assets and resources for self-care and mental health promotion (CNA, 1997, p. 68).
3. Makes discretionary clinical decisions, using knowledge of client's unique responses and paradigm cases as the basis for the decision, for example, frequency of client contact in the community.
4. Uses appropriate technology to perform safe, effective, and efficient nursing intervention (CNA, 1997, p. 68).
5. Administers medications accurately and safely, monitoring therapeutic responses, reactions, untoward effects, toxicity, and potential incompatibilities with other medications or substances.
6. Assesses client responses to deficits in activities of daily living and mobilizes resources in response to client's capabilities.
7. Provides support and assists with protection for clients experiencing difficulty with self-protection.
8. Utilizes therapeutic elements of group process.
9. Incorporates knowledge of family dynamics and cultural values and beliefs about families in the provision of care.
10. Collaborates with the client, health care providers, and community to access and coordinate resources.

STANDARD IV: EFFECTIVELY MANAGES RAPIDLY CHANGING SITUATIONS

The effective management of rapidly changing situations is essential in critical circumstances that may be termed psychiatric emergencies. These situations include self-harm and other assaultive behaviors and rapidly changing mental health states. This domain also includes screening for risk factors and referral related to psychiatric illnesses and social problems, that is, substance abuse, violence and/or abuse, and suicide and/or homicide (Society for Education and Research in Psychiatric-Mental Health Nursing [SERPN], 1996, p. 41).

The Nurse

1. Assesses clients for risk of substance use and/or abuse, victim violence and/or abuse, suicide, or homicide.
2. Knows resources required to manage potential emergency situations and plans access to these resources.
3. Monitors client safety and utilizes continual assessment to detect early changes in client status, and intervenes in situations of acute agitation.
4. Implements crisis intervention as necessary.
5. Commences critical procedures in an institutional setting, for example, suicide precautions, emergency restraint, elopement precautions, when necessary; in a community setting, the nurse uses appropriate community support systems, for example, police, ambulance services, and crisis response resources.
6. Coordinates care to prevent errors and duplication of efforts where rapid response is imperative.
7. Considers the legal and ethical implications of responses to rapidly changing situations; invokes relevant provisions in mental health acts as necessary.
8. Evaluates the effectiveness of the rapid responses and modifies critical plans as necessary.
9. Explores with the client and/or family the precipitates of the emergency event and plans to minimize risk of recurrence.
10. Participates in "debriefing" process with team (including client and family) and other service providers, for example, reviews of critical event and/or emergency situation.
11. Incorporates knowledge of community needs or responses in the provision of care.
12. Encourages and assists clients to seek out support groups for mutual aid and support.
13. Assesses the client's response to, and perception of, nursing and other therapeutic interventions.

STANDARD V: INTERVENES THROUGH THE TEACHING–COACHING FUNCTION

All nurse–client interactions are potentially teaching and/or learning situations. The PMH nurse attempts to understand the life experience of the client and uses this understanding to support and promote learning related to health and personal development. The nurse provides mental health promotion information to individuals, families, groups, populations, and communities.

The Nurse

1. In collaboration with the client, determines client's learning needs.
2. Plans and implements, with the client, health education while considering the context of the client's life experiences on readiness to learn. The nurse plans teaching times and strategies accordingly.
3. Provides anticipatory guidance regarding the client's situational needs, for example, assists the client in identifying living, learning, or working needs and ways in which to access available community or other resources.
4. Facilitates the client's search for ways to integrate mental illness, chronic illness, or improved functioning into lifestyle.
5. Considers a variety of learning models and utilizes clinical judgment when creating opportunities with clients regarding their learning needs.
6. Provides relevant information, guidance, and support to the client's significant others within the bounds of any freedom of information legislation.
7. Documents the teaching and/or learning process (assessment, plan, implementation, client involvement, and evaluation).
8. Evaluates and validates with the client the effectiveness of the educational process, and seeks client's input into developing other means of providing teaching opportunities.
9. Engages in learning and/or teaching opportunities as partners with consumer groups.

STANDARD VI: MONITORS AND ENSURES THE QUALITY OF HEALTH CARE PRACTICES

Clients may be particularly vulnerable as recipients of health care because of the nature of mental health problems and mental disorders. Mental health care is conducted under the provisions of provincial/territorial Mental Health Acts and related legislation. It is essential for the PMH nurse to be informed regarding the interpretation of relevant legislation and its implications for nursing practice. The nurse has a responsibility to advocate for the client's right to receive the least restrictive form of care and to respect and affirm the client's right to pursue individual goals of equality and justice.

The Nurse

1. Identifies limitations in the workplace or care setting that interfere with the nurse's ability to perform with skill, safety, and compassion, and takes appropriate action.
2. Identifies limitations at a community level that interfere with the entire health of the community, for example, poverty, malnutrition, and unsafe housing.
3. Expands knowledge of innovations and changes in mental health and psychiatric nursing practice to ensure safe and effective care.
4. Critically evaluates current mental health and psychiatric research findings and uses research findings in practice.
5. Ensures and documents ongoing review and evaluation of PMHN care activities.

6. Understands and questions the interdependent functions of the team within the overall plan of care.

7. Advocates for the client within the context of institutional, professional, family, and community interests.

8. Follows agency/institutional procedures when dissatisfied with the safety of a treatment plan and/or management interventions of other mental health care providers.

9. Uses sound judgment in advocating safe, competent, and ethical care for clients and colleagues even when there are system barriers to enacting an advocacy function.

10. Maintains and monitors confidentiality of client information.

11. Attends to changes in the mental health services system by recognizing changes that affect practice and client care, and by developing strategies to manage these changes (CNA, 1997, p. 79).

STANDARD VII: PRACTICES WITHIN ORGANIZATIONAL AND WORK-ROLE STRUCTURES

The PMHN role is assumed within organizational structures, both community and institutional, particular to the provision of health care. In PMHN, the ethic of care is based on thoughtful and wise practice judgments. As mental health care in Canada evolves into community-based care, the psychiatric and mental health nurse needs to be skilled in collaborative partnering and decision making, mental health promotion, and community development.

The Nurse

1. Collaborates in the formulation of mental health promotion, and in activities and overall treatment plans and decisions with the client and treatment team and throughout the continuum of care (primary, secondary, and tertiary).

2. Recognizes and addresses the impact of the dynamic of the treatment team on the therapeutic process.

3. Uses conflict resolution skills to facilitate interdisciplinary health team interactions and functioning.

4. Uses computerized and other mental health and nursing information systems in planning, documenting, and evaluating client care.

5. Demonstrates knowledge of collaborative strategies in working with consumer and/or advocacy groups (SERPN, 1996, p. 50).

6. Actively participates in developing, implementing, and critiquing mental health policy in the workplace.

7. Acts as a role model for nursing students and the beginning practitioner in the provision of PMHN care.

8. Practices independently within legislated scope of practice.

9. Supports professional efforts in psychiatric and mental health practice to achieve a more mentally healthy society.

APPENDIX C   References

Benner, P., Tanner, C., & Chesla, C. (1996). *Expertise in nursing practice: Caring, clinical judgement, and ethics.* New York, NY: Springer.

Canadian Nurses Association. (1997, June). *National nursing competency project. Final report.* Ottawa, ON: Author.

Society for Education and Research in Psychiatric-Mental Health Nursing. (1996). *Educational preparation for psychiatric-mental health nursing practice.* Pensacola, FL: Author.

A P P E N D I X D

Communication Techniques

Therapeutic Techniques	Definitions	Examples
Silence	Purposeful absence of verbal communication while continuing to focus on the client	Nodding; maintaining eye contact
Accepting	Indicating (verbally and nonverbally) that what is heard is acknowledged; does not necessarily indicate agreement with what was said	Nodding: Yes, um-hmm, I follow what you said.
Giving recognition	Acknowledgment, indicating awareness	I notice you've combed your hair. I see you're dressed this morning.
Giving information	Providing facts; answering questions	Visiting hours are from 2:00 to 4:00 PM. All clients are scheduled to attend the group meeting.
Offering self	Making yourself available without conditions or an expected response	I'll sit with you. I'll stay with you for 15 minutes.
Giving broad openings	Giving the initiative to the client	Where would you like to start? What is on your mind this morning?
Offering general leads	Encouraging the client to continue	And then? Go on.
Placing the event in time or sequence	Clarifying the time of an event or the relationship between events	Was that before or after ...? What happened just before that?
Making observations	Verbalizing and acknowledging what is observed or perceived about the client	I notice that you ... I sense that you ... You seem ...
Encouraging description of perceptions	Asking the client to verbalize what is perceived	What is happening? Describe what you are hearing.
Encouraging comparison	Asking the client for similarities or differences	Has this happened before? Does this remind you of anything ...?
Reflecting	Directing back to the client's thoughts or feelings	Are you wondering if ...? Do you think that...?
Exploring	Delving into an idea in more depth	Tell me more about that. Describe that to me.
Seeking clarification	Encouraging the client to make meaning more clear	I'm not sure I follow what you're saying. Do you mean to say that ...?
Presenting reality	Providing factual information in a non-threatening manner	I don't hear anyone talking. I am your nurse, this is a hospital.
Voicing doubt	Interjecting the nurse's perception of reality	I find that hard to believe. That seems quite unusual.
Verbalizing the implied	Putting into words what the client is hinting at or suggesting	*Client*: My wife pushes me around just like my mother and sister do. *Nurse*: Is it your impression that women are domineering?

(continued)

Therapeutic Techniques	Definitions	Examples
Attempting to translate into feelings	Assisting the client to identify feelings associated with events or statements	*Client*: I might as well be dead. *Nurse*: Is it your feeling that no one cares? How might you handle this next time?
Encouraging formulation of a plan of action	Giving the client the opportunity to anticipate alternative courses of action for the future	What are some safe ways you could express your anger?
Summarizing	Clarifying main points of discussion and providing closure	Today I have understood you to say ...

Nontherapeutic Techniques	Definitions	Examples
Reassuring	Indicating that there is no cause for concern	You're going to be fine. I wouldn't even worry about that if I were you.
Approving	Personally sanctioning the client's thoughts, behavior, or feelings	Oh yes, that's what I'd do. That's good.
Disapproving	Denouncing the client's thoughts, behavior, or feelings	That's bad. It's wrong for you to feel that way about your mother.
Rejecting	Refusing to listen to the client's ideas or feelings	I don't want to hear about that. Let's not discuss depressing subjects.
Advising	Telling the client what to do	I think you should ... Why don't you ...?
Probing	Asking persistent questions	Tell me your psychiatric history.
Challenging	Demanding proof from the client	*Client*: I was sacrificed by demons. *Nurse*: If that's true, how can you be here talking to me?
Defending	Attempting to dispute the client's negative statements	All the staff here are caring people. Your doctor is the best in this city.
Requesting an explanation	Asking for reasons (usually "why" questions) that are unanswerable	Why would you say a thing like that? Why do you feel that way?
Indicating the existence of an external source	Attributing the basis for the client's statements, thoughts, feelings, or behavior to others or outside influences	What made you do that? What makes you say that?
Belittling feelings	Dismissing or minimizing the importance of the client's feelings, usually an attempt to be cheerful	*Client*: I have no reason to live. *Nurse*: You have a wife who loves you. I've felt like that before.
Making stereotypical comments	Offering platitudes or trite expressions	Tomorrow will be a better day. This, too, shall pass.
Giving literal responses	Responding to the content of figurative comments, rather than the meaning	*Client*: My heart is made of stone. *Nurse*: If that were true, I couldn't hear it beating.
Introducing an unrelated topic	Changing the subject, usually because of the nurse's discomfort	*Client*: I wish my sister was dead. *Nurse*: Is she older or younger than you?

These techniques are adapted from Hays, J. H., & Larson, K. H. (1965). *Interacting with patients*. New York, NY: Macmillan, which is an original work that serves as the basis for most therapeutic communication techniques currently in use.

Defense Mechanisms

Defense mechanisms are processes by which the self deals with unacceptable or unpleasant thoughts, feelings, or actions. These mechanisms are not inherently bad or good but are often seen in everyday life and are an acceptable way of coping. However, when the prolonged or exclusive use of defense mechanisms precludes other effective ways of coping with stress and/or anxiety, the individual begins to experience difficulties in meeting the demands of life.

Name	Definition	Example
Compensation	Overachievement in one area to offset real or perceived deficiencies in another area	A student with little interest in sports works hard to be on the honor roll
Conversion	Expression of an emotional conflict through the development of a physical symptom, usually sensorimotor in nature	A child who is expected to go to college develops blindness, but is unconcerned about it
Denial	Failure to acknowledge obvious ideas, conflicts, or situations that are emotionally painful or provoking anxiety	A person with a newly diagnosed terminal illness is cheerful and makes no mention of the illness
Displacement	Ventilation of intense feelings toward persons less threatening than the one(s) who aroused those feelings	A person who is mad at the boss yells at his or her spouse
Dissociation	Dealing with emotional conflict by a temporary alteration in consciousness or identity	An adult remembers nothing of childhood abuse
Identification	Unconscious modeling of the behaviors, attitudes, and values of another person	A teenager espouses the beliefs and behavior of an admired relative, although he or she is unaware of doing so
Intellectualization	Separation of the emotion of a painful event or situation from the facts involved; acknowledging the facts but not the emotion	A person involved in a serious car accident discusses what happened with no emotional expression
Introjection	Acceptance of another person's values, beliefs, and attitudes as one's own	A person who dislikes guns becomes an avid hunter, just like a best friend
Projection	Attributing unacceptable thoughts, feelings, or actions to someone else	A person with many prejudices loudly identifies others as bigots
Rationalization	Justification of unacceptable thoughts, feelings, or behavior with logical-sounding reasons	A student who cheats on a test claims everyone does it; therefore, it is necessary to cheat to be able to get passing grades
Reaction formation	Unacceptable thoughts and feelings are handled by exhibiting the opposite behavior	A person with sexist ideas does volunteer work for a women's organization
Repression	Exclusion of emotionally painful or anxiety-provoking thoughts and feelings from conscious awareness	A student who is jealous of another student's scholarship award is unaware of those feelings
Sublimation	Substitution of socially acceptable behavior for impulses or desires that are unacceptable to the person	A person who is trying to stop smoking cigarettes chews gum constantly

(continued)

Name	Definition	Example
Suppression	Conscious exclusion of unacceptable thoughts and feelings from conscious awareness	A student decides not to think about a parent's illness in order to study for a test
Undoing	Exhibiting acceptable behavior to make up for or negate previous unacceptable behavior	A person who has been cheating on a spouse sends the spouse a bouquet of roses

Psychopharmacology

Antipsychotic medications are used to decrease the severity of psychosis, such as hallucinations, delusions, grossly disorganized thinking, and behavior seen in schizophrenia, schizoaffective disorder, and the manic phase of bipolar disorder. Off-label uses include treatment of anxiety and aggressive behavior.

Name: Generic (US Trade) *Canadian Trade	Usual Daily Oral Dosage (mg/day)	Special Considerations	Side Effects
Conventional Antipsychotics			
Chlorpromazine (Thorazine) *Chlorprom, Chlorpromanyl, Largactil	200–1,600	May impair ability to regulate body temperature. Client should avoid extreme hot or cold weather.	Drowsiness; hypotension; extrapyramidal symptoms (EPS)—dystonia; pseudoparkinsonism; involuntary motor movements; restlessness; dry mouth; blurred vision; weight gain; photosensitivity; sexual dysfunction.
Perphenazine (Trilafon) *Apo-Perphenazine, Phenazine	16–32		
Fluphenazine (Prolixin) *Apo-Fluphenazine, Moditen, PMS-Fluphenazine	2.5–20		
Thioridazine (Mellaril) *Apo-Thiothixene	200–600	May prolong QT interval leading to dysrhythmias or cardiac arrest. Client needs regular follow-up to monitor cardiac status.	
Trifluoperazine (Stelazine) *Apo-Trifluoperazine	6–50		
Thiothixene (Navane) *Apo-Thioridazine	6–30	Use with caution in clients with glaucoma, seizures, or prostatic hypertrophy.	
Haloperidol (Haldol) *Apo-Haloperidol, Novo-Peridol	2–20	Higher incidence of extrapyramidal side effects.	

(continued)

Name: Generic (US Trade) *Canadian Trade	Usual Daily Oral Dosage (mg/day)	Special Considerations	Side Effects
Loxapine (Loxitane) *Loxapac, PMS-Loxitane	60–100	Use with caution in clients with cardiovascular disease can cause tachycardia, hypertension or hypotension, syncope, and light-headedness.	
Molindone (Moban)	50–100		
Atypical Antipsychotics			
Clozapine (Clozaril)	150–500	May cause agranulocytosis. Client needs weekly WBC drawn.	Insomnia, anxiety, agitation, headache, orthostatic hypotension, nausea, vomiting, constipation, drowsiness, and sedation. Extrapyramidal side effects may occur, but are less frequent and intense than with conventional antipsychotics.
Risperidone (Risperdal)	2–8	May prolong QT interval leading to dysrhythmias or cardiac arrest.	
Olanzapine (Zyprexa)	5–20	Significant weight gain.	
Quetiapine (Seroquel)	300–600	Use with caution with clients with liver disease or seizures.	
Ziprasidone (Geodon)	40–160	Must be taken with food for maximum effect.	
Paliperidone (Invega)	6	Extended release tablet requires only one daily dose. Cannot be chewed or divided.	
Iloperidone (Fanapt)	6–24	Use with caution with clients with cardiac or liver disease.	
Asenapine (Saphris)	10–20	Taken sublingually—then nothing to eat or drink for 10 minutes.	
Dopamine System Stabilizer			
Aripiprazole (Abilify)	15–30	Primary use as adjunctive therapy in depression and bipolar disorder.	Headache, anxiety, nausea.

Antidepressant medications are used to treat major depression, anxiety disorders, and the depressed phase of bipolar disorder. Off-label uses include the treatment of chronic pain, migraine headaches, panic disorder, and eating disorders.

(continued on page 374)

(continued)

Name: Generic (US Trade) *Canadian Trade	Usual Daily Oral Dosage (mg/day)	Special Considerations	Side Effects
Selective Serotonin Reuptake Inhibitors (SSRIs)			
Fluoxetine (Prozac) *Apo-Fluoxetine, Novo-Fluoxetine	20–60	Use with caution in clients with impaired liver or kidney function.	Headache, nervousness, anxiety, sedation, tremor, sexual dysfunction, anorexia, constipation, nausea, diarrhea, weight loss.
Paroxetine (Paxil)	20–40	Use with caution in clients with impaired liver or kidney function, history of mania or seizures, or clients taking digoxin.	Dizziness, sedation, headache, insomnia, weakness, fatigue, constipation, dry mouth and throat, nausea, vomiting, diarrhea, sweating.
Sertraline (Zoloft) *Apo-Sertraline, Gen-Sertraline, Novo-Sertraline	100–150	Use with caution in clients with impaired liver or kidney function, or history of seizures.	Dizziness, sedation, headache, insomnia, tremor, sexual dysfunction, diarrhea, dry mouth and throat, nausea, vomiting, sweating.
Citalopram (Celexa)	20–40	Use with caution in clients with impaired liver or kidney function, or history of seizures.	Drowsiness, sedation, insomnia, nausea, vomiting, weight gain, constipation, diarrhea.
Escitalopram (Lexapro)	10–20	Use with caution in clients with seizures, kidney or liver impairment.	Drowsiness, dizziness, weight gain, sexual dysfunction, restlessness, dry mouth, headache, nausea, diarrhea.
Fluvoxamine (Luvox) *Apo-Fluvoxamine	150–200	Primarily used to treat obsessive-compulsive disorder (OCD). Use with caution in clients with history of mania, seizures, or liver dysfunction.	
Cyclic Compounds			
Imipramine (Tofranil) *Apo-Imipramine, Impril, Novopramine	150–200	May be used for enuresis in children.	Dizziness, orthostatic hypotension, weakness, fatigue, blurred vision, constipation, dry mouth and throat, weight gain.
Desipramine (Norpramin) *Apo-Desipramine, Novo-Desipramine, PMS-Desipramine	150–200		Cardiac dysrhythmias, dizziness, orthostatic hypotension, excitement, insomnia, sexual dysfunction, dry mouth and throat, rashes.
Amitriptyline (Elavil) *Levate, Novotriptyn	150–200	Urine may appear blue–green—this is harmless.	Dizziness, orthostatic hypotension, tachycardia, sedation, headaches, tremor, blurred vision, constipation, dry mouth and throat, weight gain, urinary hesitancy, sweating.

(continued)

Name: Generic (US Trade) *Canadian Trade	Usual Daily Oral Dosage (mg/day)	Special Considerations	Side Effects
Nortriptyline (Pamelor) *Apo-Nortriptyline, Norventyl, PMS-Nortriptyline	75–100		Cardiac dysrhythmias, tachycardia, confusion, excitement, tremor, constipation, dry mouth and throat.
Doxepin (Sinequan) *Alti-Doxepin, Apo-Doxepin, Novo-Doxepin, Triadapin, Zonalon	150–200		Dizziness, orthostatic hypotension, sedation, insomnia, constipation, dry mouth and throat, weight gain, sweating.
Mirtazapine (Remeron)	15–45	Use with caution in clients with impaired liver or kidney function, history of cerebrovascular accident (CVA), myocardial infarction (MI), or angina.	Sedation, dizziness, dry mouth and throat, weight gain, sexual dysfunction, constipation.
Clomipramine (Anafranil) *Apo-Clomipramine, Gen-Clomipramine, Novo-Clomipramine	150–200	Used primarily to treat OCD.	

Other Compounds

Bupropion (Wellbutrin)	200–300	Can cause seizures at a rate four times that of other antidepressants.	Nausea, vomiting, agitation, restlessness, insomnia, may alter taste, blurred vision, weight gain, headache.
Venlafaxine (Effexor)	75–225	Use with caution in clients with impaired liver or kidney function or history of mania.	Increased blood pressure and pulse, nausea, vomiting, headache, dizziness, drowsiness, dry mouth, sweating.
Desvenlafaxine (Pristiq)	50–100		
Trazodone (Desyrel) *Alti-Trazodone, Apo-Trazodone, Nu-Trazodone	200–300	Used primarily for sleep since sedation side effects are pronounced.	Sedation, hypotension, dry mouth, constipation.
Nefazodone (Serzone)	300–600	May cause rare but potentially life-threatening liver damage.	Headache, dizziness, drowsiness.
Duloxetine (Cymbalta)	30–90	May lower seizure threshold.	Increased blood pressure and pulse, nausea, vomiting, drowsiness or insomnia, sexual dysfunction.

Monoamine Oxidase Inhibitors (MAOIs)

Phenelzine (Nardil)	45–60	Use with caution in combination with antihypertensive drugs, including thiazide diuretics and β-blockers.	Drowsiness, dry mouth, overactivity, insomnia, nausea, anorexia, urinary retention, orthostatic hypotension.

(continued on page 376)

(continued)

Name: Generic (US Trade) *Canadian Trade	Usual Daily Oral Dosage (mg/day)	Special Considerations	Side Effects
Tranylcypromine (Parnate)	30–50	Use with caution in clients taking antiparkinsonian drugs or disulfiram, or clients with seizures, diabetes, hyperthyroidism, or impaired renal function.	Potentially fatal hypertensive crisis can result if foods containing tyramine are ingested, or if taken with a wide variety of prescription and OTC medications.
Isocarboxazid (Marplan)	20–40	Use with caution in clients with impaired kidney or liver function, cardiovascular disease, hypertension.	

Antimanic medications include lithium (a naturally occurring salt) and anticonvulsant medications used for their mood-stabilizing effects in the management of bipolar disorder.

Lithium (Lithane, Eskalith, Lithobid) *PMS-Lithium, Carbolith, Duralith, Lithizine	Dosage is individualized to maintain serum lithium level in therapeutic range of 0.5–1.5 mEq/L.	Contraindicated in clients with renal impairment or in those who develop renal impairment. Requires regular monitoring of serum lithium levels.	Hyperglycemia, weight gain, edema, thyroid enlargement, dry mouth, metallic taste. Monitor for signs of toxicity (agitation, severe nausea, vomiting and diarrhea, muscle weakness, loss of coordination).

Anticonvulsants

Carbamazepine (Tegretol) *Apo-Carbamazepine, Novo-Carbamaz	800–1,200	Can cause aplastic anemia and agranulocytosis.	Dizziness, hypotension, ataxia, sedation, blurred vision, leukopenia, rashes.
Divalproex (Depakote) *Alti-Valproic, Deproic, Epival	1,000–1,500	Can cause hepatic failure, life-threatening pancreatitis, or teratogenic effects such as neural tube defects.	Ataxia, drowsiness, weakness, fatigue, menstrual changes, dyspepsia, nausea, vomiting, weight gain, hair loss.
Gabapentin (Neurontin) *PMS-Gabapentin	600–1,800	Use with caution in clients with renal impairment.	Dizziness, hypotension, ataxia, sedation, headache, fatigue, nystagmus, nausea, vomiting.
Lamotrigine (Lamictal)	100–200	Use with caution in clients with impaired renal, hepatic, or cardiac function. Serious rashes can occur.	Dizziness, hypotension, ataxia, sedation, headache, weakness, fatigue, menstrual changes, sore throat, flu-like symptoms, visual disturbances, nausea, vomiting, rashes.
Topiramate (Topamax)	300–400	Use with caution in clients with impaired renal or hepatic function.	Dizziness, hypotension, anxiety, ataxia, incoordination, confusion, sedation, slurred speech, tremor, weakness, visual disturbances, nausea, vomiting.

(continued)

Name: Generic (US Trade) *Canadian Trade	Usual Daily Oral Dosage (mg/day)	Special Considerations	Side Effects
Oxcarbazepine (Trileptal)	900–1,200		Ataxia, sedation, dizziness, fatigue, confusion, fever, headache, tremor, visual disturbances, nausea, vomiting, rashes, hyponatremia.

Anxiolytic agents are used for the treatment of anxiety and anxiety disorders, insomnia, and for the management of alcohol withdrawal.

Benzodiazepines (Used for Anxiety)

Alprazolam (Xanax) *Apo-Alpraz, Novo-Alprozol, Nu-Alpraz, Xanax TS	0.75–1.5	Benzodiazepines have a high potential for misuse and abuse. Clients can become psychologically dependent on these medications.	Dizziness, clumsiness, sedation, headache, fatigue, sexual dysfunction, blurred vision, dry throat and mouth, constipation.
Chlordiazepoxide (Librium) *Apo-Chlordiaze-poxide, Corax	15–100		
Clonazepam (Klonopin) *Apo-Clonazepam, Clonapam, Gen-Clonazepam, Rivotril	1.5–20		
Chlorazepate (Tranxene) *Apo-Chlorazepate, Novo-Clopate	15–60		
Diazepam (Valium) *Apo-Diazepam, Diazemuls, Vivol	4–40		
Lorazepam (Ativan) *Apo-Lorazepam, Novo-Lorazem, Nu-Loraz	2–8		
Oxazepam (Serax) *Apo-Oxazepam, Novoxapam	30–120		
Benzodiazepines (Used to Treat Insomnia) Flurazepam (Dalmane) *Somnol	15–30		
Temazepam (Restoril) *Apo-Tenazepam, Novo-Temazepam	30–120		
Triazolam (Halcion) *Apo-Trizo, Gen-Triazolam	0.25–0.5		

(continued on page 378)

(continued)

Name: Generic (US Trade) *Canadian Trade	Usual Daily Oral Dosage (mg/day)	Special Considerations	Side Effects
Nonbenzodiazepine Buspirone (BuSpar) *Apo-Buspirone, Buspirex, Gen-Buspirone, Lin-Buspirone, Novo-Buspirone, Nu-Busprione, PMS-Buspirone	15–30		Dizziness, restless, agitation, drowsiness, headache, weakness, nausea, vomiting, paradoxical excitement or euphoria.

Anticholinergic, antiparkinsonian, and antihistamine medications are used to treat extrapyramidal side effects that can occur when taking antipsychotic medications.

Anticholinergics

Trihexyphenidyl (Artane) *Apo-Trihex	6–15	Use with caution in clients with arteriosclerosis.	CNS stimulation (restlessness, insomnia, agitation, delirium), dizziness, orthostatic hypotension, gastrointestinal (GI) upset, constipation, impaired perspiration.
Benztropine (Cogentin) *Apo-Benztropine, PMS-Benztropine	2–6	Use with caution in geriatric or emaciated clients.	Excitation, urinary retention, constipation, vomiting, orthostatic hypotension, temperature intolerance, sedation.
Biperiden (Akineton)	6–8		Constipation, GI upset, decreased perspiration, urinary retention, dry mouth.
Procyclidine (Kemadrin) *PMS-Procyclidine, Procyclid	7.5–15	Contraindicated in clients with glaucoma, bladder neck obstructions, or prostatic hypertrophy.	GI upset, sedation, dry mouth, constipation, decreased perspiration.
Carbidopa/Levodopa (Sinemet 10/25, 25/100, or 25/250) *Apo-Levocarb, Endo Levodopa, Nu-Levodopa	For Sinemet 10/25, one to eight tablets per day	Contraindicated in clients with glaucoma or history of melanoma. Use with caution in clients with renal, hepatic or cardiac impairment.	Orthostatic hypotension, headaches, insomnia, nightmares, confusion, blurred vision, constipation, nausea, vomiting.
Amantadine (Symmetrel) *Endantadine, Gen-Amantadine	200–300	Use with caution in clients with hepatic or renal disease, seizures, congestive heart failure.	Nausea, vomiting, constipation, dizziness, confusion, orthostatic hypotension, peripheral edema, urinary retention.

Antihistamine

Diphenhydramine (Benadryl) *Allerdryl, Allernix	75–200	Contraindicated in clients with glaucoma, bladder neck obstruction, prostatic hypertrophy, asthma, peptic ulcer.	Dizziness, drowsiness, tachycardia, blurred vision, nausea, epigastric distress, thickened bronchial secretions.

Psychostimulants and a selective norepinephrine reuptake inhibitor (SNRI) are used to treat attention deficit/hyperactivity disorder (ADHD).

(continued)

Name: Generic (US Trade) *Canadian Trade	Usual Daily Oral Dosage (mg/day)	Special Considerations	Side Effects
Stimulants			
Methylphenidate (Ritalin) *PMS-Methylphenidate, Riphenidate	10–60 (in divided doses)	Stimulants have the potential for abuse, i.e., by adult care-givers of the child, or through distribution to other children or adults.	Appetite suppression, growth delays, therapeutic effects of drug.
sustained release (Ritalin-SR, Concerta, Metadate_CD)	20–60 (single dose)		
Dextroamphetamine (Dex-edrine)	5–40 (in divided doses)		
sustained release (Dexe-drine-SR)	10–30 (single dose)		
Amphetamine (Adderall)	5–40 (in divided doses)		
sustained release (Adder-all-SR)	10–30 (single dose)		
Selective norepinephrine reuptake inhibitor (SNRI)			
Atomoxetine (Strattera)	0.5–1.5 mg/kg/day		Decreased appetite, nausea, vomiting, fatigue, and upset stomach.

Medication Side Effects and Nursing Interventions

Side Effect	Nursing Interventions
Extrapyramidal symptoms (EPS)—pseudoparkinsonism	Administer benztropine (Cogentin) or other anticholinergic medication as ordered by the prescriber.
EPS—acute dystonia	Administer benztropine (Cogentin) IM (lorazepam or diazepam may be ordered). Monitor the client for 1 to 2 days for continued need for oral medication, e.g., Cogentin, due to longer half-life of antipsychotic medications.
EPS—akathisia	Administer PRN benztropine (Cogentin) PO if ordered, or seek an order from the prescriber. If client remains on the antipsychotic medication, seek and order for regularly scheduled benztropine or suitable substitute.
Tardive dyskinesia abnormal, involuntary movements	Monitor all clients on long-term antipsychotic medications using a standardized assessment tool such as Abnormal Involuntary Movement Scale (AIMS). Report any changes or indications of a movement disorder to the physician.
Neuroleptic malignant syndrome (NMS)	Stop all psychiatric medication immediately.
	STAT call to physician as this is a medical emergency.
Orthostatic hypotension	Rise slowly from sitting or lying position.
	Do not begin to ambulate until dizziness subsides.
Weight gain	Prevention of weight gain through nutritional diet, portion control, and exercise is best. These same measures are used to lose the weight that is gained.
Sexual dysfunction	Lubrication may ease female discomfort from dry mucus membranes.
	Assist the client to express concerns to his or her physician for possible changes in dose or medication.
Anticholinergic effects: • Dry mouth • Constipation • Blurred near vision • Urinary retention	 • Use only ice chips, calorie-free beverages, or hard candy • Increase fluid intake and dietary fiber; stool softener • If persistent, see physician about medication change • If persistent, see physician about medication change
Photosensitivity	Use sun block, wear hat; cover arms and legs.
Insomnia	If possible, take medication upon rising (such as once-daily dose of antidepressant).
	Sleep hygiene measures including bedtime routine, warm milk, quiet, low stimulus activity, and environment.
Drowsiness to sedation	Take scheduled dose in evening or bedtime if possible.
	Do not engage in activities requiring quick reflexes and action, e.g., driving a car.

(continued)

Side Effect	Nursing Interventions
Nausea to vomiting	Take with food—at least 200 to 300 calories—unless prohibited by type of medication. Best taken at mealtime if possible.
Constipation	Increase intake of fluids and high fiber foods, use stool softener, increase physical exercise, and avoid stimulant laxatives.
Headache	Use physician-approved OTC medications, report to physician if headaches persist.
Alcohol interaction—potentiates medication effects	Avoid alcohol; discuss ability to drink alcohol with provider.
Serotonergic syndrome	Do not discontinue antidepressant medications abruptly or without consultation with provider; need to taper dosage to discontinue safely.
Appetite suppression	Monitor weight (especially in children), eat before taking medication if possible, keep a food diary to document actual food intake.
Weakness or fatigue	If mild—get more rest until it subsides; if pronounced or persistent, report to prescriber.
Elevated blood pressure, tachycardia, bradycardia	Report to prescriber.
Rashes	Report to prescriber for evaluation.
Ataxia, clumsiness	Report to prescriber.

APPENDIX H

Care of Clients Receiving Electroconvulsive Therapy

Electroconvulsive therapy (ECT) may be used to treat depression in select situations, such as with clients who do not respond to antidepressant medication or those who experience intolerable side effects at therapeutic doses of medication (this is particularly true for older adults). Pregnant women can safely have ECT with no harm to the fetus. Clients who are intensely suicidal may have ECT if there is concern about their safety while waiting for the therapeutic benefits of medication, which can take weeks (Videbeck, 2011).

ECT involves the application of electrodes to the client's head to deliver an electrical impulse to the brain, which causes a seizure. It is believed that the electrical shock and subsequent seizure stimulates brain chemistry to correct the chemical imbalance of depression.

Historically, ECT was administered without anesthetic or muscle relaxants, resulting in a full-blown grand mal seizure. At times, client would be injured or break bones during the seizure. ECT was rejected as a treatment for a period after psychotropic medications became available in 1950. Today, even though ECT is administered in a safe and humane way, there are still critics of the treatment.

Clients usually have a series of 6 to 15 treatments, given three times a week. ECT is often given during hospitalization, although the client may finish a series of treatments as an outpatient if adequate home and community support is available.

Preparation of the client for ECT is similar to preparation for an outpatient surgical procedure:

- Signed informed consent for the procedure
- NPO (nothing by mouth) after midnight
- Prescribed benzodiazepines, especially diazepam (Valium) or clonazepam (Klonopin) may be held the day before ECT due to their anticonvulsant properties
- Removal of fingernail polish in order to visualize nailbeds and capillary refill
- Removal of metal objects such as piercings, jewelry, hair clips
- Insertion of IV line for administration of medication
- Empty bladder just before the procedure

Medications administered to the client include the following:

- Anticholinergic medications such as Robinul or atropine to dry secretions
- Ultrabrief anesthetic, such as Brevitol or Pentothal
- Neuromuscular blocking agent, usually succinylcholine (Anectine) to reduce clonic-tonic muscle contractions

The procedure is implemented by a board-certified psychiatrist with an anesthesiologist or anesthetist to monitor the client's respiratory and cardiac status. An EEG is used to monitor and measure seizure activity in the brain during the treatment. Electrode placement can be bilateral (one on each temple) or unilateral (one electrode on a temple and one by the mastoid process on the same side). Bilateral ECT produces positive results more quickly but has more intense side effects. Unilateral ECT produces milder side effects and is used more frequently than the bilateral method. The client is given oxygen and assisted to breathe with an Ambu bag. The client generally awakens in a few minutes. It is important to monitor vital signs until stable and observe the client for the return of a gag reflex.

Following the treatment, the client may exhibit many behaviors that are observed after any person has a seizure. Postictal (after seizure) symptoms include the following:

- Headache
- Mild confusion
- Brief disorientation
- Feeling tired
- Memory loss

Immediately after ECT (when vital signs are stable and gag reflex is present), the client can eat if he or she is hungry. The client can be given medication such as acetaminophen for headache, and he or she is allowed to sleep until rested. It is not advisable for the client to attempt to attend groups or participate in activities, due to fatigue, headache, and memory loss.

The client will have some short-term memory loss following ECT, such as inability to remember the morning's events. This is generally mild, and once treatments are complete, memory becomes stable again. It is important to educate the client and his or her family or significant others about the memory loss before initiation of ECT so no one is surprised if it occurs.

ECT is sometimes continued on an outpatient maintenance basis to sustain the improvements gained with ECT treatment series or to prevent relapse. This often consists of one ECT treatment per month. Other clients may maintain mood improvement following ECT treatment with a maintenance dose of antidepressant medication therapy.

Schizoid, Histrionic, Narcissistic, Avoidant, and Obsessive-Compulsive Personality Disorders

A personality disorder is evidenced by a client's enduring pattern of thinking, believing, and behaving that deviates markedly from the expectations of his or her culture. The *Diagnostic and Statistical Manual of Mental Disorders Text Revision* (*DSM-IV-TR*) organizes personality disorder diagnoses into three clusters, based on the primary features of the group (APA, 2000):

- Cluster A includes three disorders with odd, eccentric, aloof behaviors: paranoid, schizoid, and schizotypal.
- Cluster B includes four disorders with erratic, impulsive, dramatic, and often manipulative behaviors: borderline, antisocial, histrionic, and narcissistic.
- Cluster C includes three disorders with anxious, fearful, or worrying behaviors: avoidant, dependent, and obsessive-compulsive.

Section 12 of this *Manual*, entitled Personality Disorders, provides care plans for paranoid, schizotypal, borderline, antisocial, and dependent personality disorders. The remaining personality disorders are summarized below. Clients with these personality disorders do not seek, nor do they desire, mental health treatment. The nurse will certainly encounter these clients in a variety of settings, for example, clinic or office, emergency room, or medical-surgical acute care settings. The following suggested interventions may help the nurse to provide the care needed without being distracted or impeded by the client's behavior.

Personality disorder	Characteristics or Behaviors	Nursing Interventions
Schizoid—social detachment and restricted emotions	Indifference to praise or criticism; preference for solitary activities; prefers "things" to people; emotional coldness; lack of desire or pleasure in social relationships; flat or blunted affect	Use a serious, straightforward approach; eliminate "social" conversation; assist the client to increase skills to function in the community or self-care skills depending on the circumstances
Histrionic—excessive emotionality, dramatic, attention- seeking	Rapidly shifting and shallow emotion—not genuine, yet theatrical; exaggerated expressions of emotionality; seductive or provocative; uses physical appearance and manner of dress to gain attention; excessive need to be the center of attention; craves excitement and stimulation	Provide factual feedback and information; keep directions short, clear, to-the-point; don't respond to emotional drama, but stay focused on the task at hand
Narcissistic—grandiose, entitled, lack of empathy, need to be admired	Grandiose sense of self-importance and specialness; arrogant and haughty attitude; exploits others for own benefit; rejects any feedback or criticism; preoccupied with fantasies of own power, success, brilliance, and so forth	Use a matter-of-fact approach; gain cooperation with needed treatment; teach necessary self-care skills if needed; do not respond to critical or condescending remarks

(continued on page 384)

(continued)

Personality disorder	Characteristics or Behaviors	Nursing Interventions
Avoidant—excessive hypersensitivity to negative evaluation, social inhibition, feelings of inadequacy	Fears criticism, rejection, disapproval, or embarrassment, yet expects those responses in almost all social interactions; avoids social and occupational situations involving many or new people unless convinced of being liked; may be socially isolated while craving interaction; fearful of change	Provide realistic support and reassurance; promote self-esteem through positive feedback for task or self-care completion; be patient when introducing new concepts
Obsessive-compulsive—preoccupation with perfection, order, and control at the expense of flexibility, cooperation, and efficiency	Preoccupied with lists, details, rules, order, organization; perfectionism that interferes with task completion; rigid; stubborn; excessive devotion to work and productivity at the expense of interpersonal relationships when unnecessary; one right way to do things which is their way	Encourage negotiation when appropriate; teach self-care skills; assist to make timely decisions and complete tasks

APPENDIX J

Case Study and Care Plan

Jane Brown is a 33-year-old woman who comes to the mental health walk-in clinic accompanied by her husband. Her appearance is disheveled, posture is stooped, movements are very slow, and she makes no eye contact with staff as she enters the clinic. Her husband approaches the desk and says, "I have to get some help for my wife. I don't know what's wrong. I practically had to drag her out of bed to get her to come here."

The nurse helps Jane to an interview room and begins the initial assessment. Jane's answers are very short, consisting of "I don't know" or "I guess so." Since Jane is providing little information, the nurse interviews Jane's husband and discovers that Jane has been eating and sleeping poorly, is fatigued all the time, and has no interest in any of her previous activities. Jane's husband also describes two previous episodes when Jane felt sad for several weeks, but her mood improved in time, and she had still been able to function in her daily routine and responsibilities. The nurse believes that Jane is depressed.

1. What will the nurse need to assess about Jane at this point?

   • It is essential that the nurse ask Jane about any suicidal thoughts or ideas. If Jane has suicidal ideas, the nurse must determine if Jane has a plan, has access to the means to carry out the plan, and any other details Jane will provide.
   • Jane tells the nurse she is too tired to go on, that her life is empty. She cries when telling the nurse that she is a horrible wife and mother, and she strongly believes her family would be better off without her, since she is such a worthless burden. Based on the initial assessment data, the psychiatrist decides to admit Jane to the hospital.

2. What nursing diagnosis would be the priority for Jane?
   • Risk for suicide.

3. Identify an immediate outcome for Jane.
   • The client will not harm herself.

4. Identify nursing interventions that will achieve the outcome.
   • Institute suicide precautions per agency policy (e.g., visually observing the client at least every 10 minutes).
   • Remove any potentially dangerous objects from the client's possession.
   • Regularly reassess the client's lethality potential; that is, Is she having suicidal ideas? Does she have a plan?
   • Ensure that the client takes all prescribed medication and does not "cheek" them or save them.
   • Encourage the client to express feelings verbally, or through writing or crying.
   • Offer support for the client's verbal expression of feelings.
   • Encourage the client to remain out of her room to engage in activities or interaction with others.
   • Assess and document any sudden changes in mood or behavior that may indicate an increase in lethality.

5. Identify two additional nursing diagnoses that are supported by the assessment data, outcomes for each diagnosis, and appropriate interventions.

Ineffective Coping

• *The client will express feelings in a safe manner.*
• *The client will identify alternative ways of coping with stress and emotional problems.*
• Spend time with the client even if her verbal responses are minimal.
• Use silence and active listening skills.
• Ask open-ended questions that require more than yes-or-no answers.
• Avoid being overly cheerful or trying to "cheer her up."
• Encourage ventilation and identification of feelings.
• Encourage the client to identify issues or problems.
• Teach the client the problem-solving process.
• Help the client apply the problem-solving process to identified concerns or issues.
• Help the client identify activities that are enjoyable to her, such as spending time with her husband and children, work, hobbies, or physical activities.
• Encourage the client to begin to resume activities gradually.
• Give the client support for plans and efforts toward resuming activities.

Chronic Low Self-Esteem

• *The client will verbalize increased feelings of self-worth.*
• *The client will evaluate own strengths realistically.*

385

- Encourage the client to engage in activities and interactions with others.
- Give the client positive feedback for completion of daily activities, interaction efforts, and participation in activities or groups.
- Limit the amount of time the client spends talking about her shortcomings.
- Redirect the client to explore her strengths; suggest making a written list.
- Encourage the client to set small goals that are reasonable to achieve, for example, giving compliments to others, starting a conversation with another person.
- Support the client's efforts to make progress toward goals, validating that this is hard work for her.
- Teach the client that one must begin to do things to feel better, rather than waiting to feel better before doing things.

INDEX